THE BIOFUELS DECEPTION

THE BIOFUELS DECEPTION

Going Hungry on the Green Carbon Diet

by OKBAZGHI YOHANNES

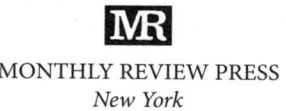

MONTHLY REVIEW PRESS
New York

Library of Congress Cataloging-in-Publication Data
available from the publisher

ISBN: 978-158367-702-5 (paper)
ISBN: 978-158367-703-2 (cloth

Typeset in Minion Pro

MONTHLY REVIEW PRESS, NEW YORK
monthlyreview.org

5 4 3 2 1

Contents

Acknowledgments | 7

1. The New Geoeconomics of Biofuels | 9
2. The Biofuel Industrial Complex and Its Migration
to the Global South | 71
3. Biofuels and the Transformation of the
Metropolitan State | 133
4. The Three Deceptions: Abundance, Green Environment,
and Blue Skies | 205
5. In Place of a Conclusion: Can We Overcome the
Planetary Emergency? | 245

Notes | 299
Index | 333

To Tamara with gratitude and love

Acknowledgments

THIS WORK HAS TAKEN THE EFFORTS of so many people, some of whom deserve particular mention. The support of the University of Louisville Department of Political Science was instrumental in providing the necessary support, particularly during my trip to Africa to study the extent of biofuels on that continent. Special thanks go to the late Laurie Rhodebeck, who passed away in fall 2017, who made an enormous contribution to this work as director of the Graduate Program providing me with highly skilled graduate research assistants. Also, my thanks go to Professors Chuck Ziegler, Roger Payne, and Dewey Clayton for their years of encouragement and support. In addition, Isabelle Christensen was very helpful in editing some of the chapters.

My special thanks go to Dr. Michael Yates of Monthly Review Press for his faith in the project and to Erin Clermont for her clear and helpful editing.

Finally, huge thanks go to my wife, Tamara. Without her diligent and persistent participation, this work could not have been done.

1

The New Geoeconomics of Biofuels: Lessons Still Unlearned

Since the 1992 Rio summit on the environment and climate, the subject of biofuels has shadowed the global debate on the triple crises of global energy insecurity, global climate change, and global poverty. This has created a gaping hole that has allowed transnational corporations to step in to shape the contours and direction of the debate. Indeed, the corporate world saw the triple crises as heaven-sent. They reassured the world that the gains from the new life-science revolution would solidify the geopolitical and energy security of nations, substantially reducing greenhouse gas (ghg) emissions and stabilizing the global climate, creating millions of green jobs, and lifting up billions of people from grinding poverty through the promotion of rural development and income generation.

According to the transnationals, the post-petroleum bio-economy will usher in a new era where all countries will rely on green liquid and solid sources of energy without fear of causing anthropogenic climate change, without fear of vulnerability to supply disruptions or global energy price volatility, and without fear of the political use of energy. The imagery and the propaganda that followed led to the global transport ethanol production soaring from 17 billion liters in 2000 to 52 billion liters in 2007, and biodiesel production growing from less than 1 billion to over 11 billion liters.[1] Indeed, the euphoric excitement in the potential of biofuels was such that the International Energy Agency (IEA, the international propaganda mouthpiece for industrial countries) projected that biofuels could constitute 23 percent of global transport fuels by 2050 through the conversion into biofuels of 1,500 metric tons of crop and forest residues per year, plus bioenergy crops grown on 375–750 million hectares of land (a hectare equals about 2.47 acres). This would be a necessary precondition to stabilize atmospheric carbon concentration at 450 parts per million (ppm) and keep global warming increases below 2 degrees Celsius by 2050.[2] Of course, this conjectural projection tells us nothing about the effects of such enormous production of biofuels on biodiversity, environment, and the atmosphere or on human food and animal feed production.

In any event, for those who must focus on capital accumulation, their obsessive preoccupation has been on how to adroitly create the subjective conditions that will combine with the urgency of the very real environmental crisis in such a way that biofuels will be seen as the way to solve the crisis but will also allow capital to solve its own crisis of overaccumulation. One objective factor facing industry is the presumed oil peak. Ever since the oil shocks of the 1970s, the bourgeois world has been haunted by the prospect of fossil resource depletion, something that found empirical expression in what is known as the "Hubbert peak." In 1956, Royal Dutch Shell geologist King Hubbert developed a useful mathematical model that allowed him to assess the length of time it would take for the United States to use its petroleum resources before the resources begin to decline. In its simplest form, the hypothesis Hubbert formulated states that the duration of the supply of petroleum depends on the rates of discoveries, production, consumption, and the delivery infrastructure put in place. During the pre-peak period, production increases in a linear fashion because of new discoveries and the increasing deployment of capital to extract and deliver the resources. However, because petroleum resources are nonrenewable and finite, maximum production eventually peaks at a given point in the extraction process. Then, during the post-peak period, production of petroleum begins to gradually decrease, threatening the fossil-based economy. Interestingly, Hubbert's depiction of the rates of discoveries, production, and consumption of petroleum in the United States was almost so precise that American petroleum production peaked at 9.6 million barrels a day in 1970, and then steadily declined to 5.1 million barrels a day in 2006, transforming the United States from having been a net exporter of oil in the 1950s to being a net importer of oil since the 1970s, importing 63 percent of its petroleum requirements by the turn of the century, even though shale oil discoveries and the fracking boom have now temporarily created illusionary abundance.[3]

The politicization of petroleum by Arab and other radical regimes in the 1970s, coupled with supply disruptions owing to natural conditions or social instability, as in Nigeria in the early 2000s, has strengthened the Hubbert peak hypothesis. Indeed, it has acquired such status that it haunts petroleum-importing OECD countries. These countries have now come to grudgingly view the Hubbert peak as the essential expression of the limits of nature to supply ever greater quantities of the hydrocarbons demanded to match limitless capitalist growth. Even the IEA acknowledges this reality. In its 2013 World Energy Outlook, the agency notes that its own investigation of more than 1,600 fields confirmed that, once production has peaked, the annual decline in output from a conventional oil field is around 6 percent on average. As a result, the output of conventional crude oil from existing fields worldwide is projected to fall by over 40 million barrels a day by 2035, requiring exploitation of shale oil and tar sands; more than half of the unconventional production is projected to offset the decline in conventional oil supply.[4] This projection should be situated within the fact that by 2006 the world had used up half of the two trillion barrels of proven petroleum reserves. At the 2006 rate of annual consumption of 31 billion barrels, the world will exhaust all proven oil by 2042.[5] It is the adroit orchestration of this ready-made objective condition that the Transnational Corporations (TNCs) have employed to win over industrial countries to the notion of biofuels as the answer to the actual and potential oil crisis. Undeveloped countries have also been brought on board with the promise of huge gains from specializing in bioenergy crop and biofuel production, in terms of both reducing their oil import bills and generating precious hard currency by exporting feedstocks to the Global North. The corporate promise that the specter of the Hubbert peak can be exorcised through a combination of synthetic substitutes for hydrocarbons and migration to bioenergy production has crystallized. The conventional discourse now is not so much about whether the Hubbert peak hypothesis is empirically supportable as it is about how to quicken the migration to renewable sources of energy, or how to move from fossil-based "black" energy to carbohydrate-based "green" energy. The financial crisis of the new century has provided additional momentum to the dogged determination of capital accumulators to quicken the migration to the biotic realm for biofuels, biochemicals, and biomaterials.

Anthropogenic-driven climate change is the second Trojan horse that TNCs have cleverly used to market biofuels as the long-awaited answer to the crisis of overaccumulation. Even a multitude of bourgeois non-governmental organizations, which long had fought for reduction in ghg emissions, have been won over to biofuels as the palpable solution, even though some of them have now backed off from their earlier enthusiasm. Former U.S. vice president Al Gore, through his well-received documentary *An Inconvenient Truth*, has been the leading spokesperson for various environmental groups that saw biofuels as climate- and environment-friendly.

The elimination of global poverty is the third Trojan horse. The TNCs have linked biofuel production to global poverty eradication. A sinister machination is at work here. Since most of the required feedstocks, either through the commercial enclosure of forests, savannahs, and grasslands or through direct conversion of existing agricultural land to feedstock production, are found in the Global South, specialization in biofuel production must be conveniently linked to poverty eradication. As the corporate narrative goes, developing nations could avoid importing costly petroleum by simply producing biofuels domestically to run their transport vehicles. Moreover, they could significantly increase precious foreign exchange by exporting feedstocks, and the rural population would immensely benefit since they are the real producers and suppliers of these resources. The employment multiplier effect could be enormous as feedstock growers, rural workers, transporters, and processers could increase in parallel with the expansion of the biofuel sector.

The counter-narrative I have developed in this book posits that the contemporary debate over the role of biofuels in the global economy is not about global energy and food security or about the challenges of global climate change. The biofuels revolution now being advanced by global corporations, their supporting governments, and corporate researchers will not produce national or global energy security, nor will it reduce global emissions or alleviate poverty anywhere. The underlying motivation of those who call for biofuels is not to solve energy and food shortages or reduce climate change. Rather, the goal is to resolve the anarchy of agricultural production in the Global North, brought about by the green revolution and the consequent transformation of agriculture into a food-manufacturing system during the second half of the twentieth century—a transformation made possible by integration with the petroleum industry. After all, the original pioneering champions of biofuels were not petroleum corporations or even governments concerned about disruptions in petroleum supply conditions, but rather global grain-trading corporations bedeviled by surplus grain on the world market causing extreme price volatility. Until the beginning of the new century, the major global grain-trading corporations had been befuddled by a perplexing paradox in the global food market. There was more food than needed by the affluent people in the rich nations, and much less than needed by those in the poor countries, where purchasing power was too low to buy the surplus food.

It was in this context that the idea of converting grain to biofuels was born. The overarching aim of agribusiness corporations, like Archer Daniels Midland (ADM), Cargill, Bunge, and Louis Dreyfus, was to make all grains flexible. Grains could be used as human food and animal feed when prices are high enough to sustain corporate profit, or as feedstocks for biofuel production when global grain market conditions experienced fluctuations. Thus the competition between grains for human food and animal feed, on the one hand, and grains for biofuels on the other, could eliminate extreme volatility in prices. It must be borne in mind that the crises of industrial overcapacity, overaccumulation, and mass unemployment have not been confined to manufacturing. Metropolitan agricultural interests have long experienced similar secular stagnation in grain markets due to surplus production, while people in the Global South continue to endure stark poverty, hunger, and malnutrition. To state it differently, the origins of agricultural surplus production in North America and Western Europe are rooted in the transformation of agriculture into food manufacturing, wholly dependent on the petroleum industry for external inputs such as synthetic fertilizers, pesticides, and fossil fuels for trucks, tractors, water pumps, and heating and cooling facilities. The European aphorism of "lakes of milk and mountains of cheese" tells the whole story of the crisis in agricultural overproduction. It was no accident that the original notion of converting grains into biofuels arose in the headquarters of ADM, when corporate managers urged policy makers to induce transitioning from petroleum dependency to biofuels under the rubric of the urgent need to diversify the country's energy portfolio in light of the oil shocks of the 1970s.

An important upshot of the drive for biofuels has been the coalescence of the global grain-trading oligopolies and the emergent biotechnology corporations, which boosted grain production in the Global North on an unprecedented scale, resulting in the crisis of agricultural surplus production, and market volatility for grain traders. At the same time, people in the Global South lacked purchasing capabilities to absorb the surplus food, compounding the crisis of overproduction. In this context, the diversion of the surplus grain into liquid biofuel production would transform all grains into flexible raw materials that could be used for either food or fuels, thus overcoming the crisis of agricultural surplus production. Biotechnology corporations, however, found the stiff opposition by the public to engineered crops a formidable impediment to accumulation. Therefore, they found it convenient to link genetically manipulated (GM) crop production to the growing requirement of feedstocks for biofuel production. In addition, the competition between food and the supposed green fuels was expected to engender scarcity, thereby creating propitious conditions for using the emergent scarcity as a way to penetrate the global food market.

The convergence of interests between the grain-trading oligopolies and the biotech corporations led to the formation and consolidation of the biofuel-biotechnology industrial complex. This entity was determined to employ the triple crises in global poverty, global energy uncertainty, and global warming to shape and reshape the global food manufacturing system in ways that could purportedly solve the crisis of agricultural surplus production and, at the same time, find new outlets for the deployment of the overaccumulated capital. To effectively market this overarching corporate aim, the biofuel-biotechnology peddlers continued to refine their presentation of biofuels as offering climate mitigation, poverty alleviation, and energy security.. To do so, they not only rely on the mobilization of internal propaganda and financial resources but also on a galaxy of researchers, social climbers, academics, and opinion-molders. The latter, with unpardonable vanity, economic opportunism, and cravings for social recognition, had no difficulty transforming intellectual promiscuity into fungible equity, perpetually nurtured by towering expectations of promotion and pecuniary reward. The biofuel-biotechnology schemers are also aided by the ascendency of counterrevolutionary neoliberalism, which has effectively extended the commodification and marketization of nature to the reconfiguration of social power and state institutions, in effect transforming the state qua state as a geo-economic agent in the service of accumulation. The romantic illusion that the biofuel-biotechnology complex and its supporters portray is that we can only solve the triple crises by speeding up the transition of the green revolution to the gene revolution in order to produce resources in sufficient quantities to satisfy the competing demands for food, feed, fiber, and green fuels.

Concomitant with the consolidation of the biofuel-biotechnology industrial complex has come a climactic confrontation between two powerful visions of the future of the global food ecology—indeed, the future of humanity and nature itself. For analytical simplicity, I cast these as agroecology versus the green/gene revolution–driven agri-food complex. Agroecology juxtaposes the advantages and the development and sustainability goals that could be had from preserving and promoting regional and locally based strategies of diverse agriculture against the homogenization of the global food ecology, foundational to food security. On the other hand, the new global bio-masters boldly propose that the only way to feed the growing global population is through the acceleration of the green and gene revolutions, the requisite condition for generating surplus grains to produce biofuels that will simultaneously meet global energy requirements and contain global climate change.

Fewer things today make one cringe more than hearing advocates of biofuels invoke the image of inexhaustible biotic resources for making a smooth transition to a post-petroleum bio-economy with no harmful long-term consequences for the environment, climate, and the livelihoods of billions of people. The endless barrage of corporate propaganda tells us that, once the transition is made from the mechanical revolution that gave us the fossil-based capitalist civilization to the new frontier of green capitalism, the world will have continuous supplies of food, biofuels, biochemicals, bioplastics, and other varieties of biomaterials. The truth, however, is that these conditions are precisely what will make competition between food and biofuels unavoidable, worsening, not alleviating, the plight of the global poor. What looms even larger is the fact that the price hikes for grains, ineluctably arising from the competition between food and biofuels, will mean the dispossession of the land of large numbers of peasants and indigenous peoples in the Global South, to make way for large-scale commercial monocultivation.

The historical lesson to keep in mind is that the reason why billions of people in the Global South cannot access the world's food surplus is that they have neither the purchasing capabilities nor the land resources to produce their own food because they have been stripped of their biosocial spaces. In this sense, inequality and poverty are historically and socially constructed. The crocodile tears that corporate managers shed for the plight of the global poor are simply public relations ploys. The corporate claim that biofuels will mitigate climate change is equally facile. As we shall see in later chapters, biofuels and the use of biomass for electricity and heat generation will not reduce global climate change. The conversion of forests, savannahs, grasslands, and wetlands into cropland to produce more grain to satisfy the competing demands for biofuels and human food requirements, the massive application of synthetic fertilizers to boost grain production, the processing of the grains using massive quantities of energy, the transportation of the biofuels to the market, and burning the biofuels in vehicles will aggravate, rather than ameliorate, emissions of CO_2, nitrous oxide, and other gasses into the atmosphere. The constant invocations of global energy insecurity, global food shortages, and looming climate change are simply aimed at deflecting popular resistance to and intellectual contestation of the conversion of grains to liquid fuels to grease and run the machine of capitalism. Thus my purpose in this book is to closely examine the ideological foundation and empirical presentations of what the proponents of the post-petroleum bio-based capitalist civilization call a paradigm shift in world energy production and consumption. My purpose is not revelation, for there is nothing left to reveal, but rather interpretation and refutation of the dangerously faulty ontological description and gross epistemological misrepresentation of nature's biocapacity to furnish what the peddlers in biofuel production and biotechnology propose. My intention is to make a modest contribution toward the development and refinement of the counterhegemonic epistemology of agroecology, a crucial precondition for food security and climate change reduction.

Admittedly, the difficulties of doing so are compounded and confounded by the fact that the global bio-masters have adroitly integrated global food, biofuel, and biopharmaceutical production as the indivisible components of a singular bio-revolutionary process. The corporate anthem of the Biotechnology Industry Organization (BIO) promises to "feed, fuel and heal the world" by unlocking the biological mystery of nature, using new bio-inventions and bio-innovations.[6] Representing over 1,100 biotech organizations, BIO has been feverishly busy selling the idea of a world with infinite potential to produce food for everyone, green fuel to drive all stationary or moving machines or flying vehicles, and drugs to treat and cure all kinds of diseases. To this end, the biotech industry has deployed large brigades of bio-evangelists of enormous pedigrees to bring the new tidings to all.

This is how the corporate managers shed their crocodile tears: Worrying about starving future generations won't feed them. Food biotechnology will. The world's population is growing rapidly, adding the equivalent of a China to the globe every ten years. To feed these billions more mouths, we can try extending our farming land or squeezing greater harvest out of existing cultivation. With the planet set to double in numbers around 2030, this heavy dependency on land can only become heavier. Soil erosion and mineral depletion will exhaust the ground.

Land such as rainforest will be forced into cultivation. Fertilizer, pesticide and herbicide use will increase globally. At Monsanto, we now believe food biotechnology is a better way forward. Our bioseeds have naturally occurring beneficial genes inserted into the genetic structure to produce—say—insect or pest resistance crops. The implications for sustainable development of food production are massive; less chemicals use in farming, saving scarce resources, more productive yields, disease resistance crops. While we have never claimed we have solved world hunger at a stroke, biotechnology provides one means to feed the world more effectively.[7]

The biofuel-biotechnology industrial complex and their corporate intellectuals have woven a tapestry of falsehoods into a seemingly coherent body of enticements, intent on presenting food crop cultivation and biofuel production as complementary processes mediated by the gene revolution. They tell us ad nauseam that genetically manipulated seeds will be immune to biotic and abiotic stressors since they will be drought and cold tolerant and disease-resistant; that they can produce bountifully greater yields of high nutritional value crops while conserving soil and using less fertilizers and pesticides; that the resistance to weeds contained within the GM seeds themselves will decrease the need for repeated application of chemical herbicides; and the resistance to pests will enable farmers to avoid the application of costly pesticides that may otherwise contaminate the environment. They even promise to engineer seeds and plants that can directly fix nitrogen from the atmosphere, thereby eliminating the need for synthetic fertilizer application altogether. Given this master narrative, it should not come as a surprise that biotech corporations acquired, between 2008 and 2010, sixty-one patents for drought-tolerant crops.[8] However, the underlying reason for all of this is the unyielding necessity for capital accumulation, with all that implies for workers and peasants. Against the backdrop of the corporate effort to reduce the crisis of capital overaccumulation to the triple crises in food, energy, and climate change, it is crucially important to point out the singular fact that these crises are only a microcosmic manifestation of the general crisis of what David Harvey calls the crisis of overaccumulation in the core capitalist countries. So a focus on the food, energy, and climate crises can only serve as a segue into the examination of capitalist production itself and its nefarious consequences.[9]

Since the biofuel-biotechnology peddlers have cleverly presented food and fuel production and climate change mitigation as indivisible goals, any scrutiny of their claims must be grounded in a larger epistemological framework. A focus on biofuels as antithetical to food production alone could be diversionary and reductionist unless the counter-epistemology is anchored in the larger context of capitalist civilization. Therefore, I will challenge the bedrock ideological foundation of capital accumulation to inquire into the structural drivers of accumulation, and to question the intellectual and professional integrity of those who readily lend their imprimatur to the process of accumulation. I will show how the supposed synthetic biological revolution, within which the prospects for an infinite supply of biofuels are subsumed, is pregnant with profound contradictions, as well as unforeseen consequences and perils for nature and society, which could be exceedingly difficult to cope with once the synthetic biological revolution becomes a reality. Biofuel production is simply a small piece of a larger agenda. The linchpin of the synthetic biological revolution is the development of biorefineries with multiplier force to produce all kinds of bioproducts, presumably replacing or displacing petroleum refineries.

In short, the overarching aim of my work is twofold. The first is to understand and explain the driving socioeconomic forces behind the rush to universalize the commodification and commercial enclosure of nature in search of bio-based products, inclusive of biofuels, biochemicals, bioplastics, and biomaterials. The second is to unravel the tapestry of mass deceptions, distortions, obfuscations, misrepresentations, and miscomprehensions woven together by the powerful mega-corporations and their intellectual defenders in the interest of global capitalist accumulation.

TOWARD A RADICAL ECOLOGICAL POLITICAL ECONOMY

The Chinese ideogram of crisis has two characters: one for danger and the other for opportunity. This is akin to the Polanyian conceptualization of the double moments in the evolution of capitalist civilization that consist of a series of negations and affirmations, contradictions and revelations. According to Karl Polanyi, neoclassical economists, known more for their ferocity than their cogency, have succeeded in producing the utmost theoretical perversion of the capitalist economy by placing it above society and politics. This perverted laissez-faire doctrine of capitalism represents a utopian attempt to endow capitalism with natural principles of self-direction and self-regulation, a project that has sown the seeds of the system's own ultimate destruction, since the consequent creation of market oppression and the social resistance to it have become the defining feature of this system. The resulting expansion of internal crises of accumulation impels owners of capital to attempt to overcome the perpetual internal crises through doing more of the same thing: overcoming the institutional barriers to their utopian goal of limitless growth through further market deregulation and trade liberalization, coupled with unbridled competition and capital market liberalization, ultimately reducing the state to a mere agent of accumulation.[10]

Granted, owners of capital have hitherto proved resilient in transforming crises into opportunities for fresh sources of accumulation through constant reorganizing of capital and restructuring of the global economy. Given the historical record, contemporary owners of capital do not see the socially constructed global hunger, the prospects of fossil fuel shortages, and looming climate change as signs of danger but as opportunities to expand the scope of accumulation as well as to reconfigure the structure of global capitalism in ways that strengthen its stranglehold on nature and society. To counter this perspective, let us look at some principles of radical ecological economics.

With respect to the organic nexus between the fundamental laws of motion governing the economy and those of nature, the French chemist Frederick Soddy (1877–1956) vigorously challenged the dominant neoclassical economic belief as one of the most dangerous formulations of our time. As he presciently argued, neoclassical economists, steeply socialized in Newtonian mechanics, had succeeded in giving the process of capitalist accumulation a pseudoscientific depiction by linking the economy to the laws of perpetual motion. With this profoundly insightful formulation, Soddy sowed the first seeds for the conception and birth of modern ecological economics.[11] Picking up where Soddy left off, others took his formulation to its logical terminus by demonstrating the ontological connection of the principles of evolutionary biology with the laws of motion governing the movement of geophysical forces, warranting the need for a biophysical theory of economics.

In his widely celebrated 1971 *The Entropy Law and the Economic Process*, Nicholas Georgescu-Roegen systematically and meticulously exposed the ideological foundation of neoclassical economists who present the economy as being in a state of perpetual motion. By refuting the neoclassical notion that the economy could grow indefinitely without encountering contraction and dissipation of the matter/energy flow, he developed a pioneering work on ecological economics. Georgescu-Roegen maintains that production processes are invariably governed by the laws of thermodynamics; as such, they are subject to the entropy law by which matter/energy dissipates once work is performed. This is so because natural resources flowing into the production system are transformed into commodities and wastes, suggesting simultaneous depletion of low-entropy resources and increased generation of high-entropy wastes.[12]

Other writers have further enriched Georgescu-Roegen's contribution to ecological economics. Herman Daly, for example, posits that understanding the economy as a subsystem of the earth's ecosystem is a priority of the first order if human beings are to adequately grapple with issues of social equity, conservation, and sustainability. In his view, since the economy is an open subsystem of the total environment, entirely depending on it for the inflow of matter and energy and for the outflow of its wastes, the continuous physical expansion of the economy entails more demand for throughput to increase production and more sink to dispose of the generated wastes. In other words, since the earth's environment is finite and non-growing, short of establishing an optimal scale of the economy at which the demand of the economy for flow throughput and sink is equal to nature's capacity to renew itself and to absorb the wastes, the end result could be a catastrophe of the highest order for the total environment on which the reproduction of the economy depends. To avert the materialization of this scenario, Daly proposes a steady-state economy, one that neither depletes natural resources nor pollutes the environment beyond its ability to regulate and control ecosystem dynamics, hydrological processes, and biogeochemical cycles. This requires placing the total biomass extraction within the carrying capacity of the environment in which harvesting rate would not exceed the existing regeneration rate, and emissions would not exceed the assimilative capacity of the present environment.[13]

This formulation is consistent with the laws of thermodynamics. The first law of thermodynamics states that matter or energy can neither be created nor destroyed; it can only be transformed from useful and available to perform work to nonuseful and unavailable and is thus unable to perform further work. Here the second law provides extremely useful insights into the functions of ecosystems by highlighting the general irreversibility of energy once it is released to the environment in the form of heat after performing work.

According to this second law, entropic processes are bound to entail continuous reductions of low-entropy throughputs and corresponding increases in high-entropy wastes. The difficulty in reversing the dissipated energy to low entropy makes the entropic process in principle unidirectional. Even though recycling may serve as a palliative, 100 percent reversion of the original state is impossible in most cases. Suppose that Alex filled his gas-guzzling car with twenty gallons of gasoline in New York, but halfway to Washington his car ran out of gas. Where did the gas go? The answer is simple, it went up into the atmosphere in the form of emission as useless and unavailable energy. However desirous Alex was to recycle the dissipated gasoline, there was no means for doing so; he had to refill his car with fresh gasoline, repeating the cycle.

The point is that if the export of high-entropic wastes to the environment is greater than the ecological system's capacity for processing and assimilating the wastes, increases in entropic dissipation inevitably accelerate.[14] Human extraction of low-entropy throughputs from the environment, and transformation of those throughputs by economic institutions into goods and wastes beyond the equilibrium point, could disrupt the natural evolutionary processes or accelerate the dissipation matrices. One of the results could be erosion of the atmosphere's ability to cleanse itself through the natural oxidation process. The erosion of this self-cleansing and self-renewing capacity generally results from human alteration of the biochemical cycles. After all, life is supported by how nitrogen, phosphorus, hydrogen, oxygen, carbon, and sulfur are combined in the right proportions and cycled, since these six elements make up 95 percent of all living things on earth.[15] Thus human appropriation or synthetic mobilization of these elements to produce vast varieties of goods, such as biofuels, wood pellets, wood pulp, bio-based goods and bioplastics, could affect the biochemical cycles in ways that would impact climate and hydrology. Through reactive nitrogen mobilization to make fertilizer, for example, we change the nitrogen cycle by generating nitrous oxide, which contributes to the thickening of atmospheric greenhouse gases and results in climate change since nitrous oxide is 300 times more potent than carbon dioxide in trapping heat.

The crucial point here is that the global physical system is thermodynamically closed in the sense that the global environment exchanges energy in the form of solar radiation but does not exchange matter with the solar system. However, the economy is open as a subsystem of the global environment, exchanging both energy and matter. The economy continuously receives throughput from the environment on one end of the loop and exports waste to the environment on the other end of the loop. As environmental economist Charles Perrings put it, the first interaction entails extractions from the environment in terms of depletion of virgin resources, and the second interaction involves general degradation of natural resources or insertions of pollution into the ecological system.[16] Since the economy entails continuous material transformations, it thus stands to reason that ecological sustainability becomes a function of the difference between ecological capacity to provide goods and services and the quantity of insertions of high entropic wastes into the environment. This epistemological position is sound when considering how the hyperacceleration of capitalist growth in the last half-century gutted the biocapacity of the earth. Jeffrey Sachs[17] recently calculated that the gross products the world is poised to produce by 2050 could be between $380 and $420 trillion compared to the $67 trillion produced in 2007 or to the $5 trillion produced in 1950. The global ghg emissions could be equally staggering, growing from 36 billion metric tons in 2007 to 87 billion metric tons by 2050. Sachs's computation bears a powerful validation, supported by empirical evidence from China and India. The Chinese economy grew by 1,400 percent between 1980 and 2006 reaching $4.4 trillion by devouring massive quantities of virgin resources. At the same time, China's emissions of CO_2 from burning fossil fuels went up from 407 million metric tons in 1980 to 1,665 million metric tons in 2006. Similarly, India's GDP grew by 600 percent to $1.2 trillion over the same period, while its output of ghg emission increased from 95 million metric tons in 1980 to 411 million metric tons in 2006.[18]

What emerges from the preceding discussion are three cardinal principles for observing the laws of evolutionary biology and thermodynamics: sustainable scale, allocative efficiency, and social justice, which together define the organic compatibility between nature's biocapacity and human needs. A violation of any of these principles will throw the relationship into fundamental disequilibrium, eventually resulting in an ecological system crash. How sheepherders in Iceland resolved a potential tragedy of the commons that was destroying their livelihoods should illuminate the point.

Several hundred years ago, the herders saw that grassland was on the verge of total collapse due to overgrazing by too many sheep. To save their collective welfare from utter destruction, the sheep owners took a decisive action to limit the number of the sheep by assigning quotas to all sheep herders in what they considered was compatible with the grassland's carrying capacity. The grassland was restored to its previous state; so were the sheep wool and wool goods industry, with each sheep owner handsomely benefiting from the result.[19] This is a vivid illustration of how a given mode of production to meet human needs must come to congruity with nature's capacity to provide the needed throughputs and sinks if potential collapse of the system is to be averted. However, in the capitalist mode of production an unresolvable dilemma is that comporting with the natural order of things is as antithetical to capital's endless growth mandate as it is beyond the moral scope of owners of capital.

The fundamental question that arises here is the extent to which the substitution of biofuels for fossil fuels could either halt or simply accelerate the metabolic transformation of natural resources and hence entropic degradation. This question invokes a note of caution in that the role of biofuels in the ecological balance is not monocausal, but rather additive to the causes of ecological depletion, degradation, and pollution from all sectors of the system. So giving material basis to the answer to the question requires situating the drive for biofuels in the ecological relations of production. As sociologist Lakshman Yapa correctly points out, the proper point of departure in the ontological recognition of the primacy of the environment begins with a focus on the ecological relations of production. Ecological relations of production are dynamic and complex relationships that exist between humans and nature, mandating a clear understanding of nature as a self-organizing, self-directing, and self-regulating living system, on the one hand, and as a "transformation of material into use values through the application of information, energy, and labor," on the other. Furthermore, "Production uses the ecosystem not only as a source of energy and matter but also as a repository of waste products, thus continually defining a myriad of interactions within the biophysical environment."[20]

Thus the imperative to understand and protect the biophysical conditions of production becomes the first order of importance, as preservation of the biophysical conditions are central to the ecology's continuous regeneration through self-fertilization, biological control of natural enemies, and self-cleansing, following the dictates of its own natural rhythm of temporal and spatial evolution. If collective human demands on the ecology for throughputs and sinks overwhelm and undermine its biocapacity to regenerate and self-cleanse in accord with the laws of evolutionary biology and thermodynamics, the result is the degradation of the biophysical conditions of production as has happened in the past. The reason for the demise of the Mayan civilization was the overuse of natural resources, leading to the complete deforestation and disintegration of their life-supporting ecology. To the same degree, the reason for the decay of the Sumerian civilization, the grain basket of antiquity, was the mismanagement of the irrigation system, which was once the envy of the world.[21] The unfortunate thing is that we do not seem to have learned from the experiences of ancient civilizations. As Herman Daly[22] poignantly notes, the resource depletion-driven decay of ancient civilizations had little or no long-term impacts in terms of global environmental destruction and atmospheric deterioration, because those civilizations were largely local. Furthermore, there was still ecological room for people to move elsewhere, giving their original biosocial spheres ample time for natural restoration. But humans have long crossed the Rubicon from the empty world to the full world where every aspect of the ecological relations of production is adversely affected by the ever-growing wants for throughputs and sinks. The interpenetration of ecological spaces and the hydrometeorological conditions makes the full world a single unit, where the effect of one ecological component reverberates in other components of the living system. When Brazil cuts down Amazon forests to make wood pellets for electricity and heat generation in Great Britain, the consequent deforestation disrupts the carbon balance, eroding the Amazon forest ecology's capacity to sequester carbon dioxide and regulate the climate, hence increasing global warming. When Indonesia converts millions of hectares of peatland into oil palm plantations in order to satisfy European demand for biodiesel, an inordinate amount of carbon dioxide is emitted into the atmosphere that affects every nation. When Ecuador converts tens of thousands of mangrove forests into industrial fish farms to raise shrimp for export to North America, the liquidation of the mangrove forests entails subtraction of invaluable natural assets from the global stock of forests that provide crucial ecosystem services, including carbon sequestration, shoreline stabilization, coastal protection against erosion, and critical habitat and food for a galaxy of species.

During the second half of the twentieth century, demography and the hyperacceleration of the capitalist transformation of use value into exchange value conspired to break up the homeostatic interactions between human societies and nature. Demographically, when Thomas Robert Malthus revised his essay in 1825 on the relationship between population and food supply, the number of humans on the planet barely graced the one billion mark; one hundred years later that number doubled; today we have crossed the 7 billion threshold, projected to reach over 9 billion by 2050. This means that the aggregate demands that humans are making on the ecology of the already full world to meet our nutritional needs and dispose of our waste have exponentially grown, undermining nature's biocapacity for regeneration and self-cleansing. For example, at the turn of the nineteenth century, forests had covered 5 billion hectares, which dropped to less than 4 billion hectares by the turn of the twentieth century, as the expansion of agriculture, pasture, firewood, lumber, and paper production took heavy tolls on forests. The growth of the pulp and paper industry, in particular, doubled down on the destruction of the global forest ecology, regardless of territorial boundaries, as global paper consumption increased by 423 percent between 1961 and 2002, with far-reaching implications for the livelihoods of forest-dependent people, ecosystem integrity, and the carbon balance.[23]

The most destructive force, however, has been the capitalist transformation of use value into exchange value, not necessarily to satisfy human needs but to further strengthen the process of accumulation. This phenomenon has led to the hyper-acceleration of production, whose demand for throughputs and sinks has proved beyond nature's biocapacity to supply food, feed, fiber, and other throughputs. For example, the near exhaustion of nonrenewable resources is the background to the contemporary rush to divert more and more grains and oilseeds into biofuel production. This has led to the bifurcation of agriculture into chemical-dependent industrial agriculture, which produces most grains and commodities, and the agroecological mode of cultivation that supports the dispossessed mass farmers. Today, there are 500 million smallholder farmers in developing countries whose food production accounts for 15 to 20 percent of overall food production and yet feeds nearly 80 percent of the world's population.[24] These small farmers, for the most part, do not infringe upon the ecological relations of production, since they closely follow nature's biocapacity to regenerate, employing practices such as retention of vegetation, integration of agroforests, integration of livestock into their farms, and reliance on organic inputs. Of course, the growth in their number, coupled with the fact that they are continually being pushed off to marginal areas by big industrial farmers, is interfering with the operation of the ecological relations of production.

To illustrate the extent of the migration of capital to biofuel, biochemical, and biomaterial production, following is a brief review of the impacts of industrial agriculture on the ecological relations of production from the perspective of ecological economics. The aim is to elucidate whether biofuels could contribute to poverty alleviation, climate change mitigation, and energy security without impacting the ecological relations of production.

Following the Second World War, the mechanical revolution in manufacturing was exported to the agricultural sector via capital's increasing appropriation of land and water resources and the mechanization of agriculture. As a result, the conversion of forests, savannahs, grasslands, and wetlands into croplands, supported by extensive irrigation works and intensive use of synthetic inputs, grew to an unprecedented scale. Worldwide, the area put under cultivation between the 1950s and the turn of the century quadrupled, as a result of which overall annual world food production increased by 44 percent, while growth in cereals increased by 59 percent; of the 1,600 million hectares under production at the beginning of this century, 302 million hectares were equipped with irrigation, accounting for 40 percent of overall food production. The total area under cultivation is projected to increase by another 235 million hectares by 2050 (all of it in the Global South), which will produce 1 billion metric tons of additional cereals that will be needed to feed the new human arrivals, and grow the feedstocks that will be required to produce biofuels. Even though agribusiness interests and their supporters attempt to reassure us that 80 percent of the additional food production increases will come from intensification of production in the form of higher yield productivity and intensity of cropping, the projected additional grain supply would come only by converting more and more forests, savannahs, and grasslands into cropland. The reason is simple: the rates of growth in yield of the major food crops have long been falling alarmingly. For example, growth in wheat yields declined from about 5 percent a year in 1980 to 2 percent in 2005; yield growth in rice and maize dropped from more than 3 percent a year to 1 percent during the same period. Projecting into the future, yields of the major food crops will fall further to 0.8 percent per year by 2030 and to 0.5 percent per year by 2050. Owing to temperature warming, the overall agricultural output in developing countries could fall by 9 to 21 percent. The secular stagnation in the yields of the major crops is projected to result in real price increases of 59 percent for wheat, 78 percent for rice, and 106 percent for maize during the period between 2010 and 2050.[25] Considering this objective reality, can the world produce sufficient biofuels to make a difference in the overall mix of energy without affecting global food supply and global food price? The answer is, of course, no.

In addition to the secular stagnations in yield productivity, the imponderable magnitude of the impacts of climate change and uncertainty in the patterns of rainfall on global food production still await a reckoning. Projections suggest that there could be a shortfall of 350 million metric tons of food grain by 2025 due to water shortages—a loss of grain equal to the total U.S. food grain produced in 2005.[26] In addition to the decline in food grain production, another result of water shortages could be the disappearance of many species of grain and plants, representing substantial reductions of ecological resources with serious implications for the temporal and spatial evolution of nature. During the twentieth century alone, around 75 percent of plant genetic resources are estimated to have been lost, and a third of today's diversity could be entirely wiped out by 2050. Between 1970 and 2010, the populations of freshwater, marine, and territorial vertebrate species were reduced by 52 percent.[27]

Notwithstanding the serial liquidation of ecological resources and the inexorable reduction of species populations, today 1.25 billion people live in absolute poverty; 768 million people have no access to safe and clean water; and 162 million children under five years of age are stunted or wasted.[28] There is dark irony in this situation in that the proponents of biofuel-biotechnology use this grim reality to justify the further enclosure of nature, arguing for the production of more grain and feedstock through the gene revolution, which will then miraculously result in poverty alleviation and climate change mitigation. The truth is that the logic of capitalist accumulation and the resultant unequal distribution of resources and purchasing capabilities are responsible for the deplorable maelstrom of material deprivation, malnutrition, starvation, and hydro-destitution of hundreds of millions of people in the Global South (with growing numbers in the Global North). For instance, even though in 2010 the world had a food surplus that could have fed the entire human population one-and-a-half times, the FAO reported that there were 925 million people who were going to bed hungry every night. In 2011, there were forty-five countries with per capita yearly food consumption under $1,000, and fifteen of them were projected to remain stuck in stagnant poverty with less than $1,000 per capita yearly food consumption by 2050.[29] This peculiar conundrum of concurrently having too much food and having too many hungry people who lack purchasing capabilities for the surplus food is a perfect illustration of the gross incongruity that exists between the capitalist mode of production, geared to the maximization of exchange value, and the imperatives of the ecological relations of production. Yet, agribusiness and metropolitan countries still intend to solve this fundamental contradiction in capitalist agriculture by diverting the surplus food to biofuels production. Of course, the hidden purpose masked by this rhetoric is, as we have seen, that the conversion of grains to biofuel production could simultaneously resolve the crisis in agricultural surplus production in industrial countries and the crisis of global energy shortages, as a result of which the continuous expansion of accumulation by dispossession would be put on a permanent course. Meanwhile, the fate of the hungry billions shall fade into oblivion.

The new dynamic of competition between food crops and biofuel production takes on an even more obscene dimension with the growing intensification of the capitalist mode of livestock production. By the turn of the twentieth century fully one-third of world grains and oil seeds were already being fed to livestock. Indeed, the liquidation of enormous ecological resources associated with the expansion of the global industrial food manufacturing system is being aggravated by the increase in the industrialization of the livestock mode of production, creating a shift in dietary habits in the Global South as more and more people imitate the Euro-American style of meat consumption. For example, since the 1980s, meat and egg consumption in the Global South increased twofold and fivefold, respectively.[30] There is no mystery to this grim reality. Industrial mass livestock production occurring in conditions of land shortages, by definition, requires the diversion of land resources from human food crops to concentrated feed production, making food and feed direct competitors. Note that North American–style meat production requires three to four times as much land, and two to four times as much reactive nitrogen fertilizers. It was no coincidence that most of the 45 percent of temperate deciduous forests, 27 percent of tropical forests, 70 percent of grasslands, and 50 percent of the savannahs converted to agriculture during the twentieth century was accounted for by the relentless expansion of the livestock mode of production.[31]

During the second half of the twentieth century in particular, industrialization of the livestock mode of production paralleled the industrialization of the green revolution–driven production of grain cereal and oilseed. By the beginning of the 1990s, 1.7 million metric tons of grains and oilseeds were fed to livestock, augmented by the conversion of 275 million hectares of forests and savannahs to planted pastures. By the turn of the twentieth century, 70 percent of grain in the United States had already been fed to livestock. The feed crops grown on 130 million hectares of U.S. cropland could have fed 400 million hungry people. If the entire livestock sector worldwide were to revert to the natural grass-based mode of livestock production, large amounts of grain could be freed, enough to meet the nutritional needs of one billion hungry people.[32] However, doing so would be antithetical to the overriding obsession with capital accumulation by bio-vandalization and human dispossession.

The driving force behind the intensification of the capitalist mode of livestock production has been what Jeremy Rifkin calls the "steers complex," where vast swaths of forests, savannahs, and cropland are converted to planted pastures and specific feed-crop production to supply animal feed to the rapidly proliferating feedlots in the Global North.[33] The unprecedented expansion of planted pastures and soybean monocultivation in Latin America was behind this drive for centralization and concentration of the livestock mode of production. In Brazil, for example, the area under soybean monocultivation soared from 23 million hectares in 2005 to 42 million hectares in 2014, and is projected to soar to 100 million hectares at the expense of frontier forests and savannahs.[34] Bilateral and multilateral lending institutions in the Global North have aided the transformation of traditional grass-based to industrial livestock production. Between 1971 and 1977 alone, the World Bank and the Inter-American Development Bank doled out $3.5 billion in loans and technical assistance to big commercial cattle producers in Latin America. Predictably, privileging feed-crop production over human needs has had a deleterious impact on the availability and accessibility of grains for human consumption. In Mexico, sorghum (historically unknown in the country) displaced corn production in many localities in order to meet the growing demand for sorghum as animal feed. Moreover, in the 1960s, a mere 6 percent of the Mexican corn was fed to cattle, growing to 33 percent by 1990, reducing the corn available for tortilla production, the staple of Mexican diet. While the urban elite and landed aristocracy deepened their meat-based lifestyle, millions of dispossessed Mexicans found themselves thrown into the maelstrom of material deprivation and urban squalor or perilous international migration.[35]

In sum, what the migration of capital to biofuel production does is triangulate the traditional competition between human food and animal feed by adding biofuel to the mix since the amounts of grains and oilseeds going into biofuel production must be subtracted from food and feed, or more forests, savannahs, and grasslands must be converted to cropland to grow feedstocks. Even worse, the simultaneous diversion of food crops and conversion of virgin ecological resources to biofuel production could grow exponentially just as the demand for the same resources by the global livestock sector is projected to grow exponentially. According to the FAO, global meat production is expected to grow from 229 million metric tons in 2001 to 465 million metric tons by 2050, while that of milk is projected to grow from 580 million metric tons to 1.043 billion metric tons. Correspondingly, the additional demand for feed crop is expected to increase by over one billion metric tons by 2050, and the additional pastures required to support the growing number of the livestock population will be 5.4 million square kilometers.[36]

From the point of view of the ecological relations of production, the rise in the global livestock population, the methods by which livestock is raised, the amount of plant biomass appropriated for the livestock sector, and the services required to support them will have severe implications for the state of climate, environment, and hydrology. As bio-economists Nathan Pelletier and Peter Tyedmers computed, if the current trends in industrial livestock production continue until 2050, the safe operating space for greenhouse gas emissions occupied by the livestock sector will increase by 70 percent, while biomass appropriation for the livestock population will increase by 88 percent and synthetic nitrogen mobilization by 294 percent, expressed in a cascade of deforestation, environmental degradation, ghg emissions, and freshwater depletion.[37] These conditions are bound to worsen as many developing countries continue to imitate the patterns of advanced countries in industrial livestock production and heavy meat consumption, entailing conversion of forests, savannahs, grasslands, and wetlands into cropland for commercial concentrate animal feed production. The 1,543 million metric tons of grain cereals, pulses, brans, oil cake, oil crops, and roots and tubers that were fed to livestock in 2005 are projected to double by 2050.[38] The amount of cereals and coarse grains directly appropriated to feed the additional global livestock population in 2050 is an amount that could be enough to feed an extra 4 billion people.[39] Thus, analysis of the livestock mode of production relative to the ecological relations of production supplies additional evidence to illustrate how the dynamic interactions between economic forces and the laws of evolutionary biology and thermodynamics operate. As the first law of thermodynamics states, nothing is created out of nothing; to create something, a given unit of throughput must be taken out of the general stock of natural resources for conversion into goods and wastes. The scale of the throughput taken out of the general stock of natural resources determines whether the sustainability and status of the general ecological stock is maintained. If the unit of throughput being used falls within the regenerative capacity of the natural environment, then the law of sustainable scale is respected. However, as noted earlier, in addition to worsening the triangulation of competition for grains and oilseeds and hence for land and water resources, the industrial livestock revolution has already contributed immensely to the erosion of the ecological relations of production. This violates the fundamental principle of sustainable scale in three crucial ways.

First, to set up animal farm operations, land must be cleared of vegetation; the sorts of ecosystem services provided by the natural vegetation are discounted in terms of the future or not counted at all. Today, livestock grazing already occupies 26 percent of the earth's ice-free land surface, while 33 percent of agriculture is devoted to feed-crop production, well beyond sustainable scale. This suggests that the ecological impact per unit of livestock production must be cut by 50 percent just to decrease the damage to the ecology beyond the present level. Note that the livestock revolution is responsible for converting 70 percent of previously forested land in the Amazon to pastures. Worldwide, 20 percent of pastures and 73 percent of rangelands had already been degraded by the turn of the twentieth century due to overgrazing, livestock action, and soil compression or compaction. In the United States, for example, the livestock sector is responsible for 55 percent of all soil erosion and sedimentation, 37 percent of pesticide use, 50 percent of antibiotic use. and 33 percent of freshwater pollution and contamination with nitrogen and phosphorus loads. All told, over a period of forty-four years since 1962, 270 million hectares of forests were converted to pastures, and 120 million hectares more are projected to be converted to pastures before 2050.[40] The expansion of the livestock sector above the level of sustainable scale has no doubt immensely contributed to the radical alteration of the ecology. It is no surprise that the livestock sector is recognized as the major driver of biodiversity loss through deforestation, fragmentation, land degradation, pollution, livestock-induced climate change, sedimentation of wetlands, and the facilitation of invasive species. In fact, 306 of the 825 ecoregions in the world across all biomass and biogeographies are said to be threatened by livestock. Of the thirty-five global areas in significant danger for biodiversity loss, twenty-three are said to be adversely affected by livestock production.[41]

Second, the livestock sector puts too much waste into the environment and the atmosphere, far beyond the waste-processing capacity of nature. In part, this stems from the industrial intensification of livestock production, resulting in the excessive concentration of their waste in limited areas instead of being usefully spread as fertilizer across scattered grasslands and cropland. For example, one giant farm in Utah with 1.5 million head of hogs was found to have a sewage problem larger than that of the city of Los Angeles. Likewise, a mega-farm in central North Carolina, where hogs outnumber people, was found producing more fecal waste than the states of California, New York, and Washington combined.[42] Moreover, since the livestock revolution denotes a transition from the extensive grazing system to industrial livestock concentration and operation in limited areas, industrial livestock production unavoidably fosters the acceleration of the demand for more animal feed and the mobilization of more reactive nitrogen required to boost production of feed crop. Since industrially fixed nitrogen determines the productivity of cropland dedicated to animal feed, more of it must be synthetically fixed, with disturbing implications for the natural carbon cycle. It is no accident that the global amount of reactive nitrogen generated by humans is more than the amount provided by all natural terrestrial systems. What the livestock revolution does is increase reactive nitrogen mobilization, most of it eventually ending up in water bodies and the atmosphere. Livestock manure by itself accounts for two-thirds of anthropogenic nitrous oxide emission, which is 300 times more potent in trapping heat than carbon dioxide.[43] Emissions result not only from animal manure, urine, and other animal wastes, but also from clearing forests to create pasture, the application of nitrogen and phosphorus to boost animal feed production, the intensive use of fossil energy to transport animal feed, the transportation of processed animal products to markets, and fossil energy used for heating and cooling animal operation facilities.

By the turn of the twentieth century, the world was producing 100 million metric tones of petroleum-derived reactive nitrogen annually to grow livestock feed alone. Unsurprisingly, livestock populations are responsible for emissions of 2.4 billion metric tons of carbon dioxide per annum, from combinations of live-stock-driven deforestation, soil cultivation, land deterioration, desertification, and reactive nitrogen mobilization. Again, it is no accident that the current mode of livestock production accounts for 65 percent of anthropogenic nitrous oxide emissions 37 percent of methane emissions, and for 64 percent of anthropogenic ammonia emissions, which generates acid rain and causes acidification of vast areas in the world. The anthropogenic disturbance of soils related to the expansion of feed-crop production in particular has far-reaching ramifications for the earth's carbon balance, since soils are the largest reservoir of carbon, storing between 1,100 billion and 1,600 billion metric tons, compared with 560 billion metric tons contained in living vegetation and 750 billion metric tons in the atmosphere. It is estimated that pasture production–induced oxidation alone results in 100 million metric tons of CO_2 emissions per annum, accompanied by 3 billion metric tons of CO_2 emissions from the respiratory processes of livestock production, 86 million metric tons of methane from enteric fermentation, and 17.4 million metric tons of methane emissions from manure decomposition.[44]

The ecological and atmospheric impacts of industrial livestock are compounded by a global meat manufacturing system that is fully integrated into the agrochemical and pharmaceutical manufacturing systems. In the United States, 37 percent of pesticides and 50 percent of antibiotics are consumed in the livestock sector. The amounts of the chemical compounds, antibiotics, and growth hormones not assimilated by livestock and their feed crops are put back into the environment; 50 percent of synthetic nitrogen applied to crop production is released and enters downstream natural assets with far-reaching impacts on ecosystem functions. Since capital accumulation in the livestock sector and accumulation in the chemical/pharmaceutical manufacturing system have now become coterminous, the combined effects of production in the two realms will continue to have a force multiplier effect of degradation on ecosystem functions. For example, the annual global emissions of air-polluting ammonia grew from 18.8 million metric tons at the beginning of the twentieth century to 56.7 million metric tons by the 1990s and is now conservatively projected to increase to 116 million metric tons by 2050.[45]

Third, the livestock revolution exerts enormous pressure on the ecological relations of production relative to ever-diminishing freshwater resources. Water withdrawals are already intensively used for animals, for growing and processing animal feed crops, cleaning and cooling farm animal facilities, and for processing livestock products. As Colin Tudge has trenchantly pointed out, today's average farmer uses 500 liters of water to grow 1 kilo of potatoes, 900 liters to grow 1 kilo of wheat, and 2,000 liters to grow 1 kilo of rice. In contrast, the same farmer uses 3,500 liters of water to raise a kilo of chicken and 100,000 liters of water to obtain a kilo of beef. In addition, the multiplication of animal farm operations will grossly interfere with the processes of hydrological circulation and regulation, making the natural replenishment of water systems difficult due to the compaction of soil, reduction in infiltration, degradation of river banks, salinization, depletion of floodplains, and the lowering of water tables.[46]

There is also the problem of quality. The livestock revolution will continue to compromise the integrity of the global hydrology through pollution, contamination, and eutrophication of freshwater bodies, following the insertions of animal waste, reactive nitrogen, phosphorus, pesticides, antibiotics, countless growth hormones, and other synthetic agents into natural water systems. In the United States, the livestock sector is responsible for 33 percent of the synthetic nitrogen and phosphorus load inserted into freshwater bodies, causing nitrate contamination, acidification, and eutrophication of immense proportions. The quantitative diminution and qualitative deterioration of water supplies will occur in the alarming context of the fact that, by 2025, 64 percent of human population will be living in water-stress basins, and 1.4 billion people will be living in water-scarcity regions. By 2014 two billion people were already living in river basins where they experienced water scarcity at least one month in a year.[47]

What all of the preceding means is that the principles of sustainable scale, efficient allocation, and social justice have long been violated by the hyper-acceleration of resource extraction and waste production. The regenerating and self-cleansing capacity of nature has been hollowed out in the past fifty years because too much raw material has been taken out of nature to keep the machine of capitalist accumulation going, and too much waste had been dumped into the environment and the atmosphere. The overextraction of forest resources compounded the erosion of the global forest ecology's capacity to provide essential ecosystem services such as temperature regulation, carbon sequestration, rainfall generation, water purification, erosion prevention, flood control, and protection of critical habitat for countless animal species. Likewise, the loss of 50 percent of global wetlands, mangroves, estuarine and deltaic resources during the past fifty years gutted the capacity of these ecosystems to provide such essential functions as carbon sequestration, shoreline stabilization, erosion and flood control, aquifer recharges, water purification, sediment detention, chemical absorption or neutralization, and the provision of critical habitat to countless terrestrial and aquatic species. It must also be borne in mind that it is estimated that the Amazon forests pump into the atmosphere 20 billion gallons each day from their stored water of 8 trillion metric tons. This is said to be equivalent to the energy of 80,000 coal-fired super-giant power stations performing the same job every day. The Amazon basin receives half of its rainfall from its own hydrologic cycle. In the Congo basin, 75 to 95 percent of rainfall comes from recycled moisture within the basin itself.[48] The natural allocative efficiency of forests as drivers of evapotranspiration, cloud formation, the hydrologic cycle, and regulation of climate is organically connected to the distributions, structures, characteristics, densities, and contiguities of forests, which determine the frequency and intensity of precipitation.

THE STRUCTURAL DILEMMA

The above broad description leads to this fundamental question: Could biofuels be produced (both first-generation and second-generation) in sufficient quantity to grease the machine of global capitalism without worsening resource depletion, environmental degradation, and atmospheric deterioration? Even though the core chapters in this book will provide the complete answer to the above question, a prefatory word is in order here. To restate the case once again, since nothing is made from nothing, it stands to reason that the throughput required to produce biofuels must come either from the diversion of food and feed crops in sufficient quantity to biofuel production or from the conversion of more and more forests, savannahs, and grasslands to cropland to grow feedstocks.

There is no other option. The emergent competition between food, feed, and biofuels occurs in the context of projected global population growth, and the rising income of the middle class in emerging markets, who demand more food and more meat products. In a nutshell, the addition of biofuels to the competition between food and feed can only worsen the stark state of the global ecology and climate. In 2005, the Millennium Ecosystem Assessment report, comprehensively and meticulously prepared by 1,300 world scientists, pointed out that fifteen (60 percent) of the twenty-four ecosystems they evaluated were being exploited at or beyond their regenerative biocapacity. The annual cost of lost ecosystems and biodiversity associated with the competition between food and feed was already in the range of $2 trillion and $4.5 trillion, a magnitude that will go up with the addition of biofuels.[49]

There are three risks associated with biofuel production as the third competitor for throughputs. First, as the land resources grow scarce because of the competition between the three production sectors, extremely valuable ecosystems will be vulnerable to commodification and commercial enclosure, short-circuiting the provision of essential ecosystem services. For the world to secure 10 percent of transport fuels from biofuel production by 2030, between 118 million and 505 million hectares of new cropland must be found to grow the required feedstocks, compared to the 38 million hectares of cropland used for feedstock production in 2008. This is equal to between 8 and 36 percent of the world's existing cropland. Note that at the current rate of cropland acquisition required to meet the growing demands for land resources, between 320 million and 850 million hectares of forests, savannahs, and grasslands would have to be converted to cropland by 2050, which is equal to the combined size of Indonesia, Ethiopia and Brazil. On top of this, other sectors of the global economy will continue to put additional pressure on the land resource base. For example, infrastructures, urban expansion, and settlements are projected to increase by between 260 million and 420 million hectares by 2050, encroaching upon agriculture. In the past, around 80 percent of urban expansion occurred at the expense of agricultural land. Furthermore, the area dedicated to biomaterial production is expected to increase by up to 215 million hectares by 2050. In addition to the stridently continuing ambition and determination of biofuel peddlers to secure ever-growing quantities of feedstocks, developing countries are desperate to secure more cropland to grow food to avoid hunger and alleviate poverty, as well as to narrow the gap in global inequality. In India, for example, where 52 percent of the population live in poverty and 45 percent of children under five are stunted or wasted, the metabolic rate of natural resource appropriation is a mere 4.6 metric tons per person per year compared with 25 metric tons in Canada. This grim reality compels India to seek more arable land to grow needed food. So the pressure of cropland expansion, land competition, land intensification, and land-use change on ecosystems and climate is not hard to imagine. Second, since the feedstocks used for biofuel production are also used to produce food and feed, the resulting competition will drive food prices upward, hurting most particularly the poor, who spend 50 to 80 percent of their income on food. Third, as we shall see in later chapters, biofuel production is water-intensive at both the cultivation and processing levels, thus competing not only with food and feed production but also with human needs for drinking and cleaning. Moreover, land-use change from clearing vegetation and reactive nitrogen mobilization to boost feedstock production present a double jeopardy in terms of ghg emissions and nitrogen pollution of water expressed in acidification and eutrophication of important hydrological systems. Note that 20 percent of carbon emissions in the 1990s were directly related to land-use change.[50]

Even though the green revolution has resulted in impressive gains, as key to the construction of the global food manufacturing system it prepared the conditions for unsustainable land competition, soil degradation, soil erosion, nutrient pollution, salinization, eutrophication, agrochemical contamination, biodiversity loss and ghg, all related to land-use change, intensification

of industrial agriculture, exorbitant reactive nitrogen mobilization, and monopolization of irrigation.[51]

As food, both feed and biofuels compete for lands and water
resources; the first casualties are forests, savannahs, grasslands, and
wetlands, which are not only repositories of ecological resources
and genetic materials, but also regulators of climate, carbon stores,
and providers of food and shelter to countless species. Indeed, the
context for the exhaustion and degradation of many ecosystems
has been that over 500 million hectares of forests, savannahs, and
grasslands were converted to agriculture and pasture between 1962
and 2006 in the Global South, at a time when industrial countries
lost 54 million hectares of cropland to urban and suburban sprawl,
as well as transportation and communication infrastructure. The
global pulp and paper industry, which still annually devours over
400 million metric tons of forest resources, has already been one
of the major drivers of deforestation, something that will grow
worse as more woody bioenergy plants are targeted by the biofuel-
industrial complex for conversion to so-called second-generation
biofuels and wood pellets.[52] The unsavory result of the increasing conversion of forests, savannahs, grasslands ,and wetlands to
cropland to grow the throughput required by food, feed, and biofuels entails the conditions of accelerating landscape denudation
and ghg emissions from both land-use change and soils carbon
oxidation.

One little understood factor is the role of soils in the sequestration of carbon. In fact, the amount of carbon stored in soils is far
greater than that stored in vegetation. When forests are clear-cut,
the soils are immediately exposed to erosion by wind and water,
as well as to compaction, solar radiation, and desiccation, inducing the release of carbon into the atmosphere. The consequent soil
degradation is reflected in a linear fashion in the degradation of
cropland, inducing more deforestation and more soil perturba-
tion. In the past half-century, 50 percent of world agriculture had
been affected by erosion, nutrient depletion, biological degradation, and compaction due to massive loss of vegetation and the

consequent soil agitation. The upshot has been doubling down on the conversion of more forests, savannahs, grasslands, and wetlands into cropland to make up for reduced soil fertility and falling crop production. This has come at the expense of further soil degradation. At the beginning of the new century, 38 percent of world agriculture, excluding permanent pastures and woodlands, was found to have been severely degraded. In all, 1.2 billion hectares of land were found to have been severely degraded and another 700 million hectares lightly degraded, leading to a loss of 75 billion metric tons of soil to erosion annually. As a result, 5–12 million hectares of cropland were abandoned every year since the 1960s due to soil degradation. Moreover, approximately 70 percent of the dry lands used for agriculture worldwide was deemed degraded and was on the verge of desertification by the turn of the twentieth century. It is estimated that soil degradation affects more than a billion people in 100 countries. Indeed, more than 135 million people could be forced to migrate elsewhere from their homelands due to soil degradation and desertification, with 60 million people in Sub-Saharan Africa alone. Between 1960 and 2000, 43 percent of Africa's cropland and 70 percent of overall economic activity were severely affected by soil degradation and desertification. Notwithstanding this deplorable reality, the biofuel hawkers see Africa as the new green oil El Dorado. The demand for land in Africa in 2009 alone, punctuated by corporate land grabbing, was equal to the cropland expansion that occurred during the previous twenty years.[53]

Against the backdrop of cropland degradation and the continuing competition between food, feed, and biofuels for new land resources, capitalists are moving to high-value ecosystems, exemplified by the grim state of peatland rainforests in Indonesia. The disruption of peat soils is particularly perilous because they consist of compressed and concentrated organic material, accumulated over centuries, and are supersaturated with carbon. Even though the area of peatlands worldwide covers 4 million square kilometers, representing only 3 percent of the earth's surface, they store approximately 528 billion metric tons of carbon, equal to 75 percent of the carbon currently in the atmosphere. Notwithstanding the dangerous consequences of converting the peatland rainforests to oil palm plantations, Indonesian elites and transnational corporations have begun plundering this delicate ecosystem, largely prompted by growing European demand for biodiesel. When the government's and corporate plans run their course, the area of peatlands and pristine rainforests converted to oil palm plantations in Indonesia will, by 2050, have grown from 9 million hectares in 2010 to 45 million hectares.[54]

For transnational corporations, however, the plunder of natural resources like the peatland rainforests is the raison d'être of accumulation, which they rationalize by reference to greater economic growth, job creation, and foreign exchange earnings. Indeed, they never run out of rationalizations to justify biofuels. For example, when the 2007–08 global financial crisis drove home the ripple effects of the competition between food, feed, and biofuels, nearly simultaneous price hikes for staple food grains and oil seeds were enacted due to the diversion of substantial quantities of food crops to biofuels.

For the fossil resources industrial agriculture depends on for synthetic fertilizers, pesticides, and fossil fuels, the biofuel peddlers and their intellectual minions refined their arguments. First, even though they partially conceded that there could be a conflict between food and fuel, they quickly adjusted their contention that such a problem could be one of management rather than scarcity. It was at this point that they brought on board the biotechnology gurus to supply more bio-rationalizations in defense of the supposed sustainability of biofuels. For the biotech companies, the "food versus fuel" debate now became a heaven-sent opportunity to penetrate the global food ecology. Presumably, genetic engineering of crops and plants could endlessly supply grains and plants that could satisfy the demand for food and green fuels without any impact on the global food ecology and global grain market. Second, when the evidence began to show the adverse relationship between food and biofuels, proponents began to argue in favor of second-generation biofuels, derived from agricultural and forest residues, nonedible plants such as eucalyptus, pines, poplars, and willows, and a vast mix of grasses. Although this book will cover their rationalizations in full in later chapters, several points must be clarified at this juncture.

First, the drive for biofuel production has already led to the ferocious expansion of giant monoculture plantations of soybeans, oil palm, sugarcane, jatropha, corn, cassava, sweet sorghum, sweet potato, and related bioenergy crops and plants, displacing tens of millions of subsistence farmers and indigenous peoples in the tropics and subtropics. The escalation of industrial monoculture has brought with it the urgency to convert forests, savannahs, and grasslands into arable land. Second, even though biotechnology corporations exuberantly and falsely try to reassure the public that biofuels derived from GE (genetically engineered) crops and GE trees would not only make the "food versus fuel" debate a non-issue but also contribute to the solution of global hunger, fuel short-age, and climate change, the recourse to GM of crops and plants under the mask of increasing production will likely be danger-ous in the long run from the standpoint of both public health and biodiversity preservation. The commercial genetic manipulation of food crops aims at the homogenization of crops to make them responsive to inputs supplied by the same companies. Moreover, the use of genetically engineered trees for biofuel production and wood pellets is likely to lead to genetic contamination of native vegetation.[55]

In summary, analysis of the ecological relations of production clearly indicates that biofuel production and pyrolysis-driven electricity generation are unsustainable. Limitless growth requires limitless supply of throughputs, but the earth's capacity to supply them is limited. Concomitant with the geometric progression of industrial production during the twentieth century, the appropria-tion of biomass increased by a factor of 3.6 per year, the extraction of ores and minerals grew by 27, fossil fuels by 12, and construction materials grew by a factor of 34. Annual natural resource extraction and use soared from 5 billion metric tons in 1900 to 55 billion metric tons in 2000, and it is projected to increase to 100 billion by 2030 and 140 billion metric tons by 2050 as developing countries continue to play catch-up with advanced countries, in an effort to eradicate hunger and alleviate poverty. The commercial appropriation of natural resources and consumption have grown in parallel with the widening and deepening of neoliberal globalization, as seen in the fact that the global trade of raw materials grew from 5.4 billion metric tons in 1970 to 19 billion metric tons in 2005. The appropriation of natural throughputs in the quantities described above not only undermines the regenerative capacity of nature but also its waste absorption capacity, because the release of waste is proportional to the natural resources processed into goods and services. For example, the extraction and consumption of 140 billion metric tons of natural resources is projected to lead to the quadrupling of carbon emissions. Note that although the total global biocapacity in 2010 was 12 billion hectares, the world's ecological footprint was 18.1 billion hectares, overshooting the ecology's capacity to regenerate, much less to supply all the throughput demanded. This means that the world has been using the equivalent of the biocapacity of 1.5 planet Earths. By the turn of the twentieth century, three of the nine planetary boundaries requisite for a fully regenerative planet—biodiversity loss, climate change, and nitrogen cycle—were considered already crossed. And while the world today needs 1.5 Earths to meet the demands that the world is currently making on the only planet we have, three or four planets will be needed by 2050 to meet the projected increases in demand for natural resources.[56] So the deployment of overaccumulated capital to bioenergy crop and plant production to generate liquid biofuels and wood pellets could potentially push nature to a tipping point. The huge investments in large-scale industrial agriculture and monoculture tree plantations have already begun to erode the global forest ecology. The long-term effect of the loss of vast tropical forests relates to their impact on ecosystem dynamics, climate, carbon sequestration, and hydrologic cycle. The interpenetration of geo-ecological spaces and meteorological conditions amplifies the negative consequences of unrestrained expansion of natural resource exploitation into virtually all components of nature. It matters little whether the harm is done in any particular country; the effects will be felt throughout the biosphere. The complex interpenetration of geo-ecological spaces and hydrometeorological conditions is such that even the Amazon and Congo basin rainforests are interconnected through biogeochemical cycles and other bio-hemispheric processes, with profound implications for climatic conditions and precipitation regimes not only on each other but also on other regions. The two tropical regions are connected by the natural back and forth oscillation of atmospheric movements across the Atlantic Ocean. As a result, heavy rainfall and floods in the Congo basin coincide with droughts in the Amazon basin and vice-versa. Moreover, these precipitation patterns affect the climate and hydrology of other regions. For example, recent observations of these weather patterns indicate the annual deforestation of the Congo basin by 1.5 million hectares resulted in rainfall decrease in the Great Lakes region of the United States by between 5 and 15 percent; a similar impact had been discerned in Ukraine and some parts of Russia.[57]

The invaluable extrapolation made from this record supports the conclusion that the 200 million hectares of tropical rainforests lost between 1950 and 1990 and the 427 million hectares of additional tropical forests that underwent significant degradation have had important bearings on local, regional, and global climate and rainfall patterns. To fully appreciate the centrality of tropical forests to climate regulation and carbon sequestration, it is useful to remember that, of the 670 billion metric tons of carbon stored in terrestrial vegetation, 86 percent is securely sequestered in the tropics and subtropics. When 100-year-old tropical trees are burned for energy or to make way for farms, they release their heavy loads of CO_2 rapidly. It will take 100 years to fully recapture the emitted carbon by growing their replacement. In the meantime, the CO_2 will still be in the atmosphere for hundreds of years, worsening climate change.[58]

It is in conjunction with these ecological relations of production that we must assess the contributions of ecological economists to the consequences of the addition of biofuel production to the capital accumulation process. Contemporary ecological economists have certainly dented the neoclassical hold on the research community in the industrial countries in four critical ways. First, ecological economists have rightly pointed out that the earth is a thermodynamically closed system in that it cannot import matter from outer space nor can it export its waste material to outer space. In this sense, our planet is physically bounded. It thus stands to reason that ecological resources become the constraining factor in an economy that is a subsystem of the ecological system. The economy has no luxury to import low-entropy throughput from outer space or to export its high-entropy wastes outside its own sphere. This supposes that the thermodynamic and biological operations of our physical world can be sustained only when there is a correspondence between the levels of available physical stocks and levels of a population whose needs must be reasonably met. In Herman Daly's formulation, long-term sustainability can be had only under steady-state conditions, in which the economy reflects the total available stocks of material wealth and the total population, all held constant at some desirable levels. This requires stringent limitations on the extraction of raw materials, such as allocation of quotas, and managed control of physical production and consumption as well as a planned population growth rate.[59] In other words, because the total basket of goods and services available to all people is a function of the physical environment's ability to supply low-entropy throughput to continue production processes and to absorb the high-entropy wastes generated by those production processes, maintenance of the total natural resource stocks at the present level or above becomes the requisite condition for sustainable development, and constancy of total natural resource stocks and commensurate population size become the minimum conditions of assuring sustainable scale.[60] Curiously, the biofuel-biotechnology hucksters, when placed under pressure, grudgingly acknowledge that all this is true. However, they hasten to add that the biophysical limitations can be overcome by further reengineering nature.

Second, ecological economists view state intermediation as crucial for bringing about a balance between the demand of individual appropriators of natural stocks and the ecological system's requirements for self-maintenance. To clarify this observation, economists Robert Costanza and Herman Daly, for example, differentiate between micro and macro allocations of ecological resources. Micro allocations are made by individual producers and consumers competing for goods and energy. Here, as individual producers and consumers compete to maximize their private benefits, there will be an overexpansion of the economy. Since natural resource stocks are vital resources held in trust by the collectivity for the benefit of present and future generations, macro or collective social decisions take precedence over private market decisions under the stewardship of the state. This is the reason why the state should have greater interest in the future of the ecological system than individuals because the integrity of the ecology and the stability of social existence of the collectivity are public goods, which only the state could provide.[61]

Third, ecological economists rightly contend that resolution of structural poverty is requisite for maintaining the integrity of the ecological system. This reasoning inheres in the contention that poor people have no stake in ecological conservation since their survival is based in the here and now. Given their wretched circumstances, the poor are likely to discount the present to the future. Therefore, it is in society's long-term interest to ameliorate the living conditions of the poor. Just distribution and sustainability are the criteria by which both social justice and sustainable scale of the economy are measured. In a nutshell, societal demand for and nature's ability to supply low-entropy throughput and sinks would not be in steady state unless a brake is put on limitless growth of resource extraction and sink utilization and unless there is just distribution of goods and services.[62]

Finally, the contribution of ecological economists to unmasking the fetishism of gross domestic product (GDP) is difficult to exaggerate. By conveniently focusing on aggregate growth of the economy, measured in terms of GDP, neoclassical economists have long masked the costs of unfettered capitalist accumulation underlying GDP growth. For neoclassical economists, anything that does not produce exchange value has no value at all. Ecosystem services are typically taken by capital free of charge, and thus have no market value because dollars are not exchanged. They confine their measurement to the natural resources that produce goods such as timber and wood pulp for which there are markets, while ignoring the non-market services provided by trees before being cut down, such as pollination services, carbon sequestration, climate regulation, water purification, storm protection, and shoreline stabilization.

In an apparent effort to demystify the position taken by orthodox economists, ecological economists have struggled for a quarter-century to put a price tag on ecosystem services in ways that are understandable to the average person, even though putting a price tag on ecosystem functions is controversial. This is because commodification and privatization of these services are associated with the valuation exercise, since some market fundamentalists have already proposed payment for ecosystem services as a solution to resource overuse. After thoroughgoing examination of seventeen ecosystem service types from sixteen biomes, Robert Costanza and his colleagues put a price tag of $145 trillion on the services that humans derive annually from the ecosystem in terms of carbon sequestration, climate regulation, water production and purification, storm protection, erosion control, shoreline stabilization, pollination, waste absorption, and provision of suitable habitats to an array of terrestrial, marine and aquatic species. If the destruction and degradation of marine and terrestrial ecosystems that took place between 1997 and 2011 had been avoided, the valuation of global ecosystem services could have been $167 trillion per annum. In other words, we have lost $22 trillion worth of crucial ecosystem services between 1997 and 2011; the destruction of coral reefs alone may have cost the global economy $11.9 trillion during that period. For reference, the gross world product of the global economy in 2011 was $75 trillion.[63]

There are also unavoidable abiotic consequences of industrial globalization, costs that are not captured by GDP. The dogged determination of capital to create a borderless world has indeed placed the fate of the biosphere on a precariously dangerous trajectory. The flows of global trade soared from $3 trillion in the early 1980s to $30 trillion in 2012, with no consideration of the environmental costs of the circulation of these goods. Almost all globally traded goods are transported by gigantic containerized cargo vessels crisscrossing the world's oceans and seas, dumping all manner of refuse and toxic fuels along the way, without anyone monitoring what they do to vital parts of the biosphere. The global circulation of goods by sea increased from 228.3 million traffic equivalent units (TEUs) in 1994 to 627.5 million TEUs in 2013; this is equivalent to 150 million trailer-size containers carrying goods across the globe.[64]

Can criticisms be made of modern ecological economics? Ecological economists are unreproachable in terms of their description of the connections between allocative efficiency, sustainable scale, and just distribution. Empirically, the market is ill-equipped to reveal the real non-market values of natural goods and services, much less to justly distribute them. Nor can the market tell us how much of the animal species, forests, and wetlands should be left intact to maintain ecosystem integrity. Additionally, since distributive equity and sustainable scale, by definition, are antithetical to the logic of capitalist accumulation, the market cannot address issues of equity and scale short of socially determined imposition of limitations and regulations on market operations. In keeping with the law of conservation of matter/energy, ecological economists are also right when they propose the paramount importance of prior determination of scale in resource extraction, since out-flow of high-entropy wastes into the environment is proportional to the inflow of low-entropy throughput from the environment into the economy.

However, when it comes to prescriptions, contemporary eco-logical economics falters. In the first place, the supposition that stocks of material wealth and levels of populations can be main-tained at some desired levels within the prevailing capitalist mode of production betrays objective understanding of how the logic of accumulation operates. The notion that steady-state conditions can be attained if people somehow temper their wants for the nearly infinite flow of goods and services smacks of religion, not of a materialist understanding of history. Because ecological econo-mists hinge their prescriptions on ethics to tame the appetites of capital accumulators and consumers, the propositions forwarded to address issues of resource conservation, poverty eradication, and climate mitigation takes on quasi-religious overtones.

Their own class limitations have, perhaps subconsciously, made ecological economists steer clear of both the reactionary stagnation of the bourgeois order and the needed revolutionary transforma-tion of it. Ecological economists forget that infinite expansion of accumulation is the heart and soul of capitalism. The prescriptive weakness of ecological economists stems from the general orienta-tion they share with all bourgeois economists on the recognition of capitalism as a system without alternative and thus incapable of qualitative change. It can only be subjected to judicious modi-fications. This requires making bourgeois ethics guide the call for reform, meaning persuading corporations, states, and consumers to recognize the singular fact that there are limits to growth, that they should be willing to trade the prevailing productionist growth ideology for an earnest commitment to sustainable development, and that consumers of all classes ought to learn how to live within their means, combating conspicuous consumption and respecting nature. But if there is anything anathema to capitalist accumula-tion, it is the combination of ethics and limits to growth. A system whose raison d'être is predicated on continuous capital expansion cannot accommodate sustainable development. The call by ecological economists to redesign capitalism in such ways as to establish a thermodynamic balance between what is biophysically possible and what is ethically, socially, and psychically desirable smacks of romantic petty-bourgeois utopianism. An effective countervailing challenge to the dominant order can succeed only if there is clarity on the epistemological understanding of the true ontological status of a system that is called into question. What has made the prevailing social order so formidably resistant to change or substantial modification is that the mastery of the chieftains of industry and corporate intellectuals over the production, control, and dissemination of information that passes for authoritative knowledge reigns supreme.

Unfortunately, this romantic petty-bourgeois intellectualism inadvertently adds another layer of confusion to the contemporary discourse on change. This kind of scholarly disquisition and the proliferation of non-governmental organizations and intergovernmental institutions, mainstreaming the concepts of ecological economics to reform the productionist growth ideology, have simply fostered the creation of the romantic illusion that meaningful change can occur by modifying the prevailing social order. For example, fully internalizing the narrative and liberally appropriating the concepts of ecological economics, the UN Environment Program (UNEP) produced a lengthy monograph in 2011 titled *Towards a Green Economy: The Pathway to Sustainable Development and Poverty Eradication*. The document never mentioned, even in a sentence, the desirability or possibility of limiting capital accumulation as a way to address the impacts on resource depletion, environmental degradation, and atmospheric deterioration. Instead, the authors wasted page after page on the purported feasibility of a green economy consistent with a hyper-accelerating global capitalism in order to convince the reader and policy makers that limitless growth could be had if corporations and government adopt ecological modernization to promote eco-efficiency and eco-sufficiency, led by the market in resource extraction and circulation. The fanciful jargon used in this exercise is dubbed "decoupling," that is, decreasing the metabolic rate of use of natural raw materials per unit of economic output. In other words, the use of less energy, raw materials, land and water resources to produce the same economic output would automatically result in eco-efficiency increases. The Pollyanna-ish consequences could be expressed as the simultaneous achievement of the goals of resource conservation, poverty eradication, climate mitigation, and green economic growth. Decoupling of natural resource use could also go hand-in-hand with negative impact decoupling, in which negative environmental impacts would decline in absolute terms, while green economic value is continuously being added.[65]

Unfortunately, the presumed correlation of efficiency with resource use reduction has long been debunked. The nineteenth-century British economist William Stanley Jevons found that efficiency in resource production actually increased consumption of the resource.[66] It must be borne in mind that efficiency in bourgeois accounting means reduction in the cost of producing and supplying a given unit of goods and services, in which case this will have a perverse impact on consumer behavior. The supply of fuel-efficient cars means that people would drive more frequently and for longer distances. It is no accident that people drive more when gasoline prices are low and drive less when gasoline prices spike. Moving of goods around the globe more efficiently because of the technological revolution in transportation and communication has not led to less extraction and use of resources. On the contrary, the efficiency gains from the technological revolution have made it easier and cheaper for consumers to use resources and goods produced in distant lands by wasting huge energy on transporting these resources and goods. The $1.6-trillion-strong global tourism industry could not have grown to the degree it has without the proliferation of air-polluting airplanes that have made global travel the most convenient and affordable mode of modern transportation.[67] To develop a keen appreciation of the extent to which the notion of decoupling is hollow, consider the fact that 320–850 million hectares of additional forests, savannahs, and grasslands are projected to be converted to cropland by 2050 in order to produce the required feedstocks, food, and feed. Could the consequences of deforestation of this magnitude, accompanied by emissions from the manufacturing and use of synthetic nitrogen, pesticides, fuels, and other agrochemicals, be decoupled from GDP? Obviously, the answer is no; to admit otherwise would represent a scornful repudiation of basic physics. The evidence-free romantic conjectures manufactured by such as the UNEP is meant not to solve the looming dangers of poverty and climate change but rather to mask their legitimation functions of neoliberal globalization.

Finally, if the aspirational project of ecological economists is too utopian to have a long-term impact on the course of history, their account of history is even weaker, because ecological economists run into serious operational difficulty when it comes to the role of the state in the economy, where they envision Keynesian eco-managerialism. The error stems from the tendency to view the state as exterior to the process of accumulation. The state is presented as a neutral force, potentially capable of objectively generating and enforcing legislation and regulation to address questions of efficiency, equity, and scale. In this sense, they share with conventional economists the state-centric approach to resource conservation and environmental protection. They thus inadvertently entertain the illusion that overexploitation of natural resources and pollution of the ecological system could be avoided if the information gaps among stakeholders are closed through state intermediation. In their view, the state can bring about a broad consensus among producers, consumers, non-governmental organizations, and all other relevant actors on the essential values of sustainable scale, just distribution, and efficient allocation of resources. As some ecological economists have argued, the processes of consensus building, ecological integrative modeling, and adaptive management could close the gaps in information and understanding. This, in turn, would yield the desired institutional framework by shaping, modifying, or altering the behaviors and attitudes of all participants in the intellectual endeavor.[68]

Let us look a little further at the ecological economists' conception of the capitalist state. In the wake of the 1970s oil shocks, the oil oligopolies have succeeded in securing radical deregulation of the fossil energy sector in the United States, cushioned by numerous exceptions, loopholes, tax breaks, and subsidies. A look at Koch Industries will serve to show how deep the political reach of corporate capital is, especially that of the petrochemical industry.

The $115 billion Koch Industries is the second largest privately held corporation in the United States after Cargill, which means that it is the sole corporate fiefdom of Charles and David Koch. Operating in over sixty countries with about 100,000 workers, Koch Industries controls four oil refineries, six ethanol plants, a natural gas–fired power plant, and 4,000 miles of pipeline within the United States. The company has prospered no matter the president or the political party in control of Congress. The two brothers saw their wealth soar from $28 billion when Barack Obama assumed office in 2009 to $86 billion by the end of 2015.[69] What matters is their capacity to relentlessly defend the extremely deregulated hydrocarbon energy sector, and to wage open war against any effort to change it. For example, when the Environmental Protection Agency moved to regulate surface ozone emission from oil refineries, the high-powered Koch lawyers argued that the EPA failed to take into consideration the immense health benefits of smog because it blocks the sun, thus reducing skin cancer. Without smog, 11,000 additional cases of skin cancer would occur annually. Remarkably, the D.C. circuit court accepted the lawyers' pro-smog arguments, even accusing the EPA of discounting the possible health benefits of ozone and overstepping its authority to regulate ozone levels. The judges had reportedly been participants in the seminars on law and economics organized by the Koch brothers.

The Koch Industries are major polluters, ranking third among the thirty worst polluters of air, water, and climate, after Exxon and American Electric Power. Its Georgia-Pacific paper mill alone was dumping more pollutants into U.S. waterways than General Electric and International Paper combined. Moreover, Koch Industries have generated more than 24 million metric tons of greenhouse gases annually. In 2012, Koch Industries was singled out to be the number-one producer of toxic waste in the United States, producing 950 million pounds of toxic chemical waste.[70]

It is this mode of accumulation by emission/pollution that makes the Koch brothers the most ubiquitous and notorious warriors against the potential resurrection of the regulatory state in America. They are exemplary capitalists, setting the standard for shaping America's domestic and foreign policy in relation to black carbon production and distribution. They have purchased the services of willing politicians, legislators, regulators, and judges to do their bidding, spending hundreds of millions of dollars in the process. Beneficiaries of the brothers' largesse must be climate change deniers and unambiguous friends of "drill baby drillers" in order to qualify for unconditional support from the Koch brothers' foundations and the synthetic front groups they finance. They have also mastered the dissemination of propaganda, internalizing Antonio Gramsci's notion of the paramount importance of ideological and cultural hegemony in the perpetuation of the status quo. Institutions of higher learning have long been among their primary targets for ideological subversion. As of 2015, Koch foundations were subsidizing pro-market supremacy, pro-disciplinary neoliberalism, and anti-tax programs in 347 institutions of higher learning, including the resource-rich Ivy League universities. Their generosity comes with strings attached. When the Koch brothers contributed more than $965,000 to the creation of the center for free enterprise at Brown University, the string attached was that the Koch foundations would participate in the selection of professors. When the brothers helped fund the creation of a freshman seminar in free-market classics at the same university, the condition was the course would be taught by a libertarian professor. Additional funding was provided to Brown graduates to do research on why and how bank deregulation would be beneficial for the poor.[71]

To boost the production of sufficient intellectual materials, the Koch brothers themselves have funneled hundreds of millions of dollars into the production and grooming of pro-market ideology scholars and researchers. Between 2007 and 2011 alone, for example, the Koch brothers gave $30 million toward the endowment of professorships, the underwritings of neoliberal economic programs, and the sponsorships of pro-market ideology conferences and lecture series. Think tanks and private policy institutions then repackage the intellectual output in a fashion that could be intelligible and accessible to the mass public. One of the most vociferous and prodigious manufacturers of Koch-inspired propaganda is George Mason University's Mercatus Center, the premier outpost of neoliberal market ideology, funded by the Koch brothers. When George W. Bush became president, the Mercatus Center recommended fourteen of the twenty-three programs in the administration's regulatory hit list, such as privatization of social security, further deregulation of taxes, deregulation of derivatives in energy, abolition of the EPA, ending the government-supported welfare system and Medicare. It was no accident that the Bush administration installed Susan Dudley from the Mercatus Center, notoriously known for her virulent anti-regulation credentials, as the top regulatory bureaucrat.

The Koch brothers have also been active in creating their own propaganda platform, organizing annual seminars on law and economics and other topics for judges, justices, senators, congressmen, scholars, and the super-rich. Even Supreme Court justices Scalia and Thomas partook of these seminars. Between 2003 and 2010 alone, 140 reactionary bourgeois foundations, spearheaded by Koch foundations, distributed $558 million to 91 different nonprofit groups, think tanks, trade associations, and academic programs to wage permanent warfare against groups that sought to promote climate change mitigation through the re-regulation of the black carbon sector, as well as to block progressive advocacy groups from gaining ground in electoral politics and democratic legislative representation.[72]

The Koch brothers have never been short of corporate allies, especially in terms of promoting climate-change denial. Exxon, Chevron, and BP have all supported the construction of what we might call the climate change denial industrial complex. No fewer than 124 organizations have received money from Exxon-Mobil to describe climate science as "junk science" and environmental activists as charlatans and fanatics. These include the Heritage Foundation, the Cato Institute, Hudson Institute, George Mason's Law and Economics Center, the Competitive Enterprise Institute, the Frontier of Freedom Institute, the Reason Foundation, the George C. Marshall Institute, and many other groups with names that make them appear as though they are grassroots citizen organizations or academic bodies, such as the Center for the Study of Carbon Dioxide and Climate Change, the National Wetlands Coalition, the National Environmental Policy Institute, and the American Council on Science and Health.[73] Two of George C. Marshall Institute's employees—the Institute received $630,000 from Exxon—wrote a long manifesto assisted by a Christian fundamentalist extolling the benefits of ghg emissions in these glowing terms:

> As coal, oil and natural gas are used to feed and lift from poverty vast numbers of people across the globe, more carbon dioxide will be released into the atmosphere. This will help to maintain and improve the health, longevity, prosperity and productivity of all people. . . . We are living in an increasingly lush environment of plants and animals as a result of the carbon dioxide increase. Our children will enjoy an earth with far more plant and animal life than that with which we are now blessed. This is a wonderful and unexpected gift from the Industrial Revolution.[74]

Taking the Senate floor, James Inhofe, Republican senator from Oklahoma who then chaired the Senate Environment Committee, echoed the climate change deniers' slogan in these terms: "The claim that global warming is caused by manmade emissions is simply untrue and not based on sound science. Carbon dioxide does not cause catastrophic disasters. Actually, it will be beneficial to our environment and our economy.... With all the hysteria, all of the fear, all of the funny science, could it be that manmade global warming is the greatest hoax ever perpetuated on the American people. It sure sounds like it."[75]

The Koch brothers and the black carbon oligopolies were not alone in their epic war to expand the privatization trajectory of sovereignty; they received perpetual reinforcement in their war against the potential return of the regulatory state, as well as against progressive pro-climate advocacy groups from other key constituencies. In particular, their alliance with agribusiness and biotechnology oligopolies had been strategic as the latter, too, had been obsessively preoccupied with defending the food manufacturing system from state regulation. Between January 1999 and June 2010 alone, the fifty largest agriculture patent holders, two of the biggest biotechnology corporations, and the agrochemical trade association together spent $572 million on lobbying Congress. In addition to using permanent in-house lobbyists, these oligopolies hired 13 former members of Congress and more than 300 former congressional and White House staffers to promote legislation in support of GM food and agricultural products or to block labeling such products. In 2010, these oligopolies had retained more than a hundred lobbying firms to descend on Congress.[76]

These examples of the power of the fossil energy, agribusiness, and biotechnology oligopolies in American politics support the conclusion that no bourgeois reform, such as those ecological economists have proposed, could occur under the prevailing system in ways that would establish sustainable scale, allocative efficiency, and social justice. It appears that contemporary ecological economists are drawing on a past that is no longer relevant, a past in which Keynesian regulation of the market was embraced, largely as a result of working-class organizations and ruling-class fear of more radical change. We live now in a world of global corporations. The state's autonomy, such as it was, has been severely compromised by capital's global power. Interventions once possible no longer are. Capital will move away from them. It is no longer bound by national territories. In addition to having lost control over domestic industrial capital, the advanced capitalist countries could no longer avail themselves of the traditional means of geopolitics to have exclusive access to spheres of influence and domination in the Global South, because most corporations have already spread their assets across the globe. The metropolitan state now sees its primary function in how to capture the larger share of global accumulation as exporting more through an integrated global market. This requires the complete demolition of trade barriers to all goods and services including high-tech GM grains where the comparative/competitive advantages of the advanced capitalist countries lie. True, state intervention in the political economy, whether national or global, has not ceased, but the form has changed, decidedly in favor of accumulation and to the exclusion of labor. Now the state intervenes in the market to foster the hypermobility of capital and to redistribute tangible and intangible resources upwardly from the taxpayer to the giant corporations, as reflected in the rescue of the super-giant banks and hedge funds during the 2008 financial crisis. Other measures include gutting social protections and social safety measures, outsourcing public services, recommodification of national assets such as parks and natural wilderness. But most important are subsidies, courtesy of the taxpayer and justified under the guise of enhancing international competitiveness, making exports cheaper vis-à-vis other countries. In 1997, the Earth Council released a comprehensive study detailing how the world was annually spending $700 billion subsidizing corporations to overuse water in countries where water tables were falling, to deplete fishery resources at a time when seventeen oceanic fishing grounds were showing signs of exhaustion, and to encourage the production and use of coal and fossil fuels at a time when climate change and sea-level rise were in evidence. Startled by the extent of the abuse and misuse of public resources, the authors of the study expressed their revulsion in these terms: "There is something unbelievable about the world spending hundreds of billions of dollars annually to subsidize its own destruction."[77]

In essence, as geographers Deborah Cowen and Neil Smith correctly identified, the metropolitan state has now become a geo-economic social agent in the service of global corporations, resulting from the prevailing structural power of corporations, the total supression of the territorial logic of the state by the market logic of global functional integration, and the relative superannuation of geopolitics as a means of creating an exclusive constellation of client states.[78] In short, the market has completely and powerfully extricated itself from the state, and the state has been reduced to the sheer provision of enabling and legitimating services to the market.[79]

Similar transformations have occurred in the Global South, where relative developmentalism has become dysfunctional. As a result, states in the South have become fully transnationalized and locked into the neoliberalized global trading system, freezing the historic global division of labor. They simply mimic metropolitan states in their attempts to induce the relocation of international capital. India offers an illustrative case. Hiding behind health concerns, in 1998 India banned the processing of oils from indigenous mustard seeds by small-scale operations and allowed free entry of foreign soybean oil. Prior to the ban, hundreds of thousands of mustard-oil processers were self-employed in rural India. Tens of thousands of small crushers used to convert locally produced mustard seeds into low-cost edible oils that accounted for 68 percent of processed oils in India. But when free imports of soybean oil became official policy, these small operations and the people who depended on them for livelihoods were no more. In addition, the free entry of soybean oil became a Trojan horse for the introduction of GM soybean cultivation as India permitted big land owners to begin GM soybean monoculture production following the ban on processing of local mustard oils.[80]

The discussion in the preceding paragraphs supports the conclusion that there is no state intermediation to speak of under late capitalism to smooth over the contradictions between the logic of accumulation and the principles of sustainable scale, allocative efficiency, and social justice. The fundamental flaw in ecological economics stems from the failure to understand that questions of allocative efficiency, sustainable scale, and just distribution cannot be isolated from the political ecology of the capitalist mode of production.

The long-term project to save capitalism from its deepening internal contradictions necessitates reframing bourgeois ideology to generate at least the illusion of consent. In the 1980s, for example, corporate intellectuals were put to work to refurbish bourgeois ideology into what has come to be known as neoliberalism. The obsessive preoccupation of neoliberalism now focused on changing the states in the Global South so that corporations from the core capitalist countries could take over assets such as state-run telecommunications, public enterprises, public utilities, etc., under the guise of promoting efficiency, accountability, and transparency through privatization, deregulation, and trade liberalization. The methodology employed in the 1980s was to remove the barriers to further accumulation in the metropolitan North. With the typical state in the Global South now subordinated to the requirements of global capitalism, the focus shifted to expanding the scope and scale of primitive accumulation through the acquisition of agricultural lands, forests, savannahs, wetlands, grasslands, and water resources, under the guise of promoting bioenergy security, poverty eradication, job creation, and rural development. If advanced capitalist states are to thwart an "Occupy Wall Street" type mass movement from escalating to full-scale social revolution, they have to devise new coping strategies. These survival strategies now come in the form of what David Harvey termed accumulation by dispossession. This involves the dispossession of millions of rural producers of their ancestral lands, and commercially enclosing forest, wetland, and water resources, followed by privatization and monopoly control over these resources, considered foundational to primitive accumulation. Where Karl Marx saw primitive accumulation as the historical precondition of capitalism based on wealth derived from non-capitalist modes of production, necessary for providing the initial yeast, David Harvey sees primitive accumulation in the Global South under late capitalism as the dominant reorganizing principle of capital, acquiring semi-permanent features, because expanded reproduction within capitalist countries through technological innovations and the social engineering of mass consumption has become increasingly problematic. The deepening crisis of overaccumulation has become a frightening prospect. So, just as early capitalist commodity production came into existence through savage dispossession, expropriation, plunder, enslavement, commercial enclosure, and colonization, contemporary capitalism has come to rely on the same means for its continued existence—by appropriating, commodifying, and marketizing hitherto uncommodified natural resources in the Global South.[81] In this view, accumulation by dispossession, i.e., the appropriation of land and other natural resources under contemporary capitalism, requires the savage expulsion of peasant producers, followed by the commodification and privatization of land and other natural resources, conversion of public properties to private corporate assets, and suppression of all forms of rights. This involves not only the commercial enclosure of nature but also the privatization of politics and culture in the sense that they serve to lubricate the deepening process of accumulation by dispossession. It logically follows that accumulation by dispossession is a politically driven process. Harvey hastens to add that if expanded reproduction (based on the exploitation of wage labor) was the dominant mode of accumulation between 1945 and 1973, accumulation by dispossession has become the primary mode of capitalist accumulation since the 1970s, involving the colonization of hitherto uncolonized social spheres in the Global South. The latter requires outright expropriation, predation, deception, intimidation, mass expulsion of peasants and violence—the primary object being the completion of the divorce of people from the means of production.[82]

THE MANNER IN WHICH THE CONTEMPORARY land grab is taking place in the Global South supports the conclusion that accumulation by dispossession has become the primary contradiction of late capitalism. Since the commercial enclosure of nature in the advanced countries is almost total, the land and water resources to be stolen are primarily located in the Global South, mostly tropical Africa, Latin America, and Southeast Asia, which are seen as the next sites for "green" oil and bio-based commodity production. The excitement in accumulation by dispossession has indeed led the biofuel-biotechnology industrial complex, global financial institutions, and corporate intellectuals to speculate that there are 445 million hectares of uncultivated land worldwide suitable for the cultivation of sugarcane, oil palm, soybeans, wheat, maize, and fast-growing, short rotation trees. Of this total, Africa is said to have 201 million hectares, Latin America 123.3 million hectares, and Southeast Asia 73 million hectares available for bioenergy and food production, enough to produce at least 245 exajoules (EJ) of energy a year by 2050. Other corporate analysts optimistically suggest that there could be as much as 2.2 billion hectares of land that could be devoted to tree plantations, perennial grasses, sugarcane plantations, and other bioenergy feedstock production with the capacity to generate many hundreds of EJ annually, replacing up to 27 percent of present global fossil energy consumption. This means conversion of at least 10 million hectares of land to bioenergy plantations every year until 2050 compared to the 4.5 million hectares of land that were put under crop cultivation every year between 1961 and 2007.[83]

It is within this context that the exceptionally ruthless land grabbing that has been occurring in the Global South since the beginning of this century must be understood. According to various sources, between 2000 and 2010, approximately 227 million hectares of land deals were struck or were under negotiation between land resource–rich countries and a constellation of corporations, hedge funds, Arab petrostates, and Asian indus-trializing countries. Of the 1,217 land deals officially registered, involving 83 million hectares, between one-third and two-thirds are estimated to have been dedicated to feedstock and biofuel production. Of these 83 million hectares, 56.6 million hectares of land auctioned off were in Africa and were equal to the com-bined cultivated area of Switzerland, Denmark, Belgium, France, Germany, and the Netherlands. By some estimates, the extent of land resources sold or leased to foreign land grabbers could feed 1 billion people. Sixty-two percent of the land deals were in Africa, a continent known for severe famine and hunger. The cruel irony is that of the bioenergy feedstocks and food crops grown on these stolen land resources are destined for export.[84]

Insofar as the spectrum of biofuels production goes, a new map of bioenergy appears to be in the making. At the top of the hierarchy are the core biofuels countries controlling the supply of finance capital, biotechnologies, and organizational power. Countries in this category include the United States, Canada, members of the European Union, Japan, and Australia. Next come the intermediate biofuels countries, which are both recipients of finance capital and biotechnologies from the core and producers of biofuels in their own right. These are the classic semi-peripheral countries that have lately joined the G7 to form the G20, such as Brazil, Argentina, China, India, South Korea, Turkey, and South Africa. The intermediate biofuels countries occupy a strategic locus in the emerging global biofuels map, finding one of their feet in the core biofuels countries as recipients of finance capital and biotechnologies to develop their domestic biofuel industry, while they opportunistically fan the idea of south-south collabo-ration to ostensibly promote the collective interest of the Global South. This allows them to develop a Janus-like strategy to align their interests with those of the core biofuel countries to further their own biofuel industry and, at the same time, compete with the core countries in the periphery feedstock-supplying nations for biological resources. In the eyes of core countries and their corporations, the intermediate biofuel countries have credibility with periphery countries because of their public pretensions to speak on behalf of the amorphous Global South. In this, the intermediate biofuels countries supply the necessary bridge for the core to the periphery, and could be used as models to be emulated by the periphery. In the end, this boils down to the singular fact that both the core and intermediate biofuel countries are equal bio-vandalizers.

At the bottom of the biofuel hierarchy are periphery feedstock-producing countries, such as Ethiopia, Mozambique, Tanzania, Ecuador, Bolivia, Cambodia, Laos, and Papua New Guinea, where capital accumulation by geoecological vandalization and human dispossession has been most pronounced. Most of the land deals made in these countries are shrouded in secrecy. In 2008 and 2009 alone, 80 million hectares of land had been auctioned off to foreign corporations and foreign governments with two-thirds of the land deals in Africa. For example, China signed a 2.8-million hectares land deal with the Democratic Republic of Congo (DRC) for oil palm plantations, while South Korea got sweet land deals of 700,000 hectares in North Sudan and the United Arab Emirates got another 750,000 hectares in the same country. More than a third of Liberia's, 48.8 percent of the DRC's, 21 percent of Mozambique's, and 10 percent of South Sudan's productive lands were auctioned off to TNCs, hedge funds, and sovereign wealth funds. Most of the grains and bioenergy feedstocks grown in these countries had been destined for export to advanced countries and emerging markets.[85] At the root of this new scramble for land resources has been the competition between food, feed, biofuel, and industrial tree plantation sectors.

---- **2** ----

The Biofuel Industrial Complex and Its Migration to the Global South

Haunted by the specter of the Hubbert peak theory, which predicted the eventual depletion of petroleum energy, George W. Bush's first act as president in February 2001was to establish a national energy task force, under the leadership of his vice president, Dick Cheney. The membership of the task force is still classified, but many analysts suspect that it was made up of high-powered oil tycoons and intellectuals from corporate-funded think tanks. The group's mandate was to identify new areas where petroleum production could be expanded. Its recommendations are contained in eight chapters. According to the group's collective speculations, by 2020 demand in the United States for natural gas, electricity, and oil would rise by 50 percent, 45 percent, and 33 percent respectively.[1] The package of recommendations included a call for the United States to accelerate domestic oil exploration and production while, at the same time, upgrading its presence in oil- producing regions, strengthening its ties with such key oil-producing states as Nigeria and Angola, and assisting U.S. oil transnationals to overcome obstacles to investment in foreign energy sectors.

Coming on the heels of the oil task force, the unprecedented global oil price hikes during the first decade of this century seemed to give some credence to the task force's overall conclusion about future fossil oil markets. It was against the backdrop of the Hubbert peak becoming a reality that the global biofuels industrial complex has given an extraordinary momentum to the expansion of primitive capital accumulation in the Global South through the conversion of living biological stocks into both liquid and solid fuels. In other words, with the apparent exhaustion of fossil fuels very much in prospect, both advanced and industrializing countries were increasingly looking to biofuels as complementary or alternative sources to fossil energy. To dramatize the long-term implications of exhaustion of nonrenewable fuels for the geo-economics of energy security, the IEA (International Energy Agency) heightened the concerns over the prospect of oil peak with the publication of *Energy Technology Perspectives 2006*, triggering a new scramble to complete the commodification of nature. Under a business-as-usual scenario, the IEA warned that by 2050 global demands for coal, natural gas, and petroleum would increase by 192 percent, 138 percent, and 65 percent, respectively. In consequence, global CO_2 emissions would increase by 130 percent by 2050. The IEA was, however, sanguine about the prospects of improving supply conditions and containing greenhouse gas (ghg) emissions by relying on nature's capacity to furnish sufficient bioenergy. According to its bold assertion, bioenergy, depending on the pace of the technological revolution, could supply up to a 26,000 million ton oil equivalent (Mtoe) by 2050. Even if the pace of technological progress lags demand, the supply of biofuels could be in the range of 6,000 to 12,000 Mtoe a year, requiring the devotion of 20 percent of world farmland to bioenergy feedstock production. If the IEA's speculations come to pass, the share of road transportation biofuels alone would rise from 19 Mtoe in 2007 to 57 Mtoe by 2015, and then to 102 Mtoe by 2030. With generous state subsidies and technological breakthroughs, the share of road biofuels could actually rise to 164 Mtoe in 2015 and then to 778 Mtoe by 2030.[2] Those were the predictions in 2007. In fact, though, the most recent IEA report shows that road biofuels consumption had exceeded predictions and had already risen to 396 Mtoe by 2015.[3]

It is against the context of such projections that countries and corporations began looking to biological resources as a source of bioethanol and biodiesel fuels, to continue limitless capitalist growth and to overcome the crisis of overaccumulation as well—effected under the veneer of emission reductions, poverty eradication, and energy independence. Indeed, the early exuberance regarding the prospects of biofuels was so irrational that the U.S. Energy Information Agency (EIA) made a projection of world liquid biofuels consumption rising to 112.5 million barrels of oil equivalent per day or 238 exajoules (EJ) per annum by 2030, of which 60 percent will be consumed by the road transport sector.[4] Buoyed by such fanciful projections, by 2010, ninety-six countries had adopted bioenergy programs, another sixty countries had instituted biofuels mandates, and thirty countries were contemplating doing the same.[5]

The 105 billion liters of biofuels produced in 2011 comprised 3 percent of global road transport fuels, produced from feedstocks grown on 3 percent of global farmland. While the United States accounted for 63 percent of global bioethanol production using corn as feedstock, Brazil was responsible for 24 percent, using sugar. With respect to biodiesel, the European Union was the leader, controlling 53 percent of total production, followed by the United States with 15 percent, and Brazil and Argentina each producing 13 percent.[6] First-generation bioethanol is produced from sugarcane, corn, sugar beets, wheat, rice, rye, sweet potatoes, sweet sorghum, cassava, and other starchy crops that must undergo fermentation and distillation. On the other hand, biodiesel is produced from soybeans, rapeseed, palm seeds, sunflowers, jatropha, as well as animal fats. Hounded by the controversy surrounding the issue of unsustainability of large-scale first-generation biofuels without jeopardizing food security, the biofuel industrial complex

has been scrambling to move up to second-generation biofuel production, using woody plants, agricultural and forest residues, or
fast-growing short rotation trees such as eucalyptus, pines, poplars, and willows as feedstocks that must undergo saccharification,
the process of converting starches and cellulose to simple sugars,
followed by fermentation and distillation into biofuels. If large-
scale second-generation biofuel production becomes feasible, the
scope for the commodification of natural resources and the biopredation of nature could be unprecedented, as will be the scope
for human dispossession.

According to the imaginations of biofuel cornucopians, because
all living biological stocks, whether crops or plants, are infinitely
renewable throughput, the world could have infinite quantities of
biofuels year after year, and, by extension, the crisis of overaccumulation of capital would be resolved. To be sure, the combination
of the fear of petroleum depletion and the overly sanguine anticipation of biofuels becoming a substitute for or complementary to
fossil fuels has been driving the growth of liquid biofuel production. Global bioethanol production rose from 38.2 billion liters in
2006 to 89 billion liters in 2008, and biodiesel production increased
from 4 billion to 12 billion liters over the same period. Early on,
energy analysts projected that the global market value for first-
generation biofuels would grow from $20.5 billion in 2006 to $80.9
billion by 2009, and then to a whopping $280 billion by 2020.[7]

If the world dream of the biofuel industrial complex stands, the
world can forever count on renewable biotic resources for 20 to
30 percent of global energy supply.[8] Other techno-optimists predict that bioenergy could supply up to 50 percent of global energy
needs by 2050.[9] But this growth requires the continuous conversion of massive amounts of arable land, forests, and wetlands to
bioenergy feedstock production as well as the use of vast quantities
of freshwater resources to grow presumably unlimited bioenergy
crops and industrial trees.

Oblivious to how the laws of evolutionary biology and thermodynamics operate, the global biofuel industrial complex is bullish

about the prospects of realizing its global dream by completing the commodification, recommodification, and commercial enclosure of nature by supplying limitless energy, eradicating world hunger, and mitigating climate change. Indeed, in anticipation of greater accumulation, the cross-pollination of investments in the emerging bioenergy sector has become unprecedented, as multifarious capitalist corporations and institutions have begun pouring their overaccumulated capital into the sector. These corporations and institutions range from hedge and pension funds to automobile, petroleum, grain, biotech, and chemical industries. These corporate oligopolies see the socially constructed crisis of global capitalism in energy and food as an opportune moment to make a profit, and they are prepared to demolish all barriers on the way to limitless expansion of accumulation.

The potential depletion of fossil fuel has also brought oligopolies and governments into ever closer union. Global corporations promise that they have unlimited biotechnological capabilities and organizational means to transform all living organisms and plants into infinite sources of food and energy. Governments, for their part, are poised to create the necessary enabling environments for totalizing the commodification or recommodification of the Commons and the extortionate exploitation of labor. Seeing biofuels as a means of overcoming their legitimation deficit in the eyes of citizens, states now pin their future on the corporate promise that the global economy can be run on supposedly low-carbon biofuels decade after decade indefinitely, thereby strengthening the corporate grip on governments, at the expense of nature and society. As global oligopolies take over the driver's seat in the commercial enclosure of nature, governments would enjoy a free ride in a run on an infinite supply of supposed renewable energy. Even more disconcerting, the socially constructed global energy crisis has brought oil oligopolies, grain corporations, and biotech companies into ever closer union through conglomerate diversification, cross-industry investment, partnerships, mergers and acquisitions, and strategic alliances, so much so that it has become impossible to make functional demarcations among them. In 1999, there were 32,000 mergers and acquisitions worldwide, valued at $3.4 trillion. By then, of the hundred largest economies in the world, fifty-one were corporations while forty-nine were countries.[10] The oligopolies in the oil, automobile, grain, and bio-tech sectors all now view biofuels as the final frontier of capitalist accumulation. As this chapter will show, the corporate transmigra-tion to the biofuels sector is not about climate change mitigation or increasing food production to feed the world, but rather about expanding the scope for capital accumulation while containing the looming crisis inherent in overaccumulation.

From Black Carbon to Green Carbon

The Hubbert peak, the potential fear of being frozen out of the heav-ily subsidized biofuel production sector, and the public relations problem facing the black-carbon economy form the backdrop for oil oligopolies to make a partial migration to the nascent biofuel sector. Public display of optimism notwithstanding, oil oligopolies have always been haunted by the specter of the Hubbert peak, and this fear has informed their decisions and moves. Even though the current technology and fracking boom has allowed oil oligopolies to venture into offshore drilling, shale, and tar sands, it is clear that the new discoveries are equally subject to depletion in the long run. In this context, biofuels are a fallback option for oil corpora-tions. To remain relevant players in the global economy, they have to reckon with the need to make a partial migration to the bio-fuel sector. However, this new vision of a bio-based direction for capitalist accumulation on a global scale is not seen as a substitute for, but rather a complement to, hydrocarbon-driven accumula-tion. Chevron's VP, Donald Paul, was frank on this point when he stated that his company did not see biofuels as a replacement for fossil fuels, but rather, as a supplement to it. As he put it, "How big is this going to be? I would have to say you don't know. When you got a new playing field with different players, the way you find

out how big it is, is you get in there and do it. We see it as an aug-
mentation strategy, quite frankly. When you look at the growth
in demand in the next 25 years in fuels, to meet some fraction of
that growth ... you're going to need to augment what we have."[11]
Shell and Exxon have even been more conservative than Chevron
over the prospects of biofuels. As Rob Routs, Shell's director for
downstream operations, notes, "We don't believe the current situation is sustainable, because if agricultural land is being picked
up for fuel production, sooner or later there is going to be a clash.
And as a fuel company, we don't want to get involved in that."[12]
This attitude has been reflected in Shell's investment priorities. For
example, Shell invested $32 billion in 2008 in fossil fuels, whereas
it allocated a mere $1.3 billion in alternative energy sources over a
five-year period.[13]

For managers of Exxon-Mobil, biofuels are "moonshine,"
believing that bio-based fuels are far into the future. In their calculation, even if production of biofuels is probable, the amount
generated would be too small to displace the hegemony of fossil
fuels. Former Exxon-Mobil CEO Rex Tillerson was candid when
he told Charlie Rose: "When coal came into the picture, it took 50
or 60 years to displace timber. Then crude oil was found, it took
60, 70 years, and then natural gas. So it takes 100 years or more
for some new breakthrough in energy to become the dominant
source. Most people have difficulty coming to grips with the sheer
enormity of energy consumption. If we look at our energy outlook,
things like renewable wind, solar, biofuels, we have those sources
over the next 30 years growing 700 to 800 percent. But in the year
2040, they'll supply just 1 percent."[14] Exxon's bearish orientation
toward biofuels is reflected in its investment priorities. In 2006, the
oligopoly allocated a mere $600 million to algae research out of its
total $23 billion capital expenditure for that year.

Among oil oligopolies, BP is more aggressive in its approach to
alternative energy. In 2006, BP announced an allocation of $8 bil-
lion for alternative energy over a ten-year period, with biofuels the
primary corporate focus. In 2007, BP led its partners, Associated

British Foods and DuPont, in a joint ethanol plant in England to jack up ethanol production from one million liters a year to 420 million liters a year, providing a third of Great Britain's ethanol demand by 2010.[15] In 2007, BP and D1 Oils also formed a joint venture to accelerate jatropha (a plant whose oil can be converted to biofuel) planting. According to the deal, while BP agreed to contribute a $160 million investment over a five-year period, UK's D1 Oils would contribute its 172,000 hectares of existing jatropha plantations in India, southern Africa, and Southeast Asia. The plan has been to plant one million jatropha uring the first four years, and 300,000 a year thereafter. However, despite its relative aggression toward biofuels, BP's investment in alternatives in 2008 was only $1.4 billion, or a mere 6 percent of its capital expenditure, demonstrating its undiminished devotion to the black-carbon economy.[16]

The fear of growing restrictions by governments on the production and distribution of fossil fuels and public support for mandated blending of biofuels with fossil fuels form another set of factors impelling oil oligopolies to grudgingly embrace biofuels. If biofuels become a viable source of energy without their participation, the biofuel sector could become a competitor with, rather than complementary to, black energy, potentially cutting deep into the market share of fossil fuels. The U.S. Department of Energy projects that the availability of biofuels in the United States alone will rise from half a million barrels a day in 2007 to 2.3 million barrels a day by 2030; for oligopolies that bank on speculations, every projection matters.[17] This potential growth could represent a significant market share loss for fossil fuel corporations. Furthermore, biofuels are heavily subsidized, courtesy of the taxpayer. None is better positioned in the corporate world than oil oligopolies to capture a lion's share of the generous public subsidies to accelerate commodifying the Commons.

There is also the issue of control. By actively participating in the biofuel sector, oil oligopolies could control the pace at which the biofuel sector grows without jeopardizing the established hegemony of fossil fuels. Therefore, oil oligopolies are establishing research centers to investigate the potential of biofuels. In June 2006, BP made the first move to establish a bioscience energy research center closely associated with the universities of California and Illinois with a $500 million initial allocation to serve its biobusiness unit. The center's primary mission has been to look at how plants could supply feedstocks for ethanol production. Three areas of investigation have been identified for the center: developing bio-based fuel additives, developing new technologies to speed up the conversion of plants into fuels, and deploying advanced plant science to develop bioenergy crops capable of producing a higher yield of energy molecules, supposedly grown on marginal land.[18]

Moreover, enticed by the potential of the genetic engineering of plants, BP has partnered with DuPont to collaborate in research on bioenergy crops. BP sees huge dividends in this partnership, as DuPont is the second-largest seed company, the sixth-largest chemical company, and the sixth-largest pesticide company in the world, and is exceptionally well positioned to be a key player in biotech, biofuels, bio-plastics, synthetic biology, and enzymes development.[19] This explains why BP became the first major oil company to join the Biotechnology Industry Organization (the trade association of biotech companies), which includes Monsanto, Syngenta, DuPont, and BASF.[20] After eyeing the potential of the Agrilife Research high-biomass energy program, BP also entered into an alliance in 2012 with Texas A&M University, the parent institution of Agrilife Research, to accelerate research into the potential of grasses for cellulosic ethanol production, specifically focusing on plant breeding and agronomics. From BP's viewpoint, this partnership with Texas A&M would strengthen its ambitious trial project in Louisiana where it has planted 100,000 acres of miscanthus to generate lignocellulosic material (dry plant matter composed of carbohydrates and polymers) for road transport fuel. BP and Texas A&M hope that the integration of plant breeding and agronomic production will allow for developing an elite genetics

and agronomic production system, considered critical to continuous production of lignocellulosic ethanol. Excited by the prospect
of the partnership, Tom Campbell, BP Biofuels technology officer,
offered a rosy commercial scenario: "Developing new varieties of
energy grass is essential for commercializing a cellulosic biofuels
industry that will enhance domestic energy security, create jobs
for Americans, and improve rural economies. Working with Texas
AgriLife Research is an important step in the process of bringing clean transport fuels to scale and to market." Craig Nessler,
Agrilife Research director, was equally bullish about the partnership's prospects: "The opportunity to collaborate with BP Biofuels
is an excellent opportunity for Texas AgriLife Research to perform
market-driven, scientific research that will create future value to
the producers of the state of Texas and beyond with an industry
leader. Renewable energy produced from dedicated energy crops
will play a vital role for the 21st century economy."[21]

Following BP's example, Chevron also announced an investment of $400 million in biofuels research and development. To this
end, it contributed $12 million to Georgia Institute of Technology
to develop technology to produce biofuels from biomass. This
involves examination of the properties of biofuel feedstocks and
the biology and chemistry of certain plants considered conducive
to ethanol production from cellulose.[22]

The urgency to green-wash the fossil fuel industry is still .
another consideration for oil oligopolies to look at biofuels as a
convenient hideout. The black carbon–based economy has long
been in deep crisis resulting from the public outcry about its climate consequences. So a "green" carbon-based post-petroleum
economy is necessary to put people at ease, and thereby ensure
the continuous reproduction of capitalism. In the view of corporate managers, the transition from a fossil-based to a biofuels-run
economy can be easily defended, as the bio-based economy can
be marketed as green and clean. This allows the oil oligopolies to
put in place enabling environments for converting more grain into
bioethanol and biodiesel or more biotic resources into biofuels. As

of now, however, oil oligopolies are determined to hang on to black carbon, because it is still the lowest hanging fruit, exemplified by the fact that the oil sector continues to enjoy heavy subsidies. In 2011, for example, the global pre-tax and post-tax subsidies for fossil fuels stood at around $5 trillion. The leading oil consumption subsidizers in 2011 were Iran and Saudi Arabia, while the United States, China, and Russia were the leading fossil fuel production subsidizers.[23]

Since 1918, oil companies in the United States received $446 billion in federal government subsidies. Even though the big five oil oligopolies—Exxon, Chevron, BP, Shell, and ConocoPhillips— together made $900 billion during the first decade of this century, and another $255 billion in profits in 2011 and 2012, they continued to sustain their addiction to the subsidies and tax breaks for the production and distribution of dirty black energy. In 2011, the effective tax rates for Exxon, Chevron, and ConocoPhillips were 13, 19, and 18 percent, respectively. Corporate managers and their congressional allies contend that the companies need public financial support to bring petroleum products to the market, even though in 2012 the oligopolies were sitting on $70 billion of idle cash.[24] In truth, the subsidies are given not because the oil and gas corporations cannot profitably operate without financial support from the state but because they control the political process. The way they do this is by controlling the electoral and legislative processes.

Between January 2009 and June 2010, for example, the oil and gas industry spent $250 million on lobbying the U.S. Congress. Trade associations spent another $290 million on lobbying Congress to squash clean energy bills, and the Chamber of Commerce spent $190 million to defeat global warming legislation during the same period. Between 1999 and 2009, oil and gas, coal, and utility companies together spent over $2 billion lobbying Congress to defeat proposed legislation whose aim was to mitigate the effects of climate change.[25] Even after a bipartisan commission recommended phasing out the subsidies to black-carbon companies in order to save $120 billion in ten years toward deficit reduction, the U.S. Congress balked at the suggestion.[26] By defeating legislation that was meant to close tax loopholes, oil and gas companies saved $45 billion. They even decisively defeated proposed legislation requiring shale gas producers to inform communities of the potential danger posed by hydraulic fracturing operations (fracking), and of the potential consequences of chemicals used in it.[27] What this type of corporate behavior suggests is that the oil oligopolies are not going to abandon fossil fuels until every available drop of black carbon is exhausted. The perils for nature and society now stem from the parallel expansion of biofuel production and the further exploration and drilling of fossil fuels. Alongside the ferocious commodification of biotic resources, tar sands, and shale formations are the new frontier of oil and gas production, which has raised the stakes for oil oligopolies to stay the course. Tar sands oil is a carbon-saturated heavy black viscous oil, composed of bitumen, clay, sand, and water, which takes a significant amount of energy to produce, presaging ecological evisceration and climate change aggravation.

In contrast, shale resources are oil and gas trapped in rocks deep in the ground. Global estimates of shale oil and gas vary significantly, making it difficult to put a handle on any reasonable figure. In May 2012, for example, the Government Accountability Office reported to Congress that the Green River formation in parts of Colorado, Utah, and Wyoming hold three trillion barrels of shale oil, half of which is technically recoverable. Shale formations in other regions of the United States hold at least one trillion barrels of shale oil.[28] If the above estimates are correct, the technically recoverable shale oil in the Green River formation alone is almost equal to the current world proven conventional oil reserves. Estimates of U.S. shale gas reserves are in the range of 870 tcf (trillion cubic feet) with the mean recoverable gas standing at 650 tcf.[29] The growing importance of shale resources is such that in 2012 shale oil accounted for 29 percent of U.S. oil production, while shale gas accounted for 40 percent of total natural gas production.[30] It is small wonder that, from 2007 to 2011, shale oil and gas production in the United States increased fivefold and fourfold, respectively.[31]

Shale formations with huge reserves outside the United States also reportedly abound. In its lengthy report of June 2013, the U.S. Energy Information Administration identified ninety-five basins with 137 shale formations in forty-one countries. According to the findings, these shale formations contain 7,239 tcf of technically recoverable natural shale gas, amounting to 47 percent of global gas reserves; and 345 billion barrels of technically recoverable shale oil, adding 11 percent to global oil reserves. Extraction of shale oil and gas requires horizontal drilling and hydraulic fracturing, followed by injections of massive amounts of water, sands, and chemicals into the wells under extremely high pressure. The prospects of having access to massive shale resources are so high that an unprecedented scale of investment is being funneled into the new frontier of black-carbon exploration and production. The estimated investment in oil and gas in the United States alone in 2012 was $302 billion, 4 percent higher than the previous year, of which $275.8 billion was for upstream oil and gas projects. As a result, drilling of new oil and gas wells has been booming in the United States in recent years with tragic ramifications for the ecology and hydrology of the country. The number of new wells drilled over the three-year period from 2010 to 2012 in the continental United States was 120,812.[32]

Other countries have also announced having huge recoverable shale resources waiting to be exploited. In addition to its proven conventional natural gas of 279 trillion cubic feet, Saudi Arabia claims that it has 649 tcf of shale gas; Algeria has over 700 tcf of shale gas; India boasts having 496 tcf of shale gas; Morocco has 266 tcf of shale gas; Indonesia boasts of having more than 1,000 tcf; and China holds 1,115 tcf of technically recoverable shale gas to go along with 32 billion of shale oil.[33] All told, the MIT Energy Initiative (2011) and the U.S. EIA (2013) speculate that the world has 20,040 tcf of recoverable shale gas, which is 150 times the current annual world natural gas consumption, and 3.12 trillion shale and non-shale oil reserves.[34]

Another country with huge shale oil and gas potential is Australia. In early January 2013, it was announced that 233 billion barrels of shale resources were discovered in the country, worth U.S.$19 trillion if all of it is exploited.[35] Chevron has reportedly found nineteen natural gas fields in Australia and is building two giant natural gas liquefaction plants with a price tag of 86 billion Australian dollars. For its part, Shell was injecting 12 billion Australian dollars into a four-soccer-fields-long offshore natural gas project in northwest Australia. All in all, 260 billion Australian dollars were injected into the country's energy sector in 2012, with seven new liquid natural gas projects accounting for 164 billion Australian dollars of the total. Completion of these seven projects will raise Australia's liquid natural gas production from 24 million metric tons to 80 million metric tons a year.[36] Australia has twelve additional liquid natural gas and coal-to-liquids projects that might add another 64 million metric tons.[37] It is thus no surprise that overall global capital expenditures on oil and gas exploration and production roared from U.S.$916 billion in 2011 to $1.08 trillion in 2012.[38]

Oil oligopolies are not limited to oil and gas production and distribution. Coal is still integral to the global energy mix as it is responsible for 50 percent of global electricity generation. In fact, in 2011 world coal consumption increased by 4.3 percent (300 million tons), accounting for half of global primary energy demand increase, and is projected to continue increasing by 2.6 percent per annum through 2017, with the increase in annual coal consumption reaching 1.2 billion tons in 2017, which is equal to the annual coal consumption in the United States and Russia combined. Never mind the much-touted commitment to green energy; even in Europe coal-fired electricity production is projected to be 4 percent higher in 2017 than in 2011.[39] The growing coal consumption in Asia is even more worrisome. China now consumes half of global coal, followed by India. These two Asian giants together are today responsible for two-thirds of global coal demand and for one-third of global coal imports. By 2017, China's coal consumption will increase by 77 percent and India's by 22 percent. China will continue to get most of its primary energy from coal; India is projected to surpass the United States as the second-largest coal consumer.[40]

As things stand now, 483 power companies are poised to build 1,200 coal-fired plants in forty-nine countries by 2017. When completed, these power plants will have over 1.4 million mw (megawatts) installed capacity, which is more than four times the total installed capacity in the United States.[41] This statistic suggests that coal is likely to remain king in the global energy mix, never mind the grandstanding "green" reiterations about reducing global greenhouse gas emissions (ghg) by 50 percent by 2050. Indeed, the IEA projects that demand for coal will rise by 21 percent by 2035.[42] To take advantage of this prospect, coal-rich countries are gearing up to boost production and export of their coal. For example, Australia is planning to triple its coal production to 900 million tons a year, just as coal-rich South Africa and Mozambique are preparing to do the same.[43] Accounting for 50 percent of global energy consumption, coal is responsible for 40 percent of global ghg emissions.[44] The peril with coal is not only that it is the dirtiest fossil fuel, but also that the market propaganda about "clean" coal technology perpetuates the myth that it can be "green" and "clean." In part, this involves conversion of coal to motor fuel. This requires heating the coal to 1,000 degress Fahrenheit to produce gas before converting it to liquid fuel. This conversion process makes coal-to-liquids even dirtier than conventional gasoline and diesel. In the United States, it takes 120 million tons of coal to generate just one million barrels of coal-to-liquids.[45]

Shale oil presents another ecological disaster in the making. The negative impacts of horizontal drilling and fracking of shale formations on hydrology and ecology are likely to be astronomical. Horizontal drilling and fracking operations generate noise, air, and soil pollution, water depletion, water contamination, and deforestation of delicate ecosystems. Even the Government Accountability Office acknowledges that shale oil and shale gas exploitation are bound to pose environmental, social, and public health risks.[46] These risks include engine exhaust from truck traffic, emissions from diesel-power pumps, gas flares, and release of pollutants from faulty equipment polluting the air; contamination of surface water and groundwater due to erosion of soil, ground disturbances, frequent spills, and releases of chemicals; underground migration of gases and chemicals, release of toxic chemicals from storage tanks, pipes and hoses; and overflow of toxic chemicals from impoundments associated with heavy rain. Finally, the use of drilling techniques in which water, sands, and chemical additives are injected under high pressure into shale oil and shale gas formations that release toxic chemicals and fluids are bound to pose risks to land resources and wildlife habitat.

Black-carbon oligopolies, however, paint a rosy picture of shale resources that they suppose can be exploited without causing environmental, hydrological, social, and health damages. To convince the public that fracking does no harm, they use the imprimatur of universities and research institutions to green-wash shale resource exploitation. For example, natural gas foundations and the oil industry sponsored the creation of the MIT Energy Initiative (MITEI), headquartered on MIT's campus, with initial donations of $125 million to make a "scholarly" case that horizontal drilling and fracturing techniques are safe and would not pose harm of any kind. BP, Shell, Saudi Aramco, and Italy's ENI contributed $25 million each to make MITEI an effective mouthpiece for the exploitation of shale formations; another ten companies agreed to pay $5 million each to win seats on MITEI's board.[47] With the urgency to counter ecological objections to hydraulic fracking in mind, the study group produced a lengthy document titled *The Future of Natural Gas*. In keeping with their mission, the authors of the document boldly assert there is no evidence that horizontal drilling and hydraulic fracking cause environmental, hydrological, and health harm. If spills or leaks occur, these are the result of "substandard well completion by some operators" rather than fracking techniques themselves.[48] The authors counsel that if these spills or water contamination occur, they are problems of management alone. Therefore, they argue, if small and big operators follow the best practices, shale gas can be safely exploited without environmental and hydrological cost. They see a big role for government to sponsor research in waste water management, reducing fracturing water use, and cost-effective waste water recycling technology in the shale gas sector, meaning heavy subsidies, courtesy of taxpayers.[49] They contend that since natural gas is inexpensive and clean, providing a bridge to low-carbon economy, shale gas resources must be part of a strategic U.S. energy policy.

The oil and gas industry has also mobilized the academic resources of Penn State, the State University of New York, Buffalo, and the University of Texas at Austin to launch a vigorous counteroffensive that uses questionable research products against environmental objections to shale fracking operations. All three institutions presented natural gas as the most essential bridge to a low-carbon world. The Penn State paper described shale gas as the dynamic engine of growth, whose operators are worthy of generous government support in the form of subsidies and relief from taxes. The Buffalo report extolled shale drillers as efficient and cautious under stringent state regulations and the vigilant supervision of regulators. The researchers at the University of Texas were even more assertive in their claim that there was no evidence of water contamination from shale drilling operations.[50]

The arguments contained in these reports are so dubious that some writers describe them as a product of "frackademia."[51] In the first place, the "frackademics" involved in shale research have brought disrepute to scientific research by overstretching credulity that shale gas is safe to extract and clean to use. Cornell University's Robert Howarth and Anthony Ingraffea have generated a study that exposed the many holes in MITEI's report. The authors of the MITEI report have conveniently glossed over the effects of methane emission from natural gas on climate, while they highlighted that natural gas produces less CO_2 than coal. The Cornell University study, however, shows that natural gas worsens climate change as much or even more than coal due to extremely high methane leaks from fractured shale gas wells. Howarth and Ingraffea estimate that the methane emission from a shale gas well is between 3.6 and 7.8 percent of its total gas content. Industry practice shows that over 80 percent of the flowback return fluids from shale gas production is vented into the atmosphere. The amount of methane that escapes into the atmosphere from fractured shale gas wells is twice as much as that from conventional gas production. Due to its potency, the effect of methane on climate is 70 to 105 times greater than from CO_2.[52] In light of the growing evidence that natural gas is hardly cleaner than other fossil fuels, many previous supporters of natural gas as a bridge to low-carbon economy are having second thoughts. The Sierra Club, for example, once among the great supporters of natural gas, has reversed its long-held position because of concerns over water contamination and air pollution from horizontal and hydraulic drilling. In fact, the organization had previously received $26 million from Chesapeake Energy to intensify its pro-natural gas campaign. In 2012, however, the Sierra Club turned down a donation of $30 million from the same company.[53]

Why the "frackademics" manufacture research products to green-wash fracking operations may come as a surprise to the casual observer with little or no understanding of how material interests often trump intellectual integrity and honesty. Opportunism, mediocrity, and manipulative salesmanship have always been well represented in academia. Since most members of the university study groups that produced the various reports are personally connected to the black-carbon companies, the research products are highly dubious. For example, MIT Professor Ernest Moniz, who chaired the study *The Future of Natural Gas*, was a member of the board of the oil company ICF from which he received $300,000 in compensation during 2011–12. Professor Anthony Meggs, who co-chaired the study, was on Talisman Energy's board. Professor John

Deutch was on the board of Cheniere Energy and owned $1.4 million in Cheniere's stocks.[54] Key members of the University of Texas study group have also been found to be hand-in-glove with oil and gas corporations. For instance, the lead author of the UT report, Professor Charles C. Groat, was paid $1.5 million over a five-year period as a member of the board of a gas drilling company, Plains Exploration and Production; moreover, he was holding $1.7 million in the gas company's stock. Shamelessly, he was still on the company's board the whole time the so-called research on the link between hydraulic fracturing and water resources was being carried out.[55] In Buffalo, John P. Martin, director of the newly created Shale and Society Institute, was heavily involved in consulting and public relations work for the oil and gas industry.

At any rate, when independent reviews of the various reports revealed countless flaws on how the research was conducted, the universities implicated in fraudulent practices began to scramble for cover. At UT, after an independent review panel found the report extremely shabby, university officials promptly withdrew the report from public circulation. The panel also discovered that other UT scholars who had done credible research work on the health effect of hydraulic fracking were deliberately excluded from Groat's team. The embarrassment to the university was such that Professor Charles C. Groat was pressured into early retirement, and the director of the energy institute at UT, Raymond Orbiach, was forced to resign. On the campus of SUNY at Buffalo, faculty and students rose up demanding full accounting about the ties, funding, founding, and staffing of the new shale institute and the flawed study it generated on shale gas production. When their demand fell on deaf ears, the university community intensified their protests until the university's board of trustees was forced to take up the matter. However, before the board of trustees could make a final decision, the university president withdrew the study and closed down the shale institute for good after a mere year in existence. The president claimed that his decision to close the shale institute was motivated by the lack of faculty members with expertise in hydraulic fracking and shale gas production.[56] His post hoc reason was crass through and through. If lack of faculty with expertise in fracking was the reason for discarding the institute, one would ask why it was created without such faculty in the first place.

BIOFUELS AND THE AUTOMOBILE INDUSTRY

The automobile industry is another major driver for liquid biofuels. Automakers have always been haunted by the fear of not having a large enough market to sell all the vehicles they produce. Cars are, by definition, durables that last long once purchased. In the past, car makers, with modest success, used planned obsolescence to render old models less attractive than newer ones in order to entice consumers to exchange their old cars for newer ones. But now, concerns over rising fossil fuel prices and the public outcry about the climate impact of burning fossil fuels appear to be discouraging car buyers. For example, the growth in battery electric vehicles increased worldwide from 113,000 in 2012 to 1,209,000 in 2016.[57] Given this context, the popularization of green fuel would simultaneously counterbalance the price volatility of fossil fuels and reassure consumers about the climate benefits of the green fuels. In the minds of automakers, the use of biofuels would lure car-buyers back to the market in large numbers. Moreover, automakers had long been under sustained pressure to move up the technological ladder in such ways as to produce fuel-efficient vehicles while decreasing engine exhaust. But this would require them to increase the composition, and hence the cost, of capital, cutting deeply into their profits. The recent proactive Volkswagen commission's revelation of actions that would be considered a crime under any circumstances unmasked this reality. To avoid expenditures on improving fuel efficiency and pollution reduction, VW had installed a sophisticated software in its new fleet of cars to suppress pollution emission during the test of the cars for emission standards. The U.S. Environmental Protection Agency caught VW red-handed in early fall 2015 when it uncovered that about 11 million VW and Audi cars sold worldwide were found to produce forty times more nitrogen oxide as is allowed by U.S. law for diesel engines.

In any case, in consideration of public pressure for emissions reduction and fuel efficiency, major automakers like Ford, GM, Chrysler, Fiat, Volvo, VW, Honda, Toyota, and others jumped on the biofuels bandwagon not only as supporters but also as major investors in the biofuel sector. The substitution of dirty fossil fuels by biofuels was seen as a ready-made strategy to sidestep the pressure to design and build more fuel-efficient vehicles while, at the same time, reaping immense profits from the expansion of biofuel production.[58]

In Europe, the chief executives of automakers are even more vocal than their counterparts in the United States in their fervent advocacy for biofuels. Frustrated by the slow pace at which biofuels production and integration into conventional fuels was proceeding, a group of six major auto manufacturers and oil companies (Volkswagen, Daimler, Honda, Neste Oil, OMV, and Shell) commissioned the E4tech consultancy group in 2013 to generate a study to present biofuels in a favorable light. The sponsors of the study were not disappointed. In a fifty-five-page report entitled "A Harmonized Auto-Fuel Biofuel Roadmap for the EU to 2030," the consultancy painted a rosy picture about the prospects of biofuels within the EU. From the consultancy's viewpoint, what has been hurting investment in the biofuel sector in Europe has been the stalemate between the EU Parliament and the member countries over the direction of biofuels. If the EU could overcome this deadlock, according to the consultancy, decarbonizing road transport fuels by 12 to 15 percent by focusing on biofuels could result in greenhouse emissions reduction savings of 8 percent by 2030. Moreover, second-generation biofuels could represent 20 percent of biofuels by 2030 and could be even double if the right policies and conducive incentive structures are provided.[59]

However, EU automakers have had to reckon with strong public opposition to the conversion of crops into liquid fuels.

The opposition is glaringly omitted from the report because it is precisely its strength that has created a deadlock between the European Parliament and member countries on how to proceed with the expansion of biofuel production. European civic associations are better organized and more active than their counterparts in the United States to effectively register their opposition to biofuels production with politicians. Hounded by vocal civil opposition, even the EU Commission, one of the EU's governing bodies, eventually acknowledged that first-generation biofuels have both direct and indirect impacts on food and the environment. The strength of civic organizations in Europe is such that they have so far successfully blocked the introduction of GM crops into European agriculture. For example, of the 181 million hectares planted to GM crops globally in 2014, only 148,000 were planted to GM crops in Europe, of which 136,962, representing 94 percent, were actually in Spain, and the remaining 6 percent were in Portugal, Romania, the Czech Republic, and Slovakia. For comparison, 73.1 million hectares of agricultural land in the United States were planted to GM crops in 2014.[60]

OLIGOPOLIES AND THE BIOFUEL INDUSTRIAL COMPLEX

Historically, grain surplus production and price volatility in the global grain market have been problematic for grain-trading companies. Even though there are billions of hungry people in the Global South who can benefit from abundance of food production, they lack purchasing power large enough to influence the global demand for food. As a result, the main clients of grain oligopolies are the affluent Global Northerners, but they do not buy enough to take all the grain supply off the market. Therefore, the increasing conversion of grain to biofuels to grease the machine of capitalism averts the crisis of grain surplus production. It is no surprise that the grain oligopolies are the leading advocates of the transition to biofuel consumption. It must be borne in mind that ADM, Bunge, Cargill, and Dreyfus together control 75 percent of world grain trade, and Monsanto, DuPont, and Syngenta together control over half of the biotech crops industry. The top ten seed oligopolies controlled 75.3 percent of the 34.5 billion commercial seed market in 2011. The top ten oligopolies controlled almost 95 percent of the global pesticide market. The top ten corporations controlled $65.7 billion of the $160.3 billion synthetic fertilizer industry.[61]

From the standpoint of grain-trading oligopolies, the green revolution, long integrated into the petroleum industry for agro-chemicals, presented both moments of opportunity and danger. The opportunity was that the green revolution transformed agriculture in the Global North and in some countries, such as Brazil and Argentina, in the Global South, producing surplus food that the market could not absorb. The danger was that most people in the Global South were poor without purchasing capabilities to register effective demand for even basic foods. On the other hand, the affluent Global Northerners, with almost infinite purchasing capabilities, could not absorb the surplus food despite market-driven overeating habits. Food manufacturers continually packaged and repackaged food products in glossy ways, and restaurants enticed patrons with "all you can eat" menus. Yet all that was not enough to get rid of the surplus food. Even food waste, which accounted for 40 to 50 percent of the food produced, did not help much either.

So what emerged out of the green revolution was a global food regime defined by extreme poverty in the Global South and over-consumption in the Global North, coupled with price volatility. The underfed and malnourished Global Southerners became increasingly vulnerable to hunger-related illnesses, infections, and deaths. On the other hand, affluent Global Northerners became susceptible to lifestyle and overeating-related chronic health complications. This was the background to the notion of developing grain-based liquid fuels.

By making biofuel production a direct competitor to food consumption, grain oligopolies can manipulate upward the global demand for grain. It was during such socially manufactured scarcity that prices for basic grains doubled between January 2006 and January 2008. In March 2008, the prices for wheat, soy, rice, and maize were 137 percent, 87 percent, 74 percent, and 31 percent, respectively, higher than the year before, and even the World Bank, FAO, and IMF grudgingly acknowledged that this food inflation was in part caused by the conversion of crops into biofuels.[62] The relationship between the 2007–2008 food crisis and the conversion of grain to biofuel production became so evident that the FAO convened a global food summit in Rome on June 3–5, 2008. Meanwhile, the Bush administration made every effort to suppress the World Bank study that showed the link between the food crisis and ethanol production until the June food summit in Rome was concluded. The Bush administration was able to do so because the president of the World Bank, Robert Zoellick, was President Bush's appointee. But the U.S. Department of Agriculture's own fabricated report and the World Bank's study were at odds. Whereas the USDA claimed that conversion of grain to biofuels production might have caused only a 3 percent rise in world grain prices, the World Bank's study, leaked to *The Guardian*, showed that a 75 percent hike in world food prices was due to the conversion of large amounts of corn in the United States to biofuels production, driving an additional 105 million people to hunger and grinding poverty.[63] Note that the World Bank's secret study was completed two months prior to the June food summit in Rome. To the chagrin of the Bush administration, the FAO's own study was also widely circulating at the food summit, showing that, at the beginning of 2008, the average real prices for foods and oils were 64 percent above 2002 price levels, after declining during the previous four decades. The average prices for vegetable oils had risen by 97 percent, for cereals by 87 percent, and for rice by 46 percent, all resulting from the diversion of coarse grains and oil seeds to biofuel production.[64]

This glaring evidence notwithstanding, the U.S. Secretary of Agriculture insisted at the food summit that biofuel production was responsible for no more than 3 percent of the price spikes, which the majority of summit participants laughed away. The person who sprang to his feet like an angry tiger to defend the United States and the importance of ethanol fuels was President Lula of Brazil. As he angrily put it: "It offends me to see fingers pointing against clean energy from biofuels, fingers soiled with oil and coal. . . . Biofuels are not the villain menacing food security in poor countries. Quite on the contrary, when cultivated responsibly, in harmony with each country's reality, they can be important tools to generate income and pull countries out of food and energy insecurity."[65]

Before the summit was over, the U.S. delegation tried to change the subject by proposing universal adoption of GM foods as the long-term answer to global hunger, a posture that has continued to inform America's foreign agriculture policy. On June 13, one week after the food summit was concluded, U.S. Deputy Secretary of State John Negroponte emphatically reiterated the view already expressed at the summit in these terms:

> We must address the policies and trade barriers that increase food prices by preventing access to food and the best technologies to produce food. In the long term, we believe sustainable food security will come from advances in science and technology and the creation of an efficient global market for both agriculture products and food production technologies. We therefore are encouraging countries to remove barriers to the use of innovative plant and plant production technologies, including biotechnology. Biotechnology tools can help speed the development of crops with higher yields, higher nutrition value, better resistance to pests and diseases, and stronger food system resilience in the face of climate change.[66]

Forgetting the debate at the world food summit, the FAO later began to echo the U.S. posture. The agency tried to placate opponents of large-scale commercial biofuel production by pointing to biotechnology companies as holding the key to solving the potential competition between food and fuel. The agency attempted to assuage concerns over food shortages, arguing that biotech entrepreneurs could in the long run expedite the selection of varieties that would be suitable for biofuel production in terms of their biomass productivity and oil content, as well as their suitability for conversion to biofuels. In the agency's words: "The field of genomics—the study of all the genetic material of an organism (its genome)—is likely to play an increasingly important role. Genome sequences of several first-generation feedstocks such as maize, sorghum and soybean are in the pipeline."[67] With twisted irony, the socially constructed food crisis created a wide gaping hole through which the Trojan horse of biotechnology could enter into the global food manufacturing system.

At any rate, the Rome food summit was not meant to find an enduring solution to world hunger, but rather to stage a propaganda campaign that something was being done to address the crisis. It was part of the mass production of deceptions and manipulations to shelter global capitalism from a crisis of legitimation. Scarcity, whether naturally caused or manufactured, has always been foundational to accumulation. Bear in mind that the grain-trading oligopolies have been the chief beneficiaries of these price hikes— global sales of grain increased from $7 trillion in 2007 to $8 trillion in 2008, holding the global poor hostage to global food supply disruptions and price hikes. Monsanto saw its net earnings soar by 83 percent in the first nine months of 2008; the global grain trader Bunge saw its net revenue in the first half of 2008 balloon by 471 percent; and Cargill's net profit soared by 62 percent in the third quarter of 2008. No wonder that the number of chronically food insecure people worldwide increased from 849 million in 2006 to 982 million in 2008, which has grown to 1.2 billion as of this writing.[68]

The socially constructed scarcity of food crops was such that even banks and hedge funds subjected food crops to corrosive financial speculations. They promptly converted the supposed food crisis of 2007–2008 into lucrative source of quick profit. Bank of America, Citibank, Deutsche Bank, HSBC, Morgan Stanley, JPMorgan, and other large banks suddenly became active players in highly speculative food commodity derivatives. Goldman Sachs alone reportedly made over $1 billion from gambling on food commodity derivatives in 2009, while Barclays Bank made £300 million on food price speculation during the same year. Again in 2012, Goldman Sachs made a hefty $400 million from betting on world food prices. The aggressiveness of banks regarding speculation on food prices became so blatant that the World Development Movement (now named Global Justice Now, a membership organization that campaigns for justice in the Global South) called upon governments to place limits on how much banks could bet on food prices and to end all secret dealings surrounding food derivatives. The introduction of export restrictions on rice by India, Vietnam, and China and on wheat by Argentina and Russia reinforced the trends toward speculation on agricultural commodities. According to the Commodity Futures Trading Commission, approximately 19 percent of outstanding rice contracts were held during the crisis by non-commercial investors for purposes of speculation.[69] The introduction of derivatives into agricultural commodities has the effect of entrenching social scarcity and exclusion of the poor from the food market. For example, the global stock of grain increased by 140 million metric tons between September 2007 and September 2010; this was unsold surplus grain because prices were above equilibrium due to speculation.[70]

The combination of the increasing diversion of food crops to biofuel production and the increasing speculation in food commodity derivatives during 2007–2008 was no doubt responsible for the high food prices and the volatility of staple food, with seismic implications for the welfare of the majority of people in the Global South where people spend 50 to 80 percent of their income on food, compared to 10–15 percent in the advanced countries. It is noteworthy that, between 2006 and 2008, cravenly greedy speculators were the dominant players in food commodity derivatives, holding 65 percent of maize contracts, 80 percent of wheat, and 68 percent of soybeans. It is difficult to imagine how the impact of such speculative price rises on the poor countries and their people could not be harmful. For example, the increase of wheat imports in Ethiopia from 300,000 metric tons in 2006 to one million metric tons in 2008, eating away the country's foreign exchange earnings, resulted in the drastic rise of the import bill from $84 million to $465 million, thereby sending domestic wheat prices through the roof and thus beyond the purchasing capability of even the middle class. Nigeria sharply reduced wheat imports from thirteen million metric tons in 2006 to three million metric tons in 2008 because the price for wheat soared from $100 per metric tons in 2006 to nearly $300 per ton in 2008. Mauritania, a country that usually imports 70 percent of its food, spent a mere $15 million on 350,000 metric tons of wheat in 2004; in 2008, however, Mauritania spent $110 million on 260,000 metric tons of wheat.[71] The financialization of food commodity markets is fostered by the creation of the dangerously destabilizing mechanisms known as index funds, into which money flows, purely based on speculative future prices of commodities. In turn, the money collected this way is put into derivatives across a wide range of agricultural commodities. These index funds are created by such giant banks as Goldman Sachs, Morgan Stanley, JPMorgan, Bank of America, Citibank, and Deutsche Bank. It is small wonder that the holdings of the index funds ballooned from $46 billion in 2005 to $250 billion as of March 2008. This, of course, was unrelated to real supply and demand conditions. It must also be borne in mind that record oil prices, which soared from $20 a barrel in 2000 to $60 in 2006 and then to $147 a barrel in 2008, worsened the situation.[72] The joint oil and food price hikes had profound implications for developing countries and the global poor. For example, the progressive rise in oil prices cumulatively increased the oil import bill of developing countries by $971 billion between 2003 and 2008, eating away their export earnings and worsening their external balance of payments. Togo spent the equivalent of 19.7 percent of its GDP on oil imports and another 4.5 percent of its GDP on food imports. Moreover, the additional cost of increased international prices of maize, rice, and wheat to consumers living in developing countries in 2007 was about $324 billion.[73]

In any event, the emergence of the food commodity derivatives market has become a heaven-sent gift for grain-trading oligopolies because it mitigates or eliminates risks associated with grain over-supply. At the same time, the situation presents an opportunity for GM oligopolies like Monsanto, Syngenta, and DuPont to use the supposed food scarcity to introduce GM seeds into global agriculture. However, the agricultural boom resulting from the biotech revolution and genetic engineering can be either a source of unprecedented opportunity to make a profit or a source of danger resulting from the recurring crises of overproduction.[74] But, again, the transformation of emerging market countries as shock absorbers and the diversion of grain to the biofuels sector become a hedging strategy against the problem of grain surplus production. The current preoccupation of grain and biotech oligopolies with major emerging markets in the Global South explains the corporate fear of a potential crisis of surplus production.

In light of these developments, because the grain oligopolies have unrestrained control over the global production and circulation of grain, coupled with the recourse to biofuels, they now feel they have exorcised the specter of overproduction for good, because all crops can be flexibly used, to supply food or to convert them to biofuels production, thereby eliminating price volatility. Corn can be used as human food, animal feed, or to generate ethanol fuel; palm oil can be used as edible vegetable oil or to produce biodiesel.[75] Thanks to this new reality, the four grain-trading oligopolies (ADM, Cargill, Louis Dreyfus, and Bunge) are now in the driver's seat to control the trajectory of global trade in grain and the production of biofuels. It is no coincidence that these corporations are not only the principal grain-trading oligopolies but also among the world's major biofuel producers. In North America, the chief exponent and largest producer of ethanol is ADM, which operates 420 crop procurement centers and 270 processing plants worldwide. The oligopoly boasts that it crushes 2.4 million bushels of corn per day to produce 1.8 billion gallons of corn-ethanol per year in the United States alone. Predictably, ADM managers argue that biofuels increase and diversify the supply of clean and green fuels at lower costs. To buttress this position, the managers refer to figures from the U.S. Department of Energy. Accordingly, the price of gasoline in the United States in 2008 would have been 20–35 cents higher per gallon without biofuels, which amounts to $28–$49 billion savings for the nation. As the argument continues, U.S. ethanol use in 2007 helped to reduce ghg emissions by 10 million tons. At this rate, by 2050, U.S. use of biofuels will reduce ghg emissions by 1.7 billion tons per year, roughly equal to 80 percent of transport-related emissions.

However, despite its greenwashing, ADM is the tenth-biggest air polluter in the United States. In fact, in 2003, the Department of Justice and the EPA found ADM guilty of emitting excessive levels of pollutants from its fifty-two plants in sixteen states, including carbon dioxide, toluene, and organic volatile chemical compounds, and required the company to reduce its emissions by 63,000 tons per year after penalizing the company with a token $3.5 million fine as a warning. ADM had already been fined $2.6 million in 2001 for similar infractions. ADM's ethanol plant in Clinton, Iowa, for example, emitted 20,000 tons of pollutants in 2004, including sulfur dioxide, nitrogen oxide, and organic volatile compounds. For reference, the EPA categorizes an ethanol plant as a source of pollution if it generates more than 250 tons of any pollutant. In 2005, the Environmental Defense Fund ranked ADM's ethanol plant in Clinton as the twenty-sixth-largest emitter of carcinogenic chemical compounds. But environmental and market infractions are not new to ADM. In 1993, many top ADM officials were implicated in international price fixing; three of those officials were eventually sent to jail, including vice chairman Michael Andreas. In 1997, the company was fined $100 million for antitrust violation. In 2005, ADM averted a class action antitrust suit, and avoiding a judicial embarrassment, by paying $400 million and, in 2006, the company was battling twenty-five administrative and judicial proceedings against it.[76]

Cargill is another grain oligopoly with a checkered history. It has presence in forty-six countries operating 245 interior silos, twenty-eight import/export elevators, sixty-two crushing plants, corn ethanol plants in Iowa, Missouri, and Nebraska, two sugar mills, and an ethanol terminal in Santos, Brazil, a biodiesel plant in Argentina, an ethanol dehydration plant in El Salvador, and a 25 percent stake in UK-based Green Energy, which converts rapeseed to biodiesel.[77] Furthermore, Cargill has been climbing the biotech and biochemical ladder in partnership with other companies to produce a host of chemicals using soybean, canola, and corn as feedstocks.

Based in Paris, France, Louis Dreyfus is another giant grain-trading corporation. It claims to have a presence in ninety countries. In addition to palm oil operations in Indonesia, the company has a giant biodiesel plant in Argentina, a soybean crushing plant in Paraguay, and a cottonseed crushing plant in Brazil. But its largest biodiesel plant is in the state of Indiana, producing 88 million gallons of biodiesel per year.[78]

Finally, Bunge Limited completes the circle of the largest global grain oligopolies. Bunge has 400 facilities in forty-six countries, buying, processing, and selling all kinds of grains. Bunge is the world's largest oilseed processor, number one bottled-vegetable seller, and the largest fertilizer producer and seller in South America.[79] It seems that the grain oligopolies have expelled (at least for now) the demons of grain overproduction—thanks to biofuels, the speculative bubble, and the growing dependency of third world countries on imported food. By 2009, 55 percent of third world countries had become net food importers.[80] This explains why the grain-trading oligopolies are the most ardent advocates of deregulation and liberalization of world agriculture and biofuels, not out of concern for global climate change, energy security, or world hunger, but out of concern for the bottom line.

In sum, contrary to corporate claims, there are numerous painfully fateful ecological, economic, social, and political repercussions of the drive for biofuels. The merging of food, feed, and fuel has introduced a combustible element of competition among the three basic sectors for the same throughput that would only reinforce the boom-and-bust cycle of agricultural commodities while at the same time throwing billions of poor people into destitution. Biofuel mandates in the United States and the EU have, in particular, been escalating the price of key food crops, plaguing poor countries with rising food prices because of their dependence on imports. By the calculation of the National Academy of Sciences, global biofuels expansion was responsible for 20 to 40 percent of the price surges in 2007–2008, when prices of food crops doubled or tripled, seriously affecting the nutritional status of the global poor who depend on basic grains such as corn. For instance, the international prices for corn progressively rose from $50 per metric ton in 1985 to $350 per metric ton in 2011.[81] Because corn is the primary source of calories and nutrients for one billion people, such a price surge has had a far-reaching impact on the nutritional status of the poor. In addition, since corn is widely used in feedlots, its availability and price unavoidably have direct impacts on the price of dairy products, eggs, and meat, affecting even consumers in rich countries. The diversion of more and more corn to ethanol production worsens this situation with significant global reverberations. For instance, when the United States, once the world's largest producer and exporter of corn, diverted its corn to ethanol production, the impact on international corn prices was palpable and immediate. North African countries saw large impacts, with $1.4 billion in ethanol-related import costs; Egypt alone witnessed a $679 million price rise of its grain imports. The result of these price hikes on basic food imports was the spread of food riots. Following the 2007–2008 food crisis, there were over sixty food riots in thirty countries.[82]

At the macrostructural level, the diversion of food crops and animal feed to biofuel production has introduced a new element of structural contradiction into agricultural commodity production, with far-reaching direct and indirect impacts on the utilization of land resources. For example, because of the price rise in U.S. corn due to the growth of ethanol production, farmers converted their soybean fields to corn production. However, the substantial reduction in U.S. soybean production resulted in higher international prices for soybeans, which prompted many developing countries like Brazil and other Global South countries to convert vast swaths of forests into soybean fields, a major driver of deforestation. Soybeans, like corn, have now become one of the most flexible crops, used for the production of biodiesel, animal feed, and edible oil. Thus expanded production of ethanol and biodiesel from corn and soybean has increased overall demand for corn and soybean, displacing land area previously dedicated to production of crops for food and feed. On the other side of the ledger, rising corn and soybean prices have affected other grains. For example, higher prices for corn have led food consumers to switch to rice and wheat consumption, which, in turn, has led to higher prices for rice and wheat, freezing out the poor from the food market. The merging of food, feed, and biofuels has directed the focus of agribusiness interests, private speculators, and land-poor countries to grabbing land and water resources in the Global South. As discussed in chapter 1, in the first decade of this century, some 227 million hectares of land have been either auctioned off or been in the process of being negotiated away, the bulk of which were in Africa. More than 60 percent of the land bargained away in Africa had been for bioenergy crop and plant feedstock production for export to the Global North.[83] The eventual outcome of the competition among food, feed, and biofuel sectors cannot be anything but the evisceration of the geoecological conditions of life-supporting natural systems, accompanied by the wanton dispossession of tens of millions of powerless people in the Global South. Even more harmful is the creation of a backdoor for biotech corporations to make forays into all forms of natural systems in the guise of increasing yields in crop and plant production through genetic manipulation and transformation of seeds and plants, in ways that would supposedly produce large throughput to meet the demand from all sectors.

How the Green Revolution Led to Biofuels

The history of capitalism is a history of struggles to overcome the material and social barriers to the expansion of accumulation. The familiar means by which these barriers have historically been overcome are technical innovations and social coercion. At this juncture, at which the crisis of accumulation is threatening the prevailing social order, corporations are fiercely struggling to find refuge in biology. This involves producing and marketing genetically modified products under the veneer of boosting production worldwide to produce enough green energy, feed everyone, and improve global climate.

A complex combination of coercion and ideological attempts at social control have marked the history of capital accumulation, both in terms of internal, national operations and globally through colonialism and imperialism. In terms of social deception and commercial propaganda, biological arguments have been critical. Much of the early rationalizations for capital's depredations focused on the inferiority of the lower classes and the tendency for the poor to procreate too rapidly, which meant the more or less forcible reduction of poor populations. Leading capitalists and their apologists, such as the Rockefeller Foundation, feared that the United States, for example, would be overrun by hordes of poor and mentally degenerated peasants. And globally, the poor in the Global South would keep increasing in numbers, threatening the availability of exploitable resources, notably land for food production. The poor might also be a potent source for rebellion.

After the Second World War, the overall focus shifted somewhat away from population control (though this has remained a mainstay of capitalist thinking) to natural resources. The Rockefeller Foundation, for example, modified its approach to the question of natural resources. The strategy now became targeting food crops and livestock population for genetic manipulation and transformation, and linking food production to the oil industry, the source of Rockefeller wealth. This change in orientation was brought about in no small measure by the radically changed international power configuration. The Second World War shattered the Europe-centered multipolar balance of power system and replaced it by a rigid bipolar balance of power system in which triumphant Soviet communism in the Eurasian heartland was poised to challenge the freshly minted U.S. hegemony, not only geopolitically but also economically and ideologically. In addition, by having successfully led a peasantry-based revolution, China charted a "red" path for countries in the Global South as an alternative to capitalism. The original fears of the Rockefeller Foundation and U.S. industrialists were rooted in the threat posed by resource depletion of too many people competing with industry for the same resources, a requisite condition for social convulsion. Now the fears of the threat to capitalism assumed even greater dimensions as the prospect of permanent socialist revolutions in the Global South might completely cut off the provision of primary commodities to the rich capitalist nations.

This was the background to the shift in the Rockefeller Foundation's orientation toward the manipulation of food crops in ways that would increase production to dampen the potential effects of overpopulation. The initial focus was on wheat, maize, and rice, the three most consumed cereals, which account for 80 percent of human nutrition. There was a powerful strategic logic behind the selection of these cereals. They are amenable to concentration and centralization of production through the mediation of synthetic fertilizers, pesticides, and irrigation. Almost all other basic food crops are excluded from research and investment, which is why the twenty-five essential food crops in the Global South are called orphan crops even though they occupied 240 million hectares of land as of 2010.[84] In Sub-Saharan Africa, for example, philanthrocapitalist foundations have targeted maize cultivation for expansion by integrating the crop into the genetic modification, synthetic fertilizer, and pesticide industrial complex, even though sorghum and millet occupy as many hectares of land as maize and wheat.

Mexico became the first test case for the new orientation of the Rockefeller Foundation. Geopolitical and geoeconomic considerations, coupled with the rise of populist nationalism, made Mexico an ideal candidate to test the new orientation. Mexico was not only the gateway to the southern and northern parts of the Western Hemisphere, but there was also a temporal convergence of views between the Mexican regime and the Rockefeller Foundation over the urgent need to modernize Mexican agriculture, a convergence often fraught with problems. In the 1930s, President Lázaro Cardenas embarked upon reformist programs in industry and agriculture that struck capital as an attempt to put Mexico on a socialist trajectory. His administration organized workers and peasants at the national level and attached them to the national political party, the professed intent being the establishment of a "workers' democracy" in Mexico. The government publicly endorsed higher wages and improved working conditions for industrial workers, distribution of land to the peasantry, establishment of new welfare programs, and it instituted socialist education in public schools. With respect to agrarian reform, the extent of land Cardenas distributed to peasant families was twice the amount of land resources given to the landless during all of his predecessors' administrations combined. The agrarian reforms resulted in the creation of 10,000 prototype collective farms known as *ejidos*.[85]

Even more unnerving to Mexico's northern neighbors was Cardenas's nationalization of the assets belonging to Rockefeller's Standard Oil Company. Cardenas's succession by Manuel Avila Camacho in 1941, however, came as a relief to U.S. policy makers and the Rockefeller Foundation as he quickly reversed the agrarian reform and everything that smacked of socialist tendencies. But Camacho had not abandoned the Mexican vision to make modernization of Mexican agriculture as integral to a strategy of domestic food self-sufficiency. The Rockefeller Foundation, with encouragement from the Roosevelt administration, seized the opportunity to take its chances with Camacho, intent on thwarting the forces of internal subversion and external communist aggression from pushing Mexico toward socialist revolution. There was some material basis for the Rockefeller Foundation's fear that this could be the case since Cardenas had expropriated Standard Oil's assets in 1939. So, reversing this reality and preventing Mexico from deepening its radical orientation was the tallest order of the Rockefeller Foundation. Therefore, they dispatched a team of three agronomists to Mexico in 1943, joined by the Nobel Laureate of the green revolution, Norman Borlaug, in 1944, to begin research on Mexican agricultural resources. Maize and wheat were promptly targeted for selective breeding and hybridization. The result in wheat breeding was no less than spectacular as the U.S. agronomists made a crucial breakthrough in developing rust-resistant high-yielding varieties. By 1951, the researchers were able to widely distribute these wheat strains to breeders and farmers in Mexico. Yields of the rust-resistant wheat in newly irrigated fields in the Yaqui valley in northwestern Mexico jumped from about 770 pounds per acre in 1952 to around 2,900 pounds per acre in 1964. Increases in wheat yields and expansion of areas under wheat cultivation transformed Mexico from having been a net wheat importer in the 1940s to a net wheat exporter in the 1960s.

Excited by the prospects of globalizing the Mexican experience, the Rockefeller Foundation transformed the team-based research effort into an international research institution in 1963, known as the International Center for the Improvement of Maize and Wheat (CIMMYT, for its Spanish acronym), which commenced training hundreds of agricultural technicians from developing countries in maize and wheat breeding. The early successes of the program in Mexico prompted the foundation to duplicate the results in Colombia, Chile, India, and Pakistan. Between 1965 and 1970, the area devoted in these countries to the new wheat varieties grew from 23,000 acres to 24.7 million acres, with impressive results.[86] Indeed, the gains in wheat production in these countries, resulting from a combination of wheat species selection, hybridization, intensive irrigation, and massive agrochemical application, were impressive, as was the gene bank of CIMMYT. For example, wheat production in India soared from around 10 million metric tons in the early 1960s to 86 million tons in 2012.[87] Today, CIMMYT holds the largest plant gene bank in the world with 150,000 wheat accessions and 27,000 maize accessions. Over a period of twenty-five years, CIMMYT claims to have distributed 150,000 wheat varieties and 91,000 maize varieties to more than 100 countries.[88]

To build on the successes of CIMMYT, the Rockefeller Foundation joined the Ford foundation in 1960 to establish the International Rice Research Institute (IRRI), headquartered in the Philippines. Asia was of concern for the Rockefeller Foundation (RF) because of the entrenched perception that Asia had had all the conditions for going the Chinese road. Left-wing insurgencies in Indochina, Indonesia, Malaysia, the Philippines, and Thailand were on the rise. The foundation now saw a clear connection between a rapidly growing, poverty-stricken population in South and Southeast Asia and the inability of governments in the regions to provide enough food for their hungry millions. The growing apprehension was that hunger could be the most important cause of revolutionary upsurge in Asia and that the only way to thwart this from happening was to produce more food to fight hunger.[89] In addition, rice was of particular attraction to the scientists and researchers because 95 percent of rice production takes place in developing countries, and rice generally occupies the greater proportions of cultivated areas for cereals. Of the 147.5 million hectares dedicated to rice production in 1989, 141.4 million were in developing countries, 90 percent of which were in Asia. In any case, IRRI was so successful in identifying, developing, and hybridizing semi-dwarf rice varieties that 60 percent of the varieties grown around the world today were developed by the institute.

World rice production increased from 150 million metric tons in 1961 to 492 million metric tons in 1988, with Asia accounting for 449 million metric tons.[90]

The Rockefeller Foundation and its researchers were now confident enough to publicly announce that, through rapid industrialization of the green revolution and the consequent astronomical increases in yields, enough food would be produced to feed everyone on earth, leading to substantial reduction of hunger and poverty and the long-term increase in improvement of rural livelihoods and human health. The means chosen were selective breeding and hybridization of the major components of cereals, progressively strengthened by germplasm, mechanization, irrigation water, reactive nitrogen, insecticide, herbicide, and fungicide.

In quantitative terms, the substantial increases in aggregate world agricultural production that took place in the second half of the twentieth century did match the original corporate rhetoric, generating surplus food stock, albeit amid agro-ecological destruction and environmental devastation and uneven distribution across countries and regions. In aggregate terms, the net increase in world food availability per person rose from 2360 kcal (kilo calorie) in the 1960s to 2803 kcal per person per day in the 1990s, even though world population significantly increased during the same period. In fact, the FAO acknowledged that the world had enough surplus food by the turn of the twenty-first century to feed the human race one-and-half times, because world food production increased by 1,225 million metric tons per annum between 1961 and 2005. But here is the rub: surplus food availability in the Global North, on the one hand, and poverty and malnutrition in the Global South, on the other, came to define the green revolution. In 2005, there were thirty-two countries with malnutrition rates ranging between 29 and 72 percent. In absolute terms, there were more malnourished and vitamin A-deficient people in the world in the 1990s than there were in the 1950s. Whereas in South Asia 30 percent of the people were still living in poverty in the 1990s, in Latin America and the Caribbean, 209 million people were classified as poor, 81 million of whom lived in absolute poverty. Similarly, in Sub-Saharan Africa over 51 percent of the continent's population was mired in grinding poverty. All told, there were forty-five countries in the Global South with per capita GDP under $1,000 in 2011 and fifteen of them were projected to remain stuck in stagnant poverty by 2050, with less than $1,000 per capita GDP.[91]

Two fundamental questions arise here: If there is much surplus food available in the world and if there are that many hungry and malnourished people in the world that could use the surplus food, why can't the debilitating conditions of hunger and poverty be ameliorated? If the already existing surplus food cannot to solve hunger and poverty, how is producing more transgenic food solve them? Since these questions go to the heart of the ongoing battle between defenders of agro-ecological patterns of production and received knowledge of agriculture and the peddlers of the green/gene revolution, it is of paramount importance to recall and evaluate what was promised by the peddlers in the green revolution since the 1950s—that the gene revolution would end world hunger, malnutrition and poverty and, at the same time, solve the crises in global energy and climate change. So let me describe how the green revolution unfolded in both the core capitalist countries and selective third world countries and how it produced surplus food and reproduced poverty. I will focus on two salient aspects of the green revolution, which eventually became connected with the drive for biofuel production.

To begin with, concentration of land and water resources into large-scale operations was the preponderant objective of the proponents of the green revolution. They understood that land and water resources were the key determinants of any form of agriculture. Thus the first preconditions for the green revolution involved the identification of optimal locations for the targeted cereals, wheat, rice, corn, or soybean, in terms of land size, soil quality, water availability, and proximity to the arteries of national and international markets and communication networks. The latter was important because the monocrop production system was to be export-oriented.

In addition, contrary to the highly orchestrated corporate myth, most of the gains in food production during the second half of the twentieth century came from expanding arable land areas by drawing down forests, savannahs, grasslands, and wetlands, rather than from increases in crop yields. The arable land areas under cultivation in developing countries increased by 230 million hectares during the period of the green revolution, while agricultural land in advanced countries decreased by 54 million hectares, due to urban sprawl and the development of associated infrastructure.[92] In Latin America, two-thirds of food production between 1950 and 1980 came from the rapid colonization of new lands, as the total arable land area increased by 109 percent; similarly, the arable land area in Asia increased by 30 percent. The costs of commodifying and commercially enclosing land resources on this scale were borne by small food producers. In Brazil, for example, the regime's determination to transform small farms producing food for domestic consumption into a capital-intensive, export-oriented, largely monoculture production system to generate foreign currency resulted in the uprooting of 28.4 million people between 1960 and 1980, which was greater than the entire population of Argentina during that period.[93]

The dedication to progressive occupation by dispossession of the best land resources in developing countries was also accompanied by the increasing monopolization of irrigation water resources for monocrop production. The early leader in the promotion of giant irrigation projects was the World Bank, which funneled $75 billion into the construction of mega-dams in ninety-two countries between 1948 and the turn of the century, most of which flowed into the coffers of giant dam-building corporations.[94] As a result, between the early 1960s and the turn of the century, the agricultural area equipped with irrigation worldwide doubled, reaching 302 million hectares, of which 235 million hectares were in the Global South, compared to 68 million hectares in the

Global North. Even though the irrigated area worldwide covered only 16 percent of the 1,600 million hectares under cultivation, irrigated agriculture was responsible for 40 percent of world food crop production by 2005.[95] When the green revolution was launched in the 1950s, water withdrawal from rivers and aquifers was one-third of what it was to become half a century later when 70 percent of global freshwater withdrawal was devoted to agriculture, at a time when 1.6 billion people faced water scarcity.[96] To support the expanding monoculture production system, country after country rushed to put in place giant all-purpose dams. According to the World Commission on Dams (WCD), the number of large dams fifteen meters or higher skyrocketed from fewer than 5,000 in 1950 to over 50,000 by the turn of the century. The number of people directly displaced by these giant dams in developing countries was conservatively estimated at 80 million. However, if the number of people affected by the radical alteration of the natural flood regimes of rivers, obstruction of fish migration, and loss of recession agriculture downstream of dams are included in the figure, more than 472 million additional people were cut off from their livelihoods and income.[97] The chief beneficiaries of the giant hydrological structures have always been large agribusiness interests and big landholders. Inasmuch as the construction, operation, and maintenance costs are usually borne by public entities, the benefits from reliance on irrigation amount to permanent boondoggles of subsidies for the big farm operators. More than selective breeding and hydridization of seeds, it was the monopolization of optimal land and water resources that made the monocrop production system of the green revolution productive. In any case, what emerged in the end was a surplus food regime from the monoculture production system in the Global North and poverty and malnutrition for the vast majority of people in the Global South. This resulted from the substantial diminution of agro-ecologically diverse food sources, brought about by the alienation of land and water resources by owners of the monocrop production system.

The crisis of agricultural surplus in the Global North and the neoliberalization of the green revolution in the Global South represent the other dimension of the green revolution. It must be borne in mind that the green revolution was entirely a U.S. innovation and export. The growing dependency of agriculture on the petroleum industry for fertilizers produced a revolutionary change in U.S agriculture, allowing farmers to shorten fallow periods since reactive fertilizer, that is, synthetic nitrogen, was seen as a perfect substitute for crop rotation and organic soil nutrients. The upshot of this transformation was the concentration and consolidation of U.S. agriculture as the number of farms fell from 6.8 million in 1935 to 2.2 million in 2000. In 1900, half of the U.S. workforce was in agriculture. In comparison, barely 1.9 percent of U.S. workers were in the agriculture sector in 2002. Specialization has also hollowed out the diversity of U.S. agriculture; the average farm in 2000 grew only one crop compared with five crops in 1900.[98]

The cumulative impacts of the changes in the concentration of agriculture and specialization of crops and the consequent dependency on the petrochemical industry for fertilizers and pesticides have been to transform U.S. agriculture into a food manufacturing system, with unavoidable contradictions. The agricultural revolution was so widespread that it created its own problems in terms of price structure, since mass production could not be sustained without mass markets. The dependency on the petrochemical industry, extension of public research and development dollars to agribusiness, tax breaks, public subsidies, and massive application of irrigation water resulted in the radical transformation of modern agriculture, creating the crisis of agricultural surplus production. In Europe, the metaphor "mountains of cheese and lakes of milk" aptly captured the crisis of agricultural surplus as the EU's fifteen countries became net exporters of 25 million metric tons of wheat in 2000, up from being net importers of 21 million metric tons in 1970, and net exporters of 4.2 million tons of sugar, up from being net importers of 2.4 million metric tons of sugar in 1970.[99]

In the United States, agribusiness companies first sought overt government intervention in the food market to contain the crisis of surplus food. Producers were paid by taxpayers to take vast acreages out of production. However, this short-term measure proved inadequate to ameliorate the inner contradiction in U.S. agriculture. So the U.S. Congress passed a farm bill known as Public Law (P.L.) 480 in the early 1950s with a view to achieving twin objectives: removing surplus food from the market and then donating the food to foreign dictators to spread U.S. influence in the third world. This empowered the government to purchase surplus food from producers before it entered the market. This food would be stored, disposed of, or serve as an instrument of U.S. foreign policy in the Global South in exchange for anti-communism. Thus food aid was woven into U.S. foreign policy as an instrument against internal social subversion and external aggression in developing countries. Senator Hubert Humphrey, the fervent champion of P.L. 480, summarized the purpose of the farm bill in this way: "I have heard . . . that people may become dependent on us for food. I know that was not supposed to be good news. To me that was good news, because before people can do anything they have got to eat. And if you are looking for a way to get people to lean on you and to be dependent on you, in terms of their cooperation with you, it seems to me that food dependence would be terrific."[100] Two decades later, Henry Kissinger took the same orientation to its logical extreme when he counseled that just as the way to control global petroleum was to control countries, to control people was to control food.[101]

P.L. 480 was helpful not only to U.S. farmers but also to investors, shippers, insurers, and other actors associated with agribusiness. For example, 65 percent of U.S. food aid is usually eaten up by transportation costs, benefiting shippers, which means that only 35 out of every 100 dollars of food aid reaches the receiving country. Therefore, tying the provision of U.S. food aid to domestic considerations became damaging to food production in receiving countries. Significant amounts of food often rot along the way because of delay, or food sourced in the United States often arrives in receiving countries when local harvest has already occurred, thereby leading to oversupply and thus hurting local farmers. Genuine food aid could have been given to needy countries in the form of cash rather than in kind so that the country could promptly purchase the food locally or regionally, which would be much cheaper and culturally appropriate.[102] But that was not the objective of U.S. foreign policy architects; their overriding goal was to make the third world hospitable to U.S. capital. This became clearer in 1966 when the Johnson administration imposed new conditions on U.S. food aid. Henceforth, shipments of U.S. food aid would be conditional upon the willingness of receiving countries to privilege agricultural growth over industrialization, to institute population control programs, and to open their economies to U.S. investors. The Johnson administration seized the 1965–67 drought and famine in India to test its policy shift when it made deliveries of food conditional upon the government opening its door for U.S. capital for the construction of fertilizer plants, and removing price controls as well.[103] Since the installation of the WTO in 1995, the United States had also been using its rules to universalize the liberalization of trade in agriculture. In practice, however, this has proved a one-way street. Despite demolition of tariffs on agricultural commodities, the United States had been lavishing subsidies on agriculturalists to undercut their competitors from the Global South where farmers have competitive advantage because of cheap labor. Between 1995 and 2010, for example, the U.S. federal government spent nearly $262 billion subsidizing agriculture.[104]

Ever since Henry Kissinger articulated his now infamous counsel to control people via controlling food, U.S. policy makers appeared to be nearing the summit of their control of global food markets. Exports of U.S. agriculture grew fivefold in the 1970s, with the agricultural trade surplus making up for the growing balance of trade deficit resulting from increased petroleum imports. The volume of U.S. agricultural exports rose from 64 million metric tons in 1970, valued at $7.3 billion, to 162 million metric tons in

1980, valued at $41.2 billion. As a result, U.S. net farm export surplus grew from just $2 billion in 1970 to $24 billion in 1980. The extravagant boom in agricultural exports, largely driven by exceptionally high foreign demand for basic grains, coupled with the availability of liberal credit, stimulated further investments in U.S. agriculture as investors projected the successes of the 1970s into the 1980s and beyond. Higher net returns, low real interest rates, and inflated expectations of continued farm export growth goaded investors to pour billions into the agricultural sector, expanding production capacity to unsustainable levels. But by the beginning of the 1980s, changes in the international political economy began to impinge upon U.S. farm exports. As a result, the illusion of a permanent revolution in U.S. agriculture came to a grinding halt in response to a confluence of factors, including the third world debt crisis, strong competition from the EU, and trade barriers for agricultural products.[105]

It is noteworthy that the first factor that fostered growth in export of U.S. agriculture was the emergence of food markets in the Global South. During the 1970s when cheap petrodollars were plentiful, third world countries imported large volumes of U.S. farm products with borrowed petrodollars in order to keep their restive urban populations at bay and maintain a modicum of social stability. However, the oil shocks and the resulting global recession, along with rising real interest rates, eroded their capacity to continue servicing their debt, much less to subsidize food imports. Moreover, with global recession in the advanced Global North (the market for third world primary commodities) in full swing, prices for traditional primary commodities collapsed, making it exceedingly difficult for such countries as Mexico, Brazil, Egypt, Nigeria, Ethiopia, and India to generate foreign exchange revenue to pay for food imports and service their ballooning debt. Between 1979 and 1982, for example, the external debt of less developed countries, which were responsible for more than a third of U.S. farm exports in 1981, increased by 54 percent. Mexico and South Korea alone imported 11.2 percent of all U.S. farm exports in 1981, while their combined external debt spiraled from $53 billion in 1979 to $124 billion in 1982, impinging on their ability to import food as before.[106] Thus, against the backdrop of extremely low prices for their primary commodity exports and rising real exchange rates in the global metropolitan countries, a large number of third world countries rapidly and sharply curtailed U.S. grain imports.

Furthermore, America's closest allies—Canada, Japan, Australia, and the EU—became overly apprehensive about its control of 58 percent of the global farm export market. Their collective apprehension had security and economic dimensions, such as potential food supply disruption in the event of wars, unilateral U.S. determination of world food prices, and the impact on domestic farm employment. To preempt such possibilities, these countries embarked upon rapid scientific stimulation of domestic agriculture, using subsidies and import protection, later followed by export promotion. Canada, Australia, the EU, and Argentina increased the area for grain production from 62.3 million hectares in 1970 to 73.9 million hectares in 1980. As a result, the combined wheat and feed grain production in these countries increased from 150 million tons in 1970 to 220 million tons in 1982, with the surplus entering the world farm export market. Canada alone doubled the area under wheat production. Thus, by the beginning of the 1980s, U.S. competitors had built large grain surpluses, throwing agriculture in advanced countries into disarray. "Mountains of cheese and lakes of milk" indeed captured the European dilemma in unsold food surplus. The result was that these countries posed stiff competition to the United States, as they began to sell their grain surpluses at below world market prices. Taxpayers would cover the losses to farmers. For example, the EU subsidized grain exports in 1982 to the tune of $5 billion, in addition to the $7.3 billion extended to farmers in production subsidies. It was in this context that grain surpluses became problematic in the United States once again, as the U.S share of world grain reserves grew from 45 percent in 1970 to more than 60 percent in 1982.[107]

U.S. agribusiness corporations sought to solve the deepening agricultural crisis through an aggressive foreign policy aimed at restructuring the political economies of third world countries, using covert cajoling or open pressure to foster the free entry of subsidized U.S. grains, increasing animal feed consumption, and diverting grains to biofuels production. The extreme case where the United States used overt means to subordinate another country's agriculture to its interests is Iraq.

Before the First Gulf War, Iraq imported one million metric tons of U.S. grain annually, paid for by petrodollars. The war ended that bonanza. But the Second Gulf War presented the Bush administration with the opportunity to restructure Iraqi agriculture. The agriculture sector had already been ravaged from ten years of sanctions and a shortage of key irrigation equipment. The indiscriminate bombing during the Second Gulf War of the remaining irrigation works, fertilizer factories, cattle feedlots, and poultry farms under "shock and awe" assaults completely gutted Iraqi agriculture. The hidden purpose was to induce and accelerate the rural to urban migration of the farm population, which fostered the privatization and concentration of Iraqi farmland.

In 2002, Order 81 of the 100 orders that Paul Bremer (head of the transitional occupation regime) promulgated was to guide this process of privatization and concentration of Iraqi agriculture. It was no accident that the man put in charge of the reconstruction of Iraqi agriculture was Daniel Amstutz, who had been Assistant Secretary of Agriculture for international affairs during the first Bush administration, as well as the chief U.S. negotiator on agricultural issues in the WTO. Upon leaving government, Amstutz became Cargill's top CEO. It was during his reign that Cargill became one of the dominant grain trading corporations. By 2003, Cargill had risen to the top, controlling about 94 percent of the soybean market and more than 50 percent of the corn market in the upper Midwest, as well as controlling 40 percent of all U.S. corn exports, one-third of all soybean exports, and 20 percent of wheat exports.[108] The most nefarious aspect of Order 81 was the introduction of commercial proprietary seeds (both new varieties and GM) with no Iraqi institution or authority involved in negotiations. The order prohibits Iraqi farmers from saving and planting patented seeds, which meant they had to come year after year to U.S. corporations like Monsanto and DuPont to get new seeds.[109] The purpose of this cynical and overtly malevolent neoliberalization was to transform Iraq into a seed market for U.S. agribusiness.

When choosing Amstutz to head the reconstruction of Iraqi agriculture, the Bush administration knew that he would ruthlessly pursue the unconditional implementation of free-market shock therapy, transforming Iraq into one of the lucrative markets in which U.S. grain corporations could dump their surplus grains, paid for by Iraqi petrodollars. Amstutz lived up to expectations when he proclaimed that the sole problem in Iraqi agriculture was government intervention and unwarranted subsidies. As he stated it: "Iraqi farmers have had little incentive to increase production because of price controls that have kept food very inexpensive. With a transition to a market economy, we can see health returning to agriculture and incentives to employ good farming practices and modern techniques." [110]

Meanwhile, in North America and Western Europe, food waste, integral to accumulation, was another source for mitigating the crisis of agricultural surplus. By FAO estimates one-third of the food produced in the world for human consumption, amounting to 1.3 billion metric tons, is lost or wasted every year. Even if just one-fourth of this lost or wasted food is saved, it could feed 870 million hungry and malnourished people. Even though about 40 million Americans depend day after day on local and regional food banks for survival, between 160 billion and 290 billion pounds of the 500 billion pounds of food produced in the United States annually is wasted along the different points of production, distribution, and consumption. The estimated 100 million metric tons of food wasted in Europe alone every year could feed 200 million people. The 670 million metric tons of food lost and wasted in the Global North each year equals $680 billion. The 220 million metric tons of food that consumers alone in the North waste every year is nearly equal to the entire 230 million metric tons of net food production of Sub-Saharan Africa. In the Global North, over 40 percent of losses occur at retail and consumer levels where food is thrown away merely on grounds of less than attractive appearance. On the other side of the ledger, 40 percent of food in the Global South, amounting to 630 million metric tons, is lost every year at the post-harvest and processing levels, mainly due to insurmountable financial, managerial, and technical difficulties in harvesting techniques as well as a lack of transportation, storage and cooling facilities.[111] However, from the vantage point of agribusiness and biotech corporations, waste of food is not waste in monetary terms because profit is already realized on the wasted food; waste is just a form of removing "surplus" food from the market so that new food products can be circulated and repeat the whole cycle—and keep accumulation going.

The transition of the livestock mode of production from grazing and mixed system to one of full industrialization has become an important palliative to the structural oversupply of grains since an increasing amount of grain is diverted from human consumption to feed for livestock. While 40 percent of the world's total grain production is used as animal feed, in the United States this is almost 70 percent.[112] The development of industrial beef cattle operations in the Global South, distinct from the traditional subsistence mode of livestock production, also proved to be an important palliative to the anarchy of production as the new large-scale commercial cattle ranches incorporated feed crops into grazing pastures. Historically, most animal feed was consumed in the Global North, but as developing countries mimicked the capitalist mode of livestock production, they have been rapidly catching up, accounting for 42 percent of the 742 million metric tons of feed used globally in 2005. In this regard, China and Brazil have been the leaders in the livestock revolution. Brazil alone increased its net meat export by a factor of 10 since the early 1980s by heavily drawing down on its forest resources to make way for pasture and feed crops.[113]

Even though the export of heavily subsidized surplus food to the Global South, the waste of food, and the use of crops for animal feed, each mutually reinforcing the other, partially enabled the core capitalist countries to mitigate the anarchy of production in industrial agriculture, they could not resolve the inherent contradictions in industrial agriculture. By the turn of the twentieth century, the champions of the green revolution had to confront the extremely unpalatable contradiction between the availability of "surplus" food that could feed every human being on the planet, on the one hand, and the existence of nearly 4 billion malnourished people who could not access this food for lack of purchasing capabilities, on the other. Under these conditions, no further expansion of accumulation in world agriculture could occur without aggravating the crisis of agricultural surplus production, furnishing a powerfully new rationale for biofuel production. In the context of the contradiction between the existence of too much food and the presence of too many people without purchasing capabilities, a transformative strategy was needed, and this was the diversion of surplus food crops to biofuel production.

The Transition to a Gene Revolution

Coincidentally or fortunately for agribusiness corporations, the dread over the rapid exhaustion of nonrenewable resources such as hydrocarbons and phosphate, coupled with the clamor of global climate change, took center-stage in world affairs. This allowed agribusiness and biotechnology corporations to adroitly recalibrate their plans. Transitioning from the green revolution to the gene revolution would permit global capitalism to produce GM food, biofuels, and all conceivable bioproducts to simultaneously solve the world energy shortage, world hunger, and global climate change became the enduring mantra of the pioneers in biotechnology. Of course, this would not solve the triple crises of world hunger, energy, and climate, but it would expand the scope for the expansion of accumulation by dispossession. Capitalists always look for permanent fixes, but so long as the growth imperative of accumulation remains the dominant driver, new problems will always arise. As the late Scottish geographer Neil Smith trenchantly observed, capitalist countries have no enduring solutions for economic, social, climate and environmental crises, they simply move them around.[114] Calling for the acceleration of the transition of the green to the gene revolution is one way of doing so. It is against this backdrop that biofuel production has loomed large in the corporate vision of a restructured nature. The global bio-masters are fully cognizant that government subsidies, food waste, animal feed, and export of surplus food to the Global South are insufficient to solve agricultural surplus production in the Global North. A more radical course had to be pursued. Fear of the exhaustion of nonrenewable fossil fuels or fear of potential supply disruption due to political or natural events were found to be handy to make the case for biofuels. Therefore, while joining the government to aggressively promote global trade liberalization in agriculture, U.S. grain corporations and biotech companies aggressively sought government support to convert surplus crops to biofuel production. Transforming grains into flexible raw materials that could interchangeably be used for food and biofuel production became a way to contain the crisis of agricultural surplus production.

Unsurprisingly, the original idea of converting corn into bioethanol found a very cozy incubation apparatus in the headquarters of Archer Daniels Midland (ADM). When ADM successfully sold the notion of converting surplus corn to biofuel production in the late 1970s, the purpose was to thwart corn overproduction from threatening the trajectory of accumulation.

This was the prelude to presenting biofuels as a means to introduce genetically modified crops into the market. It was no accident that it was the grain-trading oligopoly ADM that first proposed in 1978 the conversion of crops into biofuels as a solution to the crisis of agricultural surplus production and that it actively lobbied the government to simultaneously subsidize biofuels and deregulate GM crop production. But this required control of the trajectory of the U.S. political process. No one better understood the significance of this control than Dwayne Andreas, ADM's chairman. For him, politics was a crucial subsidiary to accumulation. So he began distributing election money to politicians from both political parties in exchange for federal subsidies to support ADM's corn ethanol plants and other agricultural products, while marketing biofuels to politicians and the general public as "a service to corn growers" and "a service to humanity." Hearing from the media that he had corrupt involvement with politicians, Andreas defended himself in these terms: "I was raised to believe you're supposed to support your mayor and your congressman and your politician. . . . If a fellow is willing to devote his life to public service, and a fellow like me has more money than I ever dreamed existed in the whole world, wouldn't I be an ass if I didn't respond to requests?" Andreas was excited about the magnitude of the dividend that ADM was receiving from those politicians in the form of subsidies. James Bovard calculated that at least 43 percent of ADM products was subsidized by the federal government at the cost of tens of billions of dollars to taxpayers.[115]

Another urgent issue for Andreas was the removal of barriers to GM crop cultivation. Fortunately for Andreas, deregulation of GM crop production was in tune with the general orientation of the Reagan administration, since U.S. economic supremacy was now seen as predicated upon sharp changes in U.S. agriculture. Indeed, despite strenuous opposition from the scientific community about the unknown health effects of GM foods, the Bush administration issued an executive order in 1992 classifying GM plants and foods as substantially equivalent to organic plants and foods in terms of nutrition, health value, quality, and taste, obviating the need for a special regulatory regime. The Clinton administration became even more hospitable to GM crops when it categorized the 1990s as a decade of agro-industry and biotechnology. The Rockefeller Foundation was not far from the boardrooms of agribusiness as it poured $540 million directly into the gene revolution over the twenty-year period since 1985.[116]

Despite domestic and international resistance to genetically modified organisms (GMOs), biotech companies have found powerful allies in the biofuels sector, because chemical companies and oil oligopolies have become big investors in synthetic biology as the potential source of second-generation fuels. The genetic manipulation of biotic resources could be justified in the name of bioenergy feedstock production. Biofuels became the entry point for the invasion of the global food ecology, destroying global forests in the name of second-generation cellulosic ethanol production. Oil, grain, seed, and chemical companies formed joint ventures of all sorts to use biotechnology as the base from which to launch their offensive to convert biotic resources into infinite amounts of fuels and bioproducts. For example, the giant oil company BP joined the giant chemical and seed company DuPont to form Butamax to produce cellulosic ethanol from seaweed. DuPont and the specialty food ingredients maker Danisco had already established a partnership to produce cellulosic ethanol before DuPont absorbed Danisco in 2011. The California-based synthetic biology company Amyris became the home base for Chevron, Total, Shell, Bunge, and other food and chemical companies from which to launch a variety of biobusiness ventures. Exxon invested $600 million in Synthetic Genomics with an eye toward ethanol production from micro-algae. In 2011, Monsanto, the global leader in commercial proprietary seed, invested in Sapphire Energy to produce ethanol from algae.[117] In the United States alone, seven government labs, thirty universities, and sixty bioenergy companies were engaged in active algae research as of 2008. The lure of algae inheres in the hopeful notion that, depending on the types of strains, the oil content of algae will be in the range of 16 to 77 percent. A company involved in algae ethanol production can supposedly squeeze 58,700 to 136,900 liters of ethanol a year from one hectare of algae. In comparison, the biodiesel from jatropha trees ranges from 1,800 to 2,800 liters per hectare per year, and the yields of biodiesel from palm oil, rapeseed oil, and soybean oil are 5,950, 1,190, and 446 liters per hectare per year, respectively.[118]

The biotech revolution appears to have given the green revolution a new lease on life, presenting as the biological trail blazer for the gene revolution; the green and gene revolutions now rest on the same ideological pillars. For example, proponents of GM crops are quick to conflate the gains in rice production with the miracle of green revolution technology, setting the stage for the gene revolution. What they deliberately gloss over is that the reason why farmers experience poor rice harvests is the lack of enough good land, sufficient water resources, agricultural inputs, and proper farming implements to sustain the growth of rice. Moreover, the rise in rice production was achieved by hollowing out the rich genetic diversity of rice species. Between 1960 and 1970, the land area under rice cultivation in Asia rose by merely 25 percent, while overall rice production rose by 77 percent, with less than a dozen semi-dwarf rice varieties taking over 70 percent of the area dedicated to rice cultivation, destroying more than 100,000 traditional varieties in the process. In Indonesia alone, more than 1,500 rice varieties were wiped out between 1975 and 1990.[119] The cruel irony is that, after the universal condemnation of the destruction of traditional rice species developed over thousands of years, green revolution rice production did plateau at least ten years ago, providing agribusiness another rationale to subject rice to complete genetic transformation.

In any case, the success in selective breeding and hybridization in rice sparked further interest. Whereas in North America the work targeted GM bovine milk production, drugs that make big animals grow bigger and faster, corn, soybeans, canola, and cotton, the focus in Asia was on rice. In the early 1980s, Rockefeller Foundation scientists developed an interest in rice as a prime candidate for the application of plant molecular biology, intent on producing GE rice on a massive commercial scale. In December 1984, the foundation's governing body authorized their scientists to pursue the holy grail in rice biotechnology. With the creation of the International Program on Rice Biotechnology, rice now became the premier model for genomic research in other cereals.

Between 1984 and 2000, the foundation expended $210 million to support the application of genomics, using rice as a test case More than 400 rice researchers from developing countries were promptly trained in molecular biology to provide stewardship to the genetic transformation of rice.[120] Since rice is the staple food for nearly four billion people worldwide, a breakthrough in genetic engineering would hasten corporate control of global agriculture. However, this would erode the genetic diversity of the 300,000 varieties of rice that farmers had developed over 12,000 years.[121]

The ultimate purpose of biotechnology is to freeze in place ever-deepening geoeconomic specialization and division of labor. The global bio-masters determine the trajectory of accumulation by controlling the types and quantities of bioproducts that will become available for global distribution. This readily lends itself to the concentration of proprietary ownership of agricultural resources and monopoly control of patents.

In the 1980s, the Rockefeller Foundation could not help but be excited because the mystery box that had long eluded its scientists was unlocked. They believed that the twin achievements in green and gene revolutions would once and for all break the relationships between high population growth and social tensions, and between resource-related conflicts and social or political instabilities in the Global South. In keeping with this orientation, thirteen priority countries were targeted for the application of the green and gene revolutions, including Mexico, Brazil, Colombia, the Philippines, Indonesia, Thailand, Bangladesh, Pakistan, India, Egypt, Turkey, Ethiopia, and Nigeria. As economic researcher F. William Engdahl correctly notes, the strategy was cleverly crafted to realize two objectives: creating international markets for petrochemical fertilizers, insecticides, herbicides, and commercial proprietary seeds, and strengthening social stability in the Global South while promoting global dependency on U.S. agriculture. The thinking was straightforward. Carbonization of the global economy meant total dependency on reactive nitrogen, pesticides, and irrigation networks, tractors, water pumps, and other farm equipment that would inevitably use diesel, the main source of Rockefeller money.[122] Meanwhile, the rationalization of transgenic crops as inputs for biofuel production would ultimately weaken the stiff opposition by the public to making the transition to the gene revolution the highest stage of controlling the global food manufacturing system.

Notwithstanding the use of numerous penetration and domination techniques, the crisis in U.S. industrial agriculture continued to worsen due to the shift to production of GM crops, which soon faced stiff resistance abroad, mainly from the European Union, something that strengthened the case for biofuel production. It is useful to note here that, in 2014, the United States had planted 73.1 million hectares of GM crops, and the adoption rate across the board was 93 percent.[123] Since many sectors in the U.S. economy have suffered rising trade deficits, agriculture has been seen as a sector that held its ground regarding international trade. For example, the year 2011 was significant because U.S. exports of agricultural commodities reached a record $137.4 billion, generating an agricultural trade surplus of $42 billion. This gain was in part attributed to America's hegemony in GMOs. In 2010, revenues from GMOs were estimated at $300 billion, accounting for 2 percent of GDP.[124]

Western Europe, however, is the nemesis of U.S. GMOs-based agricultural supremacy. Indeed, frustrated by years of stubborn resistance to its GMOs by European consumers, Monsanto finally decided in July 2013 to abandon its effort to penetrate the European market with GMOs. It withdrew its pending applications for six GM corn varieties, a GM soybean, and a modified sugar beet. Monsanto's decision was prompted by the revelation of the connection between GMOs and health risk. In September 2012, French scientists released their long-awaited study, showing that rats fed on NK603 corn RR (Roundup Ready) died earlier than rats fed on a standard diet. Unable to bear the heat generated by the growing resistance from civil society in Europe, Monsanto found itself under compulsion to consolidate its natural seed market in Europe by investing $300 million a year. Monsanto's annual turnover from its natural seed business in Europe was $1.7 billion as of 2012.[125] This stiff European resistance to GMOs further strengthened the corporate advocacy of biofuel production.

If U.S. grain corporations are to effectively capitalize on the hegemony of biotechnology, and if the United States is to improve its trade deficit by exporting more GM crops, then overcoming international resistance and exporting the biotechnology itself to targeted countries of the Global South become essential. This requires identifying and cajoling compliant countries that might approve the importation or planting of GM crops. It appears that the United States is making significant progress in this area, as Brazil, Argentina, Mexico, China, India, South Africa, and fourteen other developing countries have sufficiently been cajoled to introduce GM crops. Planting 42 million hectares of GM crops in 2014, Brazil has become second after the United States in GM crop cultivation. Argentina occupies a close third position with 23 million hectares under GM crop cultivation.[126] In Asia, China and India have become eager to introduce GM crops. In South Africa, prior Western corporate domination of the country made the introduction of GM crops relatively easy. In Europe, Spain, Romania, Slovakia, and the Czech Republic had adopted GM crops on a smaller scale.

The social barriers to full globalization of GM crops, however, remain daunting. This has to do in part with international resistance to GM crops for commercial, environmental, and health reasons, especially by the EU countries, and in part for ethical reasons over the use of food crops for fuel production to run the machine of global capitalism, as billions of people in the Global South go to bed with empty stomachs. Against this backdrop, the lyrics must be changed while the melody remains the same. The new lyrics now entail designing new GM crops for biofuel production, on the one hand, and pushing for second-generation biofuels, based on non-edible woody biomass and grasses, as well as crop and forest residues, on the other. However, this requires the help of biotech companies to engineer revolutionary methods to design crops specifically for biofuel production and to convert non-edible woody crops, grasses, and agricultural residues into biofuels. Monsanto and Cargill, for example, created a joint venture called Renessen to produce and market GM crops exclusively designed for biofuels production.[127] Biotechnology companies are promising to supply unlimited amounts of jet fuel made from forests. The California-based renewable energy developer Rentech Inc. partnered with the Ontario provincial government to produce jet fuel from Canadian forests. The company planned to invest $500 million in the plant, cushioned by a $200 million interest-free loan from the Canadian government. Rentic would cut down 1.1 million cubic meters of timber annually to feed its jet-fuel plant. The forecast was that when the plant came on stream in 2016, Rentech would supply the market with 85 million liters of green jet fuel a year. However, by 2013, Rentech had completely dropped the project.[128]

A new reality has brought oil, grain, and biotechnology corporations into interlocking clusters, making biotechnology corporations pivotal not only to the conversion of woody biomass, grasses, and agricultural residues to biofuels, but also to the ability to engineer crops ostensibly designed for biofuel production. This situation is a union made in heaven, one in which biofuel producers can access a steady supply of cheaply engineered feedstocks, and biotech companies will have a ready-made market for the bioproducts they will endlessly crank out. Biotechnology companies that have hitherto been hindered by public rejection and/or international resistance to GM crops can now hide behind public pronouncements that their GM crops can be used for biofuel production. This is another backdoor for biotech companies to invade the global food system where the boundaries between GM and non-GM crops will be completely obliterated. Through aggressive genetic modification of food crops and woody plants, the abundance of biomass feedstocks will be increased exponentially; through advanced genetic engineering, new plants with desirable traits suitable for second-generation biofuel production will be developed, and the selection of new plant varieties suitable for biofuel generation will be accelerated; and through new engineered enzymes, the characteristics of plants will be altered to facilitate their conversion to biofuels. Conversion of woody biomass to biofuels requires radical biological innovations, thus enzyme engineering is needed to unlock the secrets of plant traits and characteristics. The micro-organism *Saccharomyces cerevisiae*, currently used in industrial fermentation of sugar, does not directly process starchy materials. The plant materials must first be broken down using amylase enzymes; amylases are genetically engineered micro-organisms designed to break down woody materials into fermentable sugars. Thus, using a combination of synthetic biology, genomics, nanotechnology, and bioinformatics, biotech companies now believe that they have the capacity to design new micro-organisms that break down the cellulose and hemi-cellulose of plants into fermentable sugars as crucial input for the production of limitless biofuels; they are even envisioning that they can design trees with less lignin since lignin cannot be converted into sugars prior to fermentation into alcohol. Even better, they hope to design self-engineering plants that can produce enzymes to induce lignin degradation.[129]

Such a project would require cutting-edge research which would accelerate the commodification and commercial enclosure of the 230 billion tons of biomass that the earth produces annually, which allows the clusters of oligopolies to convert all biotic resources into biofuels, biopower, biochemicals, and bioplastics. From the corporate perspective, talk of biofuels is just a small part of the general plan to transition to a bio-economy in which the production and marketing of bio-based products becomes the dominant pattern. By the estimate of the U.S. Department of Agriculture, the market value of bio-based chemicals and plastics will be $500 billion per year by 2020.[130]

Expecting a financial bonanza from switching from a fossil-based economy to a bio-economy has spurred the grain, oil, pulp, textile, pharmaceutical, and biotech oligopolies into action to complete the conquest of the remaining 76 percent of the planet's biomass, 86 percent of which is located in the tropics and sub-tropics, providing livelihoods for billions of people.[131] The artillery deployed now against nature is the adoption of synthetic biology, genomics, nanotechnology, bioinformatics, and related tech-niques, based on extremely dangerous genetic engineering. The global bio-masters use genomics to gather information about the identity, location and functions of genes germane to the applica-tion of biotechnology to a whole host of plants. Then they use bioinformatics to analyze and predict the structure, function, and behavior of organisms. They also use micro-propagation techniques to take plant tissues or whole plant structures and culture them under artificial conditions to produce completely new plants. Micro-propagation speeds up plant breeding or even entirely bypasses the relatively slow sexual reproduction of plants, with a view to producing superabundant plant materials suitable for all industries.[132] In the imagined world of a post-fossil fuels bio-economy, the production of fuels, drugs, chemicals, plastics, and other high-value bioproducts and industrial compounds is expected to be based on the supposedly infinite supply of such biological feedstocks as agricultural crops, forests, bushes, shrubs, grasses, algae, microbes, and seaweed. This invites the eruption of biological Armageddon, presaging the total commodification and commercial enclosure of nature for purposes of biofuels and bioproducts.

Given the dedication of biotech companies to endlessly crank out genetically engineered bioproducts and the commitments of governments to support them financially and politically regard-less of the cost to the environment and society, the invocation of a biological Armageddon can no longer be brushed aside as alarm-ist. The industry today boasts that the planting of GM crops has grown from 1.7 million hectares in just three countries in 1996 to more than 181 million hectares grown by twenty-eight countries in 2014. These countries, together home to four billion people, are regarded as the mainstay for the emerging bioproduct market. Of these countries that planted GM crops in 2014, twenty were developing countries, led by China, India, Brazil, Argentina, and South Africa, which planted 96 million hectares in GM crops.[133]

This new reality has created a dynamic context for grain and biotech oligopolies, not only to accelerate the conversion of more and more crops to biofuel production but also to expand their effort to commodify other biotic resources for all kinds of bio-based products and fuels. Indeed, every plant species is now subject to genetic alteration, including trees that were previously confined to the timber industry, the pulp and paper sector, and wood fuel and charcoal production.

3

Biofuels and the Transformation of the Metropolitan State

Karl Marx observed that all political decisions are, in the final analysis, economic decisions. The same observation can be inverted to state that all economic decisions are, in the last analysis, political decisions. For its continuous reproduction, capital accumulation requires favorable political contexts, whether to create the necessary social peace to avoid disruption of the supply of raw materials and labor and markets for distributing goods and services to consumers or enabling the business environment through privatization, deregulation of the market, and demolition of barriers to trade. Putting environmental and labor standards by the wayside, while lavishing tax breaks, depreciation allowances, and subsidies on owners of capital, is also important.

The performance of domestic functions by the metropolitan state in the service of corporations is reinforced by equally vigorous performance of international functions in ways that make the global market free for corporations to roam without fear of regulation or restraint in the deployment of capital, accumulation, repatriation of profit, and required adherence to environmental and labor standards. In performing these functions, metropolitan states rely on a vast international intergovernmental network of institutions, such as the World Bank, the IMF, and the WTO, as well as on such regional banks as the Inter-American Development Bank, the African Development Bank, and the Asian Development Bank in which the metropolitan states are the dominant shareholders. Pretending to be global apolitical institutions in which equality of states is respected, these institutions legitimize neoliberalism. In practice, this neoliberal macrostructure serves the metropolitan states and their corporations in a manner akin to the colonial mode of primitive accumulation in which inherited patterns in the division of labor and specialization are retained in all but in name. The recruitment, training, and promotion of staff in these intergovernmental institutions are carefully managed to ensure ideological commitment to the neoliberal order. The extraordinary power of the World Bank, the IMF, and the WTO enables their staffs to intimidate third world state bureaucrats to shape up or lose all forms of bilateral and multilateral assistance and loans from the metropolitan North. As certifiers of international credit-worthiness, these global institutions can and do, on behalf of the metropolitan states and their business oligopolies, directly or indirectly block developing countries from accessing markets and capital in the metropolitan North.

The biofuel industrial complex has become the latest beneficiary of the continuum of domestic state and global intergovernmental services to further capital accumulation without restraint. Domestically, this latest industrial complex is generously rewarded with subsidies, tax breaks, and price supports, all in the name of job creation and the provision of alternative fuels and bio-based products. Globally, the same transnational corporations use official state machinery and the institutional tentacles of intergovernmental organizations to penetrate and dominate third world markets and to dispossess millions of peasants of their landholdings, converting them into bioenergy crop monocultivation. When President George W. Bush made a pilgrimage to Latin America in March 2007, he was performing a diplomatic mission on behalf of the biofuel-biotechnology industrial complex. In visiting seven South and Central American countries, the president's overarching aim was to goad the transnationalized state bureaucrats into specializing in bioenergy crop cultivation. The visit's fruition manifested in the formation of a long-term partnership with Brazil to jointly promote the development of bioenergy crop monocultivation and biofuel production in other countries through the deployment of U.S. and Brazilian capital, technology, and expertise. Moreover, President Bush brought the Inter-American Development Bank (IDB) on board with the project. To the demonstrated satisfaction of the U.S. president, the IDB promptly dedicated $3 billion to biofuel production in the region.[1] This pecuniary generosity was made possible, not only because of U.S. predominance in the IDB as the largest shareholder, but also because of Luis Alberto Moreno's presidency of the regional bank. Colombian by origin, Moreno received all his education in U.S. institutions, where he was sufficiently indoctrinated into the make-believe world of neoliberalism. Prior to his appointment as IDB president in 2005, Moreno served as Colombia's Economic Development Minister and ambassador to Washington. Moreover, Moreno joined Roberto Rodrigues (Brazil's former agriculture minister), and Jeb Bush (former Florida governor and President Bush's brother) to form the Inter-American Ethanol Commission as a private lobbying organization.

THE GEOECONOMICS OF BIOFUELS IN AMERICA

Insofar as the role of the metropolitan state goes, the United States, dominating global corn ethanol production and consumption, has been the pioneer in the popularization of bioenergy crop monocultivation and the loudest cheerleader for the globalization of biofuels production. It all began nearly four decades ago when ADM, one of America's largest grain-trading corporations, successfully sold to policy makers the idea of corn-based ethanol as alternative or supplement to fossil fuels under the guise of the urgency to diversify the country's energy portfolio. In 1978, the U.S. Congress positively responded to ADM's proposition for energy diversification by passing the Energy Tax Act, which introduced the first major federal subsidies to ethanol with full exemption from the motor fuel excise tax, after ADM supplied the first 20 million gallons of commercial ethanol. In subsequent years, Congress doubled down on the provision of additional subsidies to corn growers and ethanol producers. The Energy Security Act of 1980, for example, extended federally-insured loans for ethanol producers, guaranteeing up to 90 percent of the construction cost of an ethanol plant. The legislation also introduced price guarantees for biomass energy projects and purchase agreements for biomass energy used by federal agencies. Thirty-eight states also began in rapid succession providing various incentives to ethanol producers. The state of Minnesota, for example, exempted ethanol producers from taxes to the tune of more than $20 million a year between 1998 and 2005.[2]

All told, twenty-two federal programs were established in rapid succession, administered by five different agencies and departments, to accelerate biofuel production. The benevolent measures taken to support the speedy rise of the biofuel industrial complex included blending and production tax credits, import tariffs to protect domestic producers from cheaper foreign-produced ethanol, loans and loan guarantees to stimulate the development of biofuel production and distribution infrastructure, and research grants for new biofuel technologies.[3]

Cushioned by taxpayers' hard-earned money, corn ethanol production took off from 83 million gallons in 1981 to over 900 million gallons in 1990.[4] Concomitant with rapidly expanding corn ethanol production came the official orchestration campaign of biofuels as a heaven-sent alternative to dirty fossil fuels. The USDA presented the consumption of biofuels as an integral expression of patriotism in terms of both reinforcing America's agricultural hegemony and climate change reduction. Sugar-coating their message, the department's chief propagandists told the public that, by 2030, the United States would be in a secure position to obtain 5 percent of its power, 20 percent of its liquid road transport fuels, and 25 percent of the fuels needed for bio-chemical production from renewable bioenergy crops and plants, which together would displace 30 percent of annual petroleum consumption.[5]

By the mid-2000s, the patriotic fervor for biofuels appeared to have reached epic proportions. Al Gore's advocacy for biofuels through his book *An Inconvenient Truth* lubricated the enthusiasm for biofuels. Even well-known environmental organizations such as the Environmental Defense Fund, the Sierra Club, the Natural Resources Defense Council, and the National Wildlife Foundation jumped on the bandwagon, treated to the melody from the bio-fuel lobby choirs. America's celebrities, ranging from Hollywood actors to musicians, also saw biofuel-driven cars as glamorously fashionable and lined up to express their green patriotism. The well-known country-western singer Willie Nelson started up his own biodiesel company.[6] For their part, car makers like Ford, GM, and DaimlerChrysler celebrated the arrival of biofuels on the market, giving them some relief from public pressure to increase fuel efficiency and reduce pollution from engine exhausts.

However, the greatest allies of the biofuel cornucopians were the key political players. Both federal and state bureaucracies became pivotal in advancing agrobusiness interests, fulfilling three crucial functions: orchestration of the public relations campaign; sub-sidies to corn growers and ethanol producers; and provision of protective tariffs against foreign competitors. Between 1995 and 2004, corn farmers received $42 billion in subsidies from twelve federal programs. In 2005, they received $9.4 billion in federal subsidies, more than all the subsidies that other sectors of agri-culture received, something that prompted many farmers to shift out of soybean cultivation to corn production, some farmers even converting dry lands deemed unsuitable for corn cultiva-tion to corn production. Subsidies to sorghum production, which accounted for only 3 percent of ethanol production, were in the range of $65 million to $101 million per annum. ADM and other corn-ethanol producers were rewarded with even larger subsidies, courtesy of taxpayers. The direct corporate capital expenditures of $11.8 billion devoted to biofuel production between 2000 and 2005 were annually augmented by over $6.5 billion of federal subsidies and were projected to add up to $92 billion between 2006 and 2012. This figure does not include the approximately $70 billion lost to the Internal Revenue Service in foregone tax receipts over the same period, or the more than $450 million that state governments lost every year in foregone tax receipts. Nor does it include the cost of free land given by state and local governments for the construction of ethanol plants or the expenditures on upgrading roads and rail lines.[7]

In 2005, amid the surging mood of optimism surrounding the prospects of biofuels, Congress established the Renewable Fuel Standards (RFS), making consumption of biofuels mandatory. A minimum of 4 billion gallons of ethanol had to be blended with gasoline and used by 2006, rising to 7.5 billion gallons by 2012. The U.S. Environmental Protection Agency (EPA) was statutorily placed on the green pedestal to determine and monitor the pace and direction of biofuel production and distribution. In 2007, Congress expanded the RFS mandate with the minimum consumption of biofuels to be 9 billion gallons by 2008, rising to 36 billion gallons by 2022, with 21 billion gallons, including 16 billion gallons of lingo-cellulosic fuels and 4 billion gallons of the so-called advanced fuels, using second-generation raw materials such as algae and grasses.[8]

Intent on reassuring the biofuel-biotechnology peddlers about the potential availability of feedstocks to produce the mandatory quantity of biofuels, the departments of Energy and Agriculture jointly prepared a lengthy document pointing to the abundance of feedstocks that would meet not only the needs of biofuel producers but also supply feedstocks for the production of a vast array of bioproducts, as well as generate heat and steam for the pulp and paper industry. According to this document, extolled as the "one-billion-ton study," the United States could conservatively produce nearly 1.4 billion dry tons of feedstocks annually, including 368 million dry tons of removable biomass from forestlands, and 998 million dry tons from agricultural lands, sufficient to produce 85 billion gallons of biofuels a year to displace more than 30 percent of present U.S. petroleum consumption by 2030.[9] Since it was assumed that 70 million gallons of ethanol per one dry ton of lingo-cellulosic biomass could be achieved at current conversion technologies, the USDA argued that 230 million to 265 million dry tons of lingo-cellulosic biomass could easily be found to produce the mandated 16 billion gallons of cellulosic ethanol, even without tapping the vastly available agricultural and forest residues, critical to organic matter formation.[10]

What the bureaucrats forgot to tell us is the other side of the ledger, the cost of removing forest and agricultural residues in the magnitude stated above. It did not occur to the preparers of the "one-billion-ton study" that agricultural and forest residues are critical to soil reformation, moisture retention, erosion prevention, and carbon sequestration. For example, numerous studies indicate that the removal of 75 million tons of corn stover alone can increase soil erosion by 84.4 million tons per year, which would cost society $327 billion a year in terms of lost environmental benefits such as erosion avoidance, crop productivity, soil carbon and nutrient enhancement, and soil carbon sequestration.[11] Agricultural and forest residues supply essential nutrients to crops and plants, thereby reducing the need for synthetic or inorganic inputs. For instance, in situations where the natural state is maintained, the organic carbon content in the top 40 inches of soil is on the order of 16 to 67 tons per acre in cropland soils; 21 to 73 tons per acre in forested soils; 19 to 65 tons per acre in rangeland soils; and 14 to 182 tons per acre in soils in other land uses.[12] Moreover, the total carbon sequestration in agriculture and forest sinks at the time when the "one-billion ton study" came out was more than 800 million metric tons of carbon dioxide equivalent, offsetting 11 percent of gross U.S. ghg emissions. In 2005, forests and harvested wood products alone had sequestered 699 million tons of carbon dioxide equivalent.[13]

In any case, thanks to public money, U.S. ethanol production soared from 1.4 billion gallons in 1998 to 9.8 billion gallons in 2008, and then to 14.34 billion gallons in 2014. In parallel with increased biofuel production, the number of ethanol plants also multiplied. By early 2008, there were 183 bioethanol plants mostly concentrated in the Corn Belt states.[14] In relation to the bioethanol industry, the biodiesel industry in the United States was slow to jump-start; in 1999, the total biodiesel production was a mere 400,000 gallons, even though its growth accelerated thereafter to reach 575 million gallons by 2005. In 2014, the 97 biodiesel plants still produced only 4.8 billion liters of biodiesel compared with the 54 billion liters of bioethanol produced.[15] Most of the soybeans produced are either processed into animal feed or exported. In 2013, for instance, the amount of soybeans exported to China raked in over $28 billion.[16] The explanation of the relatively low development of the biodiesel sector in part lies in the fact that the livestock population, comprising about 100 million head of cattle, 66 million head of hogs and pigs, and over 9 billion of poultry population are reliant on soybeans for feed. Over 98 percent of the soybean production retained for domestic uses is processed into animal feed while, of the remaining balance, 70 percent is processed into food products and edible oil for human consumption and 30 percent is converted into biodiesel.[17] However, with the growing demand for fuels, U.S. biodiesel plants may in the future process more and more soybeans into liquid fuels, which has serious implications for the global forest ecology. As U.S. soybean exports decline, countries in the Global South may convert their forest resources into soybean fields to take advantage of the rising international soybean prices. In fact, that is exactly what Latin American countries have been doing ever since the biofuel boom.

Make no mistake, the purpose of grants, tax exemptions, subsidies, credit, allotment of free land, and public expenditures on infrastructure development was not to improve the energy security of the country nor to reduce climate change but rather to boost the corporate bottom. To contextualize this point, we should pay attention to the distorted priorities of the bureaucrats. Three-quarters of the tax benefits and two-thirds of all federal subsidies allocated for renewable energy production in 2007 went to corn ethanol production. The tax credit given to ethanol producers in 2007 was more than four times the credits given to solar, wind, and geothermal power production, and hydrogen cells innovation, the authentically reliable sources of renewable energy.[18] We shall explore the reasons for this in chapter 5.

The popularity of biofuels was also stimulated by oil price hikes. It was in response to the fear of another petroleum-driven stagflation that the U.S. Congress passed the American Jobs Creation Act in 2004, providing federal stimulus for biofuel production by establishing a volumetric excise tax credit, including a tax credit of 51 cents per gallon for ethanol producers and retailers, and a tax credit of $1 per gallon for producers if they used agricultural residues for ethanol production. Those who used waste for biodiesel production were eligible for a tax credit of 50 cents per gallon. This legislation was quickly followed by the Energy Policy Acts of 2005 and 2007, establishing minimum blending and consumption thresholds for biofuels. To protect the growth of domestic biofuel production, a 54-cents-per-gallon tariff on ethanol imports was imposed, primarily targeted at Brazil's sugar ethanol, which had competitive advantage over corn-based ethanol.[19] The Energy Independence and Security Act of 2007, which President Bush signed into law in December 2007, was particularly ambitious in establishing fanciful quantitative dimensions for the production of 36 billion gallons of biofuels by 2022, of which 21 billion gallons would supposedly come from lignocellulosic and advanced fuels, supported by $118 billion in federal government subsidies during the course of the mandated period. In addition, domestic biofuel production would be augmented by the importation of 3.5 billion gallons of advanced cellulosic fuels a year by the end of this decade.[20]

The aspirational objective was to obtain 30 percent of the country's total energy requirements from biofuels by 2030. To reach this goal, increasing amounts of American corn and soybean outputs would be devoted to biofuel production. In addition, large tracts of land would have to be recalled from the 37 million acres of land held in the Conservation Reserves Program (CRP) and devoted to the monocultivation of corn and soybeans. As we shall see later, land resources held in the CRP under contractual arrangement between landowners and the government are taken out of agricultural production to protect the country's waterways, wildlife refuges, and to prevent soil erosion. To rationalize the reconversion of the natural resources held in the national reserve program to bioenergy crop production, biofuel producers in the United States have worked hard to convince the federal and state governments that they could supply up to 60 billion gallons of advanced fuels by 2030 if only more land in reserve is released and more generous public subsidies could be had.[21]

Truth to tell, devoting increasing amounts of domestic grains to biofuel production or recalling lands held in reserve for grain production is very unlikely to meet the biofuel mandates as outlined by the federal bioenergy policy. To put this observation into perspective, ecologist David Pimentel succinctly noted that the United States would need 2 billion acres of farmland to produce the claimed amounts of biofuels, which is more than five times the total arable land available in the country. One must hasten to remember here that even after biofuel producers devoted 20 percent of the 2006 corn harvest to ethanol production, it displaced only 3 percent of gasoline consumption. If the entire annual corn grown on 90 million acres is converted to ethanol fuels, the country may be able to displace only 12 percent of its annual gasoline consumption. If the country uses its entire soy production to generate biodiesel, the displacement gain will be only 6 percent of the diesel consumption. Even after doing all that, the energy gain is still negative. When including all the direct and indirect costs related to fossil energy used, fertilizer, and pesticide production used to grow corn feedstock, the fermentation and distillation processes, energy used to transport the corn feedstock to the ethanol plant, and energy expended on capital equipment, the loss is significant. By some calculations, the total energy input to produce one gallon of ethanol comes to 129,600 BTU, while one gallon of ethanol has an energy value of only 76,000 BTU, showing a net loss of 53,600 BTU. This means that it takes 71 percent more energy to produce one gallon of ethanol than the energy contained in a gallon of corn ethanol.[22] If the costs of fossil energy used in the cultivation, application of synthetic fertilizers and pesticides, harvesting, and production of the biofuels is taken into account, the displacement rate of fossil fuels by biofuels in the United States will actually be equivalent to only 2.4 percent for bioethanol and 2.9 percent for biodiesel.[23] To put this in proper perspective, currently 440,000 gallons of corn ethanol are obtained from one acre of corn in the United States. At this rate of corn yield, the United States must allocate 20 percent of its corn and pasture lands to corn production to produce 2.2 million barrels of ethanol fuel per day, which means that the United States will still use 18 million barrels of petroleum per day.[24] This hardly inspires confidence in achieving the objectives of national energy security and emission reduction. In 2008, for example, the United States consumed around 186 billion gallons of gasoline and diesel, plus 8.9 billion gallons of biofuels. Yet that year the country imported 3.7 billion barrels of crude oil in which case biofuel production made little difference.[25]

Despite the extravagant official orchestration about the geo-economic and geopolitical indispensability of biofuels, and the ceaseless showering of taxpayers' money on the industry, the production of biofuels in the magnitude envisioned by the bio-fuel peddlers is not a prospect. The biofuel industrial complex and its champions know this very well; that is why they have put the emphasis on second-generation or cellulosic biofuel production in order to blunt the contentious politics of the food versus fuel debate. In 2006 some science writers proposed that the United

States could use switchgrass, a diverse mixture of prairie grasses and woody plants grown in the 235 million hectares of grassland available in the country and use its vast crop residues to produce ethanol fuels.[26] The proposal was so outrageous that it unnerved the scientific community, because in the scale proposed it would leave the land bare, exposed to erosion whereupon loss of topsoil might increase a hundred-fold, and the increased runoff from upland landscapes would lead to nutrient pollution, siltation, acidification, and eutrophication of vital natural water systems. Furthermore, the removal of vast amounts of grasses and crop residues would foster soil-carbon oxidation, increasing greenhouse gas emissions. Even if we leave the environmental and climatic costs of the proposal unexamined, converting the entire 235 million hectares of grassland, coupled with the conversion of vast amounts of crop residues, into ethanol fuels would provide a mere 12 percent of annual U.S. oil consumption. Even if the United States converts its entire forest endowment to agro-fuels, the nation might meet only 15 percent of its energy requirements.[27]

Despite this objective reality, however, the biofuel industrial complex is determined to press ahead with the industrial biofuel revolution. Given the size of the corporate army of lobbyists descending on Congress, one would not be surprised if the entirety of land held in the CRP is called into production or if vast swaths of natural forests are converted into fast-growing tree plantations to produce the required feedstocks. Even the Pentagon has become a favorite target of biofuel producers since this mammoth military apparatus is the largest oil buyer in the world, regardless of the fact that its apparatus had come under congressional pressure to scale down its biofuel program, purely out of budgetary concerns. In reaction to the clamors from some politicians from non-corn states, biofuel companies muscled their lobbying power, raising the specter of future energy shortage. In July 2012, agribusiness dispatched a large contingent of retired military brass to Congress to warn the politicians not to mess with the Pentagon's green energy program. The military brass told senators and their staffs in no uncertain terms that purchasing expensive biofuels would in the long run pay for itself by reducing America's dependency on Middle Eastern oil, and by improving the country's national security interests as well. As Colonel Dan Bolan put it: "A small investment in biofuels could reap trillions of dollars for the country at large. What the Navy has invested in biofuels is such a small percentage of what the total investment in fuels is."[28]

What precipitated this robust lobbying campaign was the revelation that the Pentagon spent $12 million on 450,000 gallons of biofuels, at almost $27 per gallon, for its "green fleet" demonstration project.[29] Interestingly, the Pentagon had been doing the biofuel-biotechnology industrial complex's bidding since 2003 by linking biofuel production and national security. In 2003, it came up with its own secret study on the possible consequences of global warming and climate change, resulting in catastrophic wars, natural disasters, and mass dislocation and migration, with potentially far-reaching security ramifications for the United States. The authors of the study warned that climate change–driven global warming

> could potentially destabilize the geopolitical environment, leading to skirmishes, battles and even war due to resource constraints such as 1) food shortages due to decreases in net global agricultural production; 2) decreased availability and quality of freshwater in key regions due to shifted precipitation patterns, causing more frequent floods and droughts; and 3) disrupted access to energy supplies due to extensive sea ice and storminess. . . . With only five or six key grain-growing regions in the world (United States, Australia, Argentina, Russia, China, and India), there is insufficient surplus in global food supplies to offset severe weather conditions in a few regions at the same time—let alone four or five. The world's economic interdependence makes the United States increasingly vulnerable to the economic disruption created by local weather shifts in key agricultural and high population areas around the world. Catastrophic shortages

of water and energy supply—both which are stressed around the
globe today—cannot be quickly overcome.[30]

Moreover:

> With over 400 million people living in drier, subtropical, often
> overpopulated and economically poor regions today, climate
> change and its follow-on effects pose a severe risk to political,
> economic, and social stability. In less prosperous regions, where
> countries lack the resources and capabilities required to adapt
> quickly to more severe conditions, the problem is very likely
> to be exacerbated. For some countries, climate change could
> become such a challenge that mass emigration results as the
> desperate peoples seek better lives in regions such as the United
> States that have the resources to adaptation.[31]

Such foreboding discourses notwithstanding, it is important
to bear in mind that the search for alternative fuels has never
been about energy security nor job creation, but about finding
complementary sources of capital accumulation. After all, the
total employment in the U.S. biofuel sector in 2014 was a mere
282,000.[32] The hollowing out of the country's manufacturing base
or the de-industrialization of the country had long deepened the
crisis of overaccumulation, on the one hand, and the mass dislocation of the working class, on the other, portending existential
social disequilibrium. Indeed, the Obama administration exposed
the fundamental limits of biofuels to overcome the crises of overaccumulation and mass dislocation by taking the debate over
biofuels to a higher level; it is not only biofuels but an entire gamut
of bio-based products that the United States must strive to produce
and market if it is to contain the crisis of overaccumulation, and
the consequent mass unemployment-related legitimation crisis. In
this regard, the chieftains of the biofuel-biotechnology industrial
complex and the political professional class see eye to eye on the
urgency to peddle the transition to the supposedly post-petroleum

economy. The peddlers in biofuels and GM crops desperately need the economic agency and advocacy of the state to politically market to Congress and the mass public the assumed gains that can be had from swift adoption of biofuels and GE crops. On the other hand, the political class need some palpable employment gains from inducing the economy to move up to a different trajectory if the country is to avert future spontaneous Occupy Wall Street–like movements from escalating to conscious social revolution. After all, the blowback from the macrostructural changes connected with the deepening processes of globalization have long been haunting America's professional political class, as manifested in the federal government debt approaching $20 trillion as of this writing, and a trade deficit that has yet to see daylight since it hit a record high of $450 billion in 2002. In 2015, the country's international trade deficit was $505 billion, notwithstanding the fact that the average price of imported oil had fallen to $47 a barrel from $91 a barrel in 2014 and from $140 a barrel in 2008.[33] Thus the obscenely upward distribution of national income and the country's grossly distorted international economic relations have eroded the political class's ability to maintain an acceptable level of social equilibrium. Employment stagnation, erosion of family incomes, the hollowing out of social protections, and growing structural inequality have now exposed millions of Americans to material deprivations, social disorientation, and deep psychological anxieties than can supply the fuel for potential social uprisings.

Indeed, threatened by recurrent crises, the ever-intensifying global competition, and the threat of revolt from below, industry chieftains and the political class are now seeking refuge in the notion of what is called the bio-economy, calling for widening and deepening the commodification and neoliberalization of nature. The earlier faith in cellulosic biofuel production as a promising source of capital accumulation and employment has proved to be illusionary. The biofuel champions have grown hesitant to throw their capital into the cellulosic biofuel sector, whose future has become punctuated by uncertainties primarily due to the shale resource extraction boom, reflected in a cheap petroleum supply as U.S. aggregate oil production increased by 50.6 percent between 2011 and 2014, leading to crude oil price tumbling from $112 a barrel in June 2014 to $48 a barrel in January 2015. This has had some positive impact on the U.S. balance of payments. For instance, the U.S. spent $317 billion on 3.38 billion barrels of imported oil in 2014 at an average price of $91 a barrel, and it spent only $170 billion on 3.4 billion barrels at an average price of $47 a barrel in 2015.[34] Moreover, the biofuel peddlers have found the organic composition of capital in the second-generation biofuel production very high, making quick cost recovery precarious. In addition to the high initial cost of conversion technology plus the uncertain supply of feedstocks, the petroleum industry seized the moment to join livestock and poultry producers in an unholy alliance to launch stiffened opposition to the RFS as unworkable, demanding substantial modification of the program. Livestock and poultry producers resented that the diversion of corn and soybeans to biofuel production raised the price for feed. Representing the petroleum oligopolies, the American Petroleum Institute (API) was equally resentful of the mandatory blend wall that required gasoline outlets to blend a predetermined percentage of ethanol with gasoline, having the effect of reducing the consumption of petroleum. What followed was the filing of five legal challenges against the EPA and its administration of the RFS since 2010. The charge that received wide publicity, brought by the API, pertained to the cellulosic biofuel mandate. The API argued that EPA projections about cellulosic fuels were erroneous and objectionable; the courts concurred with the plaintiff, compelling the EPA to vacate its projections. The EPA had already begun to lower the statutory requirement of cellulosic ethanol production for other reasons having to do with the stagnation of the conversion technology and production capacity, and it continued to do so.

The agency justified the sharp cutback on the mandates by the lack of current and projected production capacity for advanced fuels due to the hesitancy of biofuel producers to invest in commercial-scale refineries for cellulosic biofuels. This had to do with the corporate calculation that the state of cellulosic bio-fuel conversion technologies and the cost of the biothermal and biochemical conversion processes of the biomass feedstocks into motor fuels could chip away at the expected gains, especially given cheap fossil fuels.

The crux of the problem for the EPA was that even the substantially lowered requirements could not be achieved. The structural dilemma facing the agency and the biofuel industrial complex was to either abandon the project altogether or to double down on first-generation biofuels, primarily using grains as feedstocks, heightening the competition for grains as the main source of food, feed, fiber, and feedstocks. Droughts and speculation on agricultural commodities also combined to worsen the underlying volatility of the biofuel market. This explains the stagnation in second-generation biofuels that were unable to meet the mandates required by the 2007 legislation. It was this harsh reality that forced the EPA to rely on its waiver authority to lower the statutory volume of cellulosic ethanol production. From here on, the future of biofuels would have to be coupled with other considerations.

In 2010, the chemical and plastic sectors attempted to make a case for going beyond biofuel production by switching to the production and universalization of bio-based products. In 1950, the chemical and plastic sectors employed five million workers and generated a $20 billion trade surplus for the country. By 2003, however, the United States incurred a $10 billion trade deficit in chemicals and plastics as U.S. imports of plastics increased from $10 billion in 1989 to $35 billion in 2003 and that of chemicals soared to $50 billion. Employment in chemical manufacturing facilities dropped to an all-time low of 800,000 in 2009, with further declines projected.[35] Representatives of the chemical and plastics industry now vigorously pleaded their case that only bio-based products could reverse this trend only with generous government subsidies, loan guarantees, and tax credits to expedite innovation, commercialization, and adoption of bio-based products. Industry managers liberally colored their plea by suggesting that a switch to the production of bio-based products could reduce emissions of CO_2 by up to 2.5 billion tons through 2030, in addition to creating millions of new jobs.[36]

The vanguard mouthpiece for both the biofuel industrial complex and the bio-based products sector has been the Biotechnology Industry Organization (BIO), representing 1,100 biotech corporations in the United States and thirty other countries. Such household names as Monsanto, DuPont, BASF, Syngenta, and Bayer are leading players. This is how James C. Greenwood, BIO's President and CEO, presents the marketing strategy of the biotech industry:

> The mission of the biotechnology industry is to heal, fuel and feed the world. Innovative biotech therapies, renewable energy sources and agricultural advances are helping to meet some of our most pressing global challenges. Biotech is also a rapidly growing industry that plays an important role in expanding the economy and creating high-wage, high-quality jobs. Other biotechnology innovators are developing renewable energy sources and bio-based industrial products—like plant-derived plastics— that reduce our reliance on fossil fuels. Bio-based materials and renewable products are becoming cost-effective alternatives to petroleum-based counterparts. More than 50 bio-refineries are planned, under construction or in start-up mode to produce cellulosic and algae biofuels, renewable chemicals and plastics, and other types of advanced transportation fuels. Demand is growing for bio-based ingredients in food packaging and personal care products, and once-small biotech companies are expanding production.[37]

Moreover, Greenwood continues:

> Agricultural biotechnology is increasing crop yields, improving animal health and welfare, enhancing the environment, and

contributing to agricultural sustainability. The first biotech crops were introduced in 1996. Today 14 million farmers in 25 countries grow more than 330 million acres of biotech crops. Biotech crops not only help farmers produce more food per acre, but can require less plowing, which reduces fuel use, carbon dioxide emissions, and overall environmental impact while increasing the supply of food and fiber for a growing global population.... Animal biotech is also advancing. Our companies are producing animals with improved food production traits, as well as animals that will consume fewer resources and produce less waste, helping to improve the environment and human health.[38]

The president of BIO hastens to add that the biotechnology sector has become one of the vital pillars of America's innovation economy, directly employing 1.42 million, while supporting 6.6 million indirect jobs, with average annual pay of $77,600 in 2008 compared to $45,200 in other mechanical science-based sectors.[39] The production and dissemination of such propaganda barrages have been ceaseless and continuous. For example, in June 2014, the Ohio-based BIO member Battelle produced a 72-page report, extolling the present performance and prospects of the biotechnology sector. According to the report, the biotechnology sector directly employs 1.62 million people in 2012 across 73,000 business establishments throughout the United States, augmented by the creation of 6.24 million indirect jobs through the employment multiplier effect, at a time when jobs had been disappearing in other sectors. The report claims that, despite the severe recession, the growth of economic output of the biotechnology sector expanded by 17 percent since 2007.[40]

Impressed by this, the Obama administration issued in April 2012 what it calls the "Bio-Economy Blueprint," urging public and private sectors to launch an all-out offensive to accelerate the transition to a post-petroleum bio-economy by speeding up the commercialization of bioinventions based on synthetic biology and biological research at the cellular and molecular levels. Doing so would supposedly increase the availability of such bioproducts as bioenergy feedstocks, lignocellulosic biofuels, biopower, biochemicals, bioplastics, biopharmaceuticals, biolubricants, biopolymer, and a host of others.

To make more dramatic its advocacy for industrial biotechnology, the Obama administration pointed to the importance of bio-based products. In 2010, for example, the administration reminded the public that the contribution to the U.S. economy of industrial biomaterials was $115 billion while that of the GM crops and foods was $300 billion.[41] In 2013, bio-based products reportedly contributed $369 billion to the U.S. economy and created four million direct and indirect jobs.

The "blueprint" presupposes a transformation of the state as a geoeconomic agent in the service of the bioproduct industrial complex and the transition to a post-petroleum bioeconomy. The state must perform this role by sponsoring collaboration among corporations through public/private partnerships. The goals would be to unleash the biological potential of synthetic biology, proteomics, and bioinformatics to produce unlimited quantities of commercial goods, biofuels, enzymes, and biomaterials; to educate American workers to support the objectives of the bio-economy; to support commercialization of bioinventions from the laboratory to the market; and to support R&D in synthetic biology and other emerging fields. According to the "blueprint," the promotion, synchronization, coordination, and integration of these objectives require the development and execution of a multi-agency strategy by the federal government. This includes expansion of the Biopreferred Program in which all federal government agencies are mandated to give preference to bio-based products in their procurement. The Biopreferred Program was created by the 2002 Farm Bill, which empowered the U.S. Department of Agriculture to certify bio-based products as to the amounts of biological feedstocks they contain. Subsequent farm bills strengthened and expanded the Biopreferred Program in such ways as to induce companies to shift to bio-based goods production. With this objective in mind, the 2014 Farm Bill provided loan guarantees for biorefinery projects and for biomass research and development. In 2005, the Biopreferred Program designated six product categories eligible for procurement by federal government agencies; by 2014, the designation of such bio-based products grew to 97 product categories, comprising 14,000 products on the market.

At the center of this synthetic biological revolution are biorefineries, marketed as capable of supplying such multiple bioproducts as bioplastics, biolubricants, biolatex, and biopolymers in addition to biofuels that support the bio-based products industry. The integration of biomass conversion processes and equipment to produce biofuels, biopower, biochemicals, bioplastics, and biopolymers from biomass is the contemporary analogue of the functions performed by petroleum refineries that produce fossil fuels and more than 6,000 coproducts ranging from asphalt to lubricants, solvents, plastics, and pesticides from petroleum. As of January 2015, there were 213 biorefineries in the United States, with annual production capacity of 15 billion gallons. In addition, more biorefineries were under construction to produce another 100 million gallons of biofuels per year. In a nod to the expansion of a bio-based products sector, the U.S. Department of Agriculture renamed its Biorefinery Assistance Program as the Biorefinery, Renewable Chemical, and Bio-Based Product Manufacturing Assistance Program. And the 2014 Farm Bill re-authorization provides loan guarantees of up to $250 million for the construction or retrofitting of commercial-scale biorefineries and bio-based product manufacturing facilities.[42]

The Obama administration's embrace of the synthetic biological revolution completes the most recent step in the evolution of the state as an agent in the service of corporations. The latter sets the agenda and the state provides the implementing machinery out of its own utilitarian considerations. One of these is the defense of its existence as the central actor in politics, economics, and foreign relations through the provision of economic welfare, employment, and protection of the military-industrial complex. Performing these services requires domestic revenue generation and employment creation if the state is to preempt "Occupy Wall Street"–like movements from becoming more radical. Thus, the elite who dominate the state see a future in the synthetic biological revolution. They hope it will bring a new dynamic to the U.S. economy and create new bio-based industries in place of the old industries that have migrated to China and elsewhere. According to their thinking, this revolution will also bring a cleaner environment.

THE CONSEQUENCES OF BIOFUEL PRODUCTION AND CONSUMPTION

Bent on destructive creation and dispossession, the driving need of the biofuel industrial complex has never been to improve the human condition in terms of energy security, job creation, and emission reduction, but rather to create new conditions of forever greater accumulation regardless of the immensity of hydrological, ecological and socioeconomic consequences. The corporate strivings to expedite the transition to the post-petroleum bioeconomy portends many difficulties and hazards and calls for close scrutiny and sustained examination. To do so, I shall evaluate the present and future consequences of the dreamed-up bioenergy security and bioeconomic prosperity in terms of water, land, environmental, and international impacts.

The first deleterious impacts of biofuel production are on the nation's hydrological conditions. The shift to biofuel and bio-based goods production exerts enormous pressure on the availability and use of water at both the stage of growing feedstocks and that of processing those feedstocks into liquid fuels. Hundreds of years of unrestrained capitalist industrialization have already taken a heavy toll on America's important natural water systems. The urgency to increase production of bioenergy crops and plants and the construction of biorefineries geared toward processing the feedstocks into the mandated 36 billion gallons of biofuels can only worsen the pressure on the hydrological situation in the future.

Bioenergy crops and plants like corn are water-intensive. It takes 300 gallons of irrigation water on average to grow a bushel of corn, with a good deal of variation around this average. In Nebraska and Kansas in 2003 irrigated bushels of corn each required 850 and 700 gallons of water respectively, while in Oklahoma growing a bushel of corn required 2,900 gallons of irrigation water. Refining the same bushel of corn into ethanol requires more water since each gallon of ethanol takes 5 to 7 gallons of freshwater. Thus, an ethanol plant in Oklahoma producing 100 million gallons a year uses up 500 million to 700 million gallons of water. In the town of Madrid, Nebraska, 100 residents use just 10 million gallons of water from the Ogallala aquifer each year, while the two ethanol plants in the town use more than one billion gallons of water from the same aquifer each year, enormously accelerating the depletion of the aquifer.[43]

What made America's agricultural prosperity the envy of the world was its transformation into a food manufacturing system through its integration with the petroleum industry for fuels and fertilizer and its exploitation of water resources through the construction of dams for irrigation and hydropower. The conversion of grains and plants to biofuel and bioproduct production has added new pressure to the country's hydrological resources, which had already been under stress for quite some time. Following the Second World War, the U.S. Army Corps of Engineers and the Bureau of Reclamation directed the construction of numerous multipurpose dams to harness the country's water resources; 91 percent of the river lengths in the lower United States were developed to keep up with the rapidly soaring demand for water. By 1990, the United States had 75,000 dams, holding 548 billion cubic meters of water; each of the largest 2,654 dams stored over 6 million cubic meters of water; the 50,000 smaller dams stored 60,000 to 6 million cubic meters, while the more than 2 million micro-dams stored undetermined amounts of water. The availability of freshwater of this magnitude in easily accessible locations inevitably led to the intensification of water withdrawals, which peaked at 1.7 billion cubic meters per day by 1980; by then, 517 million cubic meters of water per day was withdrawn for irrigation to sustain 57 million harvested acres. The daily water withdrawals of 1.3 billion cubic meters by 1965 had already exceeded sustainable water supply by 13 percent.[44] But today the growing demand for water for biofuel and bioproduct production is pushing freshwater extraction beyond the threshold of sustainability. Indeed, the expansion of ethanol production capacity had already begun to experience water constraints in some states. For example, ethanol plant operators in Minnesota expressed grave concerns as early as 2005 over the possibility that water could be a limiting fact as the projected water use by ethanol plants could quadruple from 2.5 billion to 10 billion gallons a year, mostly drawn from aquifers.[45]

It is important to bear in mind that the key input for ethanol production in the United States is corn, the growth of which is notorious for its water intensity. This explains why irrigation of corn nationwide grew from 8 percent in 1969 to 18 percent in 1990. Even though the largest corn-producing zone (the heartland region comprising Illinois, Indiana, Iowa, parts of Ohio, Kentucky, Missouri, Nebraska, South Dakota, and Minnesota) is responsible for 70 percent of the corn crop and relies on irrigation for only 5 percent of the corn acres, the prairie gateway comprising Colorado, Kansas, parts of Texas, Nebraska, New Mexico, and Oklahoma, the second-largest corn-producing region and where the new ethanol plants are being concentrated, relies heavily on irrigation, mostly from the Ogallala aquifer, to grow 15 percent of the country's corn harvest. In fact, the prairie gateway region contains over 60 percent of all irrigated corn acreage in the United States; 95 percent of the water pumped from the Ogallala aquifer is for crop irrigation. There were only 600 wells surrounding the Ogallala aquifer during the 1930s, which astonishingly increased to more than 200,000 wells by the late 1970s, supplying 26 billion cubic meters (bcm) of underground water per year to more than a third of the nation's irrigated fields. Small wonder that the water level in the aquifer has dropped by 100 feet in certain parts of the aquifer since 1950 and the saturated thickness has declined by 50 percent in other parts.[46]

Let us look in more detail at the hydrological situation in two regions: the High Plains aquifer, otherwise known as the Ogallala aquifer, and the Colorado River basin.

One of four critical freshwater sources in the Western Hemisphere and one of the 22 largest aquifer systems in the world, the Ogallala aquifer occupies the high plains of the United States, underlying an area of 450,000 square kilometers (173,746 square miles) in portions of the states of South Dakota, Nebraska, Wyoming, Colorado, Kansas, Oklahoma, New Mexico, and Texas. Regarded as the food basket of America (indeed of the world), the irrigated area in the region accounts for 27 percent of the total irrigated land and for 30 percent of the total groundwater used for irrigation in the United States; 40 percent of the beef cattle in the nation is fed on grains and alfalfa grown here; and three-quarters of the wheat that is traded globally is grown here as well. Because irrigated agriculture is foundational to the economy in the high plains region, 95 percent of the groundwater use in the region is for irrigation. Because 65 percent of the Ogallala aquifer is located in Nebraska, 70 percent of corn grown in the state is irrigated, accounting for 46 percent of the irrigated area in the high plains, explaining why Nebraska was the second-largest ethanol producer in the nation with over one billion gallons of ethanol production capacity as early as 2005. This was as well a powerful reason why Nebraskans have been the most vocal opponents of the Keystone oil sand pipeline, fearing that a rupture in the pipeline might destroy their treasure trove of hydrological wealth.[47] Overall, the irrigated acreage in the high plains increased from 2.1 million acres in 1949 to 15.5 million acres in 2005; correspondingly, annual groundwater withdrawals from the Ogallala aquifer for irrigation grew from under 5 bcm to 26 bcm over the same period; the aggregate groundwater withdrawals during the period were 312 bcm.[48]

This intensive water withdrawal for irrigation had already been responsible for an over 30-meter drop in water levels by 1980 in portions of the Ogallala aquifer in Texas, Oklahoma, Kansas and New Mexico, forcing farmers to revert to dry farming because their wells had dried up. Because the annual recharge to the Ogallala aquifer is minimal, it will take two thousand years to replace the amount of water withdrawn between 1950 and the turn of the century. If the remaining water is depleted, which is projected to be the case in five decades if the current irrigation trends continue unabated, it will then take six thousand years to recharge the Ogallala under relatively favorable hydro-meteorological conditions. According to a 2012 study, 3 percent of the Ogallala aquifer was used up by 1960, 30 percent by 2010, and nearly 70 percent will be gone by 2060. If water withdrawals are to approximate the natural rate of recharge, the current rate of pumping water for irrigation will have to be reduced by 80 percent, a very unlikely scenario.[49] In view of the fact that 60 percent of U.S. crop production relies on groundwater, the rate of depletion at the Ogallala Aquifer must be of grave concern; 35 percent of the southern Great Plains will not be able to support irrigated agriculture at all within the next thirty years.[50]

Another vital natural water system under severe stress is the Colorado River, whose spatial extent is 450,000 km^2. The river is the lifeblood for seven western states, reliant on its water for irrigation, hydropower generation, and drinking. Prior to human intervention in the natural flow of the Colorado River, it annually collected 21 bcm of water from its tributaries and carried the flood to the Gulf of California unimpeded, creating lush green scenes on its banks and delta while supporting countless aquatic species. But in 1922 a determination was made to divide, almost equally, the annual flows of the river between the river states, with 10.45 bcm of water going to the downstream states of Arizona, Nevada, and California, and retaining 9.25 bcm of water for the upstream states of Colorado, New Mexico, Wyoming, and Utah, and saving 1.5 bcm of water for Mexico as the lowest river country. The hydrological requirements of ecosystem maintenance and the future were discounted from consideration. The sole imperative considerations at the time were the prevention of water dispute among basin states and the creation of favorable conditions for the development of capitalist agriculture.

No doubt, the gains from the large-scale industrialization of the Colorado River were monumental. But the real issue is whether the development of capitalist agriculture, based on intensive utilization of irrigation water, and the capitalist mode of livestock production are sustainable enough to support the additional requirements of water to expand feedstock cultivation for biofuel production. By the turn of the twentieth century, the industrialization of the Colorado River had already become so total that no water reached the Gulf of California, resulting in the desiccation of the river's delta. More important, discernible change in hydro-meteorological conditions has created almost permanent drought conditions that have plagued the states in the region. For example, the 2002 river flow of 3.6 bcm was the third-lowest volume in the past 100 years, and the sharply diminished average rate of flow remained below 75 percent until 2005.[51] In fact, in the fifteen years between 2000 and 2014, there have been only three years when precipitation in the Colorado River basin and river flows had been normal; the remaining eleven years were buffeted by drought. In 2013, the water stored in Lake Mead behind the Hoover Dam was down to 12 bcm from 35 bcm and the water stored in Lake Powell behind Glen Canyon Dam was reduced to 15 bcm from 30 bcm. As a result, the hydroelectric dams operated way below capacity because of the sharp reduction in stored water levels.[52]

Evaluation of climate models inspires little confidence in the hydrological future of the Colorado River basin. The U.S. Bureau of Reclamation projects that the Colorado River basin will be much drier by the end of this century compared to the past hundred years. The occurrence, duration, and intensity of droughts, reduction in snowpacks, and evapotranspiration, associated with climate change, will likely be 50 percent higher in the future than in the past. According to the median projection, there will be 45 percent less runoff into the Colorado River from precipitation. As a result, there will be at least 3 bcm of water shortage in the basin as early as 2035. To cope with future water shortages, the Bureau of Reclamation floated a series of strategies such as desalination, elimination of water-intensive crops and plants, water recycling, reduction of water use in power plants, water banking in aquifers, importation of water from other river basins, and weather modification through cloud seeding. Detailed execution of these adaptation and mitigation options and strategies is intended to generate between 3 bcm and 11 bcm of water annually, on the assumption that maximum output from each of the proposed techniques could be realized. However, close scrutiny and realistic evaluation of the technical, economic, and climatological conditions make the expectations fanciful. Arizona has found the climate projections and the portentous water shortage so alarming that the state government has established a water banking authority, responsible for developing strategic water reserves, akin to the federal strategic petroleum reserves. By 2013, Arizona had stored some 4 bcm of Colorado River water in aquifers for use in times of future shortage. Encouraged by generous tax exemptions and long-term credit, individual water providers stored about 6 bcm of water.[53]

Compounding the emerging hydrological crisis in the Colorado River basin is the increased accumulation of salts on farms associated with increased reliance on synthetic agrochemicals, increased temperature warming, and increased evaporation. The Colorado River dumps around 10 million tons of salts on irrigated fields every year, none of which reaches the ocean. In the lower basin of the river, each square foot of acre is said to contain around 2,000 pounds of salts. In California's Imperial Valley alone, every 1.5 cubic meters of water arriving there brings with it more than one ton of salt. To remove the accumulated salt and dump it into the Salton Sea, it would take 52,000 trucks every year. The annual crop loss due to salt deposition is $350 million.[54]

The immediate casualty of this growing problem of salinization is the Salton Sea, fed principally by runoff from the irrigated agriculture in the Imperial Valley. To grow their crops, farmers are under pressure to flash the salt with increasing amounts of water year after year; but this flashed water inserts 3 million tons of salt into the Salton Sea each year, which is compounded by the deposition of harmful synthetic agrochemical residues. The relationship between the Imperial Valley's irrigated capitalist agriculture and the Salton Sea is an excellent case that illustrates the connections between geoecological spaces, biogeochemical processes, and hydrometeorological conditions. Approximately 900 km² in area, the Salton Sea is California's largest lake, created just 110 years ago by exceptionally heavy rain and snow melt that made all embarkments, impoundments and barrages on the Colorado River burst, flooding into what is today the Salton Sea region. Once created, the giant lake provided a new microclimate that made the region relatively habitable by humans and animal species. The moderating influence of the microclimate, created by the lake in a region where temperatures used to rise to 120 degrees Fahrenheit, has been crucial to agricultural production in the Imperial Valley. The presence of this giant lake reduces the average summer temperatures to 95 degrees and keeps winter temperatures above 50 degrees, making the cultivation of crops year-round possible.[55] In return, the lake has been reliant on agricultural runoff of 1.7 bcm annually from the Imperial Valley. Thus the size of the Salton Sea and the quality and chemistry of water stored therein have always been contingent on the amount and quality of the agricultural runoff. This symbiotic relationship worked well until the dawn of the green revolution. The Salton Sea had been replete with vertebrate and invertebrate aquatic species; fish production had become prolific; the abundance and diversity of avifauna were unique in California's deserts as more than 430 species of resident and migratory birds flourished there. The lake and its surrounding vegetation serve as waystations for birds from the Pacific region; indeed, the area became one of the last significant wetlands remaining on the migratory route between Alaska and Central America. Because of its beauty and bounty, more people visited the lake each year than Yellowstone National Park.[56] However, since the 1990s, the lake began to shrink due to sharp reduction in runoff from the Imperial Valley. The pressure to conserve water, the use of relatively efficient ways of irrigating farms, and change in the patterns of crops grown under recurrent drought conditions all contributed to the substantial decrease in runoff. The increase in the deposition of salt and evaporation, coupled with a reduced inflow of water, has made the lake increasingly saline, threatening birds and aquatic species. Today, most of the lake's fish species are gone; tilapia species are the only ones remaining, but they, too, may soon disappear as the lakes become ever saltier.

It is easy to surmise that these two tremendous sources of water are under extreme duress, the consequence of the normal functioning of capitalism. The scramble for more and more feedstock for biofuels can only make matters worse, markedly so. The same is true for other hydrologically well-endowed regions under severe stress. The Mississippi River Valley Alluvial (MRVA) aquifer is a case in point. It underlies the Mississippi alluvial plain in different portions of seven states: Mississippi, Louisiana, Arkansas, Missouri, Illinois, Kentucky, and Tennessee. The biofuel initiative in the Mississippi delta region triggered a reduction of harvested acreage of cotton by 47 percent in 2007, while the harvested acreage of corn increased by 288 percent and that of soybeans by 46 percent; this was in response to the growing demand for feedstock to support expansion of biofuel production. Since corn requires 80 percent more irrigation water than cotton, and takes more synthetic nitrogen than cotton, the ramifications of this shift from cotton to corn monocultivation on the quantity and quality of water in the region are unmistakable. For example, the frequent application of reactive nitrogen since the conversion to corn increased the transportation of nitrogen from the Yazoo River basin to the Mississippi River by 7 percent, thereby contributing to further eutrophication (nutrient enrichment) of the Gulf of Mexico. Since the capacity of the Yazoo River, the largest river in Mississippi, draining 34,000 km², to carry nitrogen and agrochemicals to the mainstem of the

Mississippi River is enormous, it is a major contributor to hypoxia formation in the Gulf of Mexico.[57] Because the MRVA is a thin hydrogeologic formation with an average thickness of 41 meters and an extent of 85,470 km², it is also vulnerable to evapotranspiration and overuse of water due to the growing demand for irrigation water, consistent with the urgency to expand bioenergy crop production. For example, the MRVA is the most heavily used aquifer in Mississippi; farmers withdraw around 15 million cubic meters of water per day during the May to August farming season. In 2010, farmers in eastern Arkansas were withdrawing 7,592 million gallons per day from the same aquifer compared with 1,063 million gallons per day in 1965, a 614 percent increase. As a result, between October 1987 and October 2009, the recorded average annual loss in storage from the MRVA aquifer was 355 million cubic meters due to the market-driven conversion of cotton to corn and soybean monocultivation. Water withdrawals from the MRVA aquifer for corn jumped from 219 million cubic meters in 2006 to 566 million cubic meters in 2007.[58]

What emerges from the discussion above is that water is very likely to be a major determinant in how much cropland the United States can put under cultivation to produce food, feed, fiber, and feedstocks to satisfy all competing demands, unless the country emulates China's example in transporting water from one region to another. In the western states, there are already ten interbasin water transfers. There are 38 large and small transmountain diversion systems that contribute significantly to the yearly transfer of over 802 million cubic meters of water from the basins of the Gunnison, San Juan, and Colorado rivers.[59] As noted earlier, since temperature warming in the United States is predicted to reach 2 degrees Celsius above the 1990 level, the future of interbasin water transfers will be precarious as precipitation in the western slopes declines. A corollary to this hydrometeorological condition is intensification of evapotranspiration, fostering salt accumulation on cropland that requires more water to flush it out. By 2007, saline soils had already occupied about 5.4 million acres of cropland in the coterminous United States while another 76.2 million acres were deemed at risk of becoming saline.[60]

This sobering hydrological reality must be put in the context of the fact that the spatial extent of irrigated cropland acreage in the United States has grown from 7.8 million acres in 1900 to 57 million acres by 2007; of this total, 42 million acres were in 17 western states where the competition for water resources is growing intense; it is in these states that most of America's corn, soybeans, fiber, wheat and sorghum is grown.[61] Taking into consideration all the facts and factors discussed above, are there sufficient water resources where they are needed to satisfy the competing demands for growing food, feed, fiber, and feedstock? The answer is no.

The next area of grave concern entails the impacts of biofuel production on food availability and accessibility. The 2007–2008 global price volatility involving agricultural commodities brought home the competition among food, feed, fiber, and biofuels. Governor Rick Perry of Texas made this abundantly clear in April 2008 when he asked the EPA to waive the statutory ethanol production requirement, citing escalating economic damage to the livestock and poultry industries in his state. Corn ethanol production mandated under the RFS had contributed to rising food prices and high input costs for livestock and poultry producers.[62] In 2012, following the severe drought that hit the Corn Belt, cutting the corn harvest by 28 percent and soybean harvest by 18 percent, livestock and poultry producers appealed to the EPA to waive the RFS mandate. Scores of politicians joined the chorus, including 6 state governors, 25 senators and 156 representatives, who filed formal letters with the EPA demanding waiver of the RFS mandate.[63]

Conceptually, there are two pathways to mitigate the competition among agricultural commodities: expansion or intensification. The first pathway is through expansion of existing farmland to produce the additional feedstocks demanded, in which case the demands for food, feed, and fiber remain stable. This can happen either through the conversion of forests and pastures to new farmland or by shifting existing farmland dedicated to the production of other crops to the production of the feedstocks. Recalling lands held in the Conservation Reserve Program (CRP) into cultivation exemplifies the first case, while shifting soybean fields to corn production illustrates the second option. In 2008, the spatial extent of corn production increased by 19 percent when American farmers planted 91 million acres of land to corn, up from 60.3 million acres in 1983, while the area of soybean production fell by 15 percent.[64]

However, as we shall see later, meeting the demand for bioenergy crops by expansion has both domestic and international implications. Reduction of soybean production raises the price for soybeans, giving farmers the perverse incentive to shift land dedicated to other crops such as sorghum, wheat, or rice to soybean production in order to take advantage of the new price equilibrium as happened in the United States and South American countries. The conundrum does not stop here; when soybean monocultivation displaces other crops, it triggers another cycle of competition for land. In Brazil, for example, the soaring international price for soybeans pitted soybean growers against livestock producers. When soybean growers bought pastureland to plant soybeans, the price for beef significantly rose, giving Brazilian livestock producers incentive to move to the frontier to clearcut forests for new pastures. The same thing happened in Argentina. Today, the two South American nations together have put 65 million hectares of land under soybean monocultivation, making Brazil the second-largest soybean producer and the largest exporter, surpassing the United States for the first time in 2014, and Argentina the third-largest soybean producer and the largest biodiesel exporter in the world, thanks in part for substantial reduction in U.S. soybean cultivation.[65]

The second pathway to mitigate competition involves intensification of production, which means increasing yields per acre. Since the increased yields can supposedly offset the additional demand for bioenergy crops, there will be no need to convert forests and

pastures to farmland or shift land from, say, soybean to corn production. But here is the rub: intensification of corn production
means deepening dependency on synthetic agrochemicals and
increased utilization of ever-diminishing water resources. As we
shall note later, in addition to being financially costly, synthetic
agrochemicals entail incalculable environmental and societal
costs.

What the mitigation pathways suggest is the illusionary nature
of biofuels to solve the triple objectives of energy security, emission reduction, and employment and rural development. Earlier
I discussed how the inherent limitations of biofuel production
induced corporate migration away from the use of corn starch as
feedstock for ethanol. This was why ethanol and biopolymer producers began to target other grain sources such as wheat, sorghum,
barley, and potato for starch. As the traditional sources of food
acquire a flexible character, in that they can alternately be used
for food, feed, fiber, and biofuel or biochemical production, the
competition for land resources increases, with spillover effects on
other hitherto protected natural resources. Even though America's
farmers planted 15 million acres more farmland to corn in 2007
than they did the previous year, it was not enough to meet all
competing demands; more additional farmland had to be found
elsewhere. A case in point is the CRP.

In 1985, the federal government established a framework in
which farmers were encouraged to voluntarily set aside portions of
their highly erodible and environmentally sensitive holdings from
agricultural production for purposes of conserving wetlands, soil,
water, wildlife habitat, and sequestering carbon in exchange for
annual rental payments from the government. The Conservation
Reserve Program was administered by the Department of
Agriculture at an annual cost of $2 billion. This way, the most
environmentally vulnerable landholdings would conserve vegeta-
tive covers, or be restored to their original state, such as wetlands,
which helps soil erosion reduction, sedimentation avoidance, and
nutrient and pesticide runoff prevention, as well as the creation of

valuable wildlife habitat and sequestration of carbon.[66] Since then, the CRP has worked well in realizing these objectives. In 2008, it was estimated that the 36 million acres still registered in the CRP were annually preventing 470 million tons of soil from eroding.[67] Unfortunately, the future of the CRP is far from certain. After the RFS was adopted in 2005, 2 million acres of environmentally sensitive and beneficial landholdings were excised from the CRP within two years and were brought into monocultivation, followed by the excision of another 5 million acres during the active period in this field of the first term of the Obama administration.[68]

The fateful forces at work, driving land conversion from conservation value to profit maximization, were objective material market fundamentals. Contrary to the USDA's market projections that long-term corn prices would remain below $5 a bushel until 2020, corn prices reached $7 a bushel by 2013. Indeed, the rising prices for agricultural commodities in the United States are now projected to raise the annual cost of food per capita by $10 per person by 2020.[69] There is no surprise here. Farmers are socialized to use the market and do not have a contractual obligation to the government as their sole guide in making decisions. If a price signal indicates that the monetary gains from the conversion of the land held in the CRP is greater than keeping the land in the program, large numbers of farmers will withdraw their holdings from the program for conversion to cropland. Given this utilitarian consideration, the total land acreage registered in the CRP in 2013 had fallen to 25.6 million acres from nearly 40 million acres in the pre-biofuel boom period, the lowest in twenty-six years.

This concern must be placed in the context of the fact that 30 percent of the total cropland acreage in the United States was classified as erodible in 1982, accounting for 57 percent of total cropland soil erosion.[70] There is a disturbing irony in that the Obama administration, bogusly labeled as green in outlook and purpose, did little to ameliorate the scramble for conversion of environmentally invaluable land resources to capitalist agriculture. On the contrary, the administration continued to encourage farmers to produce more bioenergy crops for biofuel production. For example, when Doug Davenport (a middle-level bureaucrat from the Department of Agriculture) counseled farmers in southern Iowa to judiciously use conservation practices and to refrain from converting fragile and erodible land into corn fields, he was put on notice that he should never contradict the department's policy or his boss, Secretary Tom Vilsack, who was reassuring the biofuel industrial complex that his department was doing everything to make biofuel production a signature component of the bioeconomy. As he told ethanol lobbyists in Washington: "We are committed to this industry because we understand its benefits. We understand it's about farm income. It's about stabilizing and maintaining farm income, which is at record levels."[71]

What emerges from the conflict between the continuous search for greater capital accumulation and the imperative of conservation of environmentally sensitive natural resources is that capital will almost always be decisive in determining the outcome. But greater accumulation requires even greater land resources to produce the feedstocks, resulting in even greater land inflation. In Wayne County, Iowa, when land speculators from the Northeast rushed to purchase tens of thousands of acres, land prices skyrocketed from $300 an acre at the beginning of this century to $5,000 an acre by 2013.[72] Factor in that the total cropland acreage in the United States declined from 420 million acres in 1982 to 357 million acres in 2007; 14 million acres of prime cropland were lost to urban and transportation development during the period, with 2 million acres of the loss occurring in the Corn Belt states.[73] Thus the competition among agricultural products is still another proxy for the competition for land and water resources with dreadfully far-reaching implications, not only for the availability and accessibility of affordable food supply but also for the ecology, most particularly for wetland ecology.

Wetlands are nature's kidneys and nature's supermarket. In the first instance, wetlands, by occupying the most delicate geoecological space between land and water, readily intercept runoff loaded with nutrients, sediments, and chemicals before it enters natural water systems. In this way, they protect natural water systems from manifold aggressions of terrestrial origin through uptake or neutralization of the nutrients. In this sense, wetlands are natural water treatment systems. If wetlands are damaged or fragmented, they cannot perform their functions properly, just as a human body with damaged kidneys cannot function well. In the second instance, wetlands are invaluable natural supermarkets where countless species gather for food, protection, breeding, and nursery. However, the invaluable functions of nature's kidneys and nature's supermarket provided by wetlands in the United States are long damaged by the capitalist quest for ever greater accumulation. This takes place through the drainage of wetlands for agriculture, construction of dams, canals, and aqueducts, channelization of river banks to widen or straighten streams for navigation, the expansion of irrigation-based agriculture, and the logging and clearing of headwaters, all of which have resulted in sweeping modifications or alterations of wetlands and, by extension, of stream ecology, with concomitant ramifications for wetlands and riverine biodiversity and sustainability.[74]

For the contiguous United States, more than half of the original 221 million acres of non-federal wetlands have been converted to various uses, but mostly to agriculture since colonial times. In the Mississippi River basin, 26 million acres of the original 45 million acres of wetlands have been converted to cropland, supported by the construction of an extensive network of surface ditches and subsurface drainage systems, intended to protect crop roots from both water-logging and salinization by regulating the flow of water. As of 1987, over 45 million acres of farms on what were previously wetlands in the corn states of Illinois, Indiana, Iowa, Ohio, Minnesota, Michigan, Missouri, and Wisconsin were being drained by subsurface drainage systems. In the Mississippi River basin alone, where 80 percent of America's corn and soybeans are grown, some 80 percent of farms, covering around 70 million acres, are equipped with surface ditches and subsurface drainage systems with concomitant radical alterations of hydrological dynamics, land-form structures, sediment movements, habitats for aquatic organisms, nutrient cycling, and floodplain and interconnection of rivers, as these surface ditches and subsurface drainage systems dump nitrogen, phosphorus, and other agrochemicals into nearby streams and rivers that are transported to the main stem of the Mississippi River and then to the Gulf of Mexico. In Iowa alone, 3.6 million hectares of cropland, accounting for 25 percent of the state's harvested acreage, are artificially drained. The reality is that destruction of wetlands has economically, hydrologically, and environmentally reduced critical functions and services such as the loss of habitat for wetland-dependent species, drastic change of biogeochemical and hydrologic cycles, loss of flood storage, impairment of water-quality functions, and elimination or neutralization of nutrients and other buffering capacities. As a result, a vast array of terrestrial and aquatic species is imperiled. Agricultural runoff and hydrologic alteration are ranked as two of the top three threats to 139 endangered freshwater fish, 4 crayfish, 70 mussels, and 23 amphibians.[75]

Thus the competition for land resources recognizes no geo-ecological boundaries; every landscape is subject to occupation, expanding the scope for greater accumulation. For instance, the construction of 14 mega-dams on the Columbia River for irrigation and hydropower generation and the consequent domestication of the otherwise rapidly flowing river, involving removal of wetlands and river vegetation, resulted in the loss of more than 108,000 hectares of fish and wildlife habitat. During the beginning of the twentieth century, the annual commercial fish harvest on the Columbia River was 24,400 metric tons, which fell to 6,800 metric tons by the early 1970s. Moreover, the industrial regulation of the river was held responsible for putting 75 percent of the native Pacific salmon stocks at the risk of extinction.[76]

From the standpoint of the biofuel-biotechnology industrial complex, there is a positive upshot of land resource scarcity. It has opened the backdoor for the introduction of ever-increasing numbers of genetically engineered crops and plants, subject to heavy doses of chemical treatment, with the promise of increasing yields, while fighting pests and resisting drought. We are repeatedly told that these new crops and plants require less land, less water, less fertilizer, fewer pesticides, and are more drought-resistant. We are frequently reminded of how the transformation of American agriculture through seed hybridization and through its integration into the petroleum industry boosted U.S cereal production in the last six decades. What the mechanical revolution did to U.S. agriculture, the gene revolution will replicate many times over with grain production. Since the global food price surges, biotechnology corporations have been cranking out engineered crops and plants. By 2008, there were more than 1,600 patent applications for engineered biological materials, including 530 for climate-ready crops.[77] By 2014, American farmers had already planted 73.1 million hectares to transgenic corn, soybean, cotton, canola, sugar beet, alfalfa, papaya, and squash. In November 2014, the USDA approved the adoption of transgenic potato, which is the fourth-largest staple after wheat, rice, and corn. Today, 94 percent of soybeans and 93 percent of corn grown in the United States are transgenic.[78]

One area where proprietary seed companies have been concentrating is the manufacturing of so-called climate-ready crops, particularly corn and soybeans, which are supposed to resist biotic and abiotic stresses such as heat waves, drought, salinity, and floods. Over half of the climate-ready patent applications belong to Monsanto and BASF, which have been collaborating on a $1.5-billion research project to manufacture the so-called drought-resistant crops, chiefly corn and soybeans. By 2010, 261 climate-ready gene patents had been awarded.[79] For its part, in 2011 DuPont announced that it had invested $930 million in such endeavors, and planned to invest twice that amount in the next five years, particularly in corn and soybean research.[80]

There are imminent ramifications from increased reliance on genetic engineering, both socioeconomically and environmentally.

America's food manufacturing system is becoming increasingly delinked from agroecology, wholly held captive to the designs and manipulations of biotech oligopolies, and the dispossession of independent farmers is becoming complete. Having lost control over their crops, farmers are increasingly under compulsion to purchase commercial proprietary GM seeds year after year from corporations. In addition, farmers' dependency on commercial seed companies is not limited to the purchase of seeds as it becomes a necessity to purchase the agrochemicals needed to support the growing of GM seeds. Thus, while the vulnerability of farmers to corporate strangleholds increases, GM seed and agrochemical companies maximize profit from double dipping.

The environmental impacts of biofuel production are another area that merit close investigation. Just as the agents of the biofuel industrial complex are eager to extol the benefits of biofuels, they are prompt in suppressing or ignoring the inconvenient environmental implications of this mammoth project. One of the most environmentally damaged regions is the Mississippi-Atchafalaya River basin, which drains 31 states that cover 40 percent of the coterminous territory of the United States. Occupying the predominant corn and soybean producing basin, the Corn Belt states of Illinois, Indiana, Iowa, Kansas, Minnesota, Nebraska, Ohio, and South Dakota produce 75 percent of corn in the country. The majority of ethanol plants are also concentrated in these states.[81] There are enormous environmental and public health costs associated with the ceaseless expansion of feedstock and biofuel production, which biofuel cornucopians readily excise from their bookkeeping. Corn is a high-maintenance crop in terms of synthetic nutrients and protective chemicals, just as it is destructive in its effects on agronomic and hydroecological conditions. America's cornfields absorb more water, more insecticides, more herbicides, and more reactive fertilizers than other common crops. Even though corn farms occupy 23 percent of America's total farms, 40 percent of reactive nitrogen is applied to corn fields. The harmful consequence of this massive fertilizer application is of equal proportion. Because corn seeds are sown in rows, the gaps between the rows are left bare for half a year after harvest and until planting the next season, exposed to direct solar radiation and to consequent desiccation and soil erosion. It is small wonder that the midwestern plains of the United States have lost 30 percent of their topsoils in the last 100 years.[82]

Spurious publicity about the environmental wholesomeness of biofuels has remained at loggerheads with the mounting empirical evidence of the negative consequences of biofuels. Contrary to the myth that ethanol plants are environment-friendly, they are just as polluting as petroleum refineries because most ethanol refineries are powered by fossil energy, mostly either coal or natural gas, emitting air contaminants and toxins, such as hydrocarbons, nitrogen oxides, acetaldehyde, and ozone concentration, as well as releasing particulate matter, ethanol vapors, carbon monoxide, volatile organic compounds, and several carcinogens, causing a slew of cancers, respiratory complications, and premature deaths. Mounting evidence shows that volatile organic compound emissions from ethanol plants are on the order of 120 tons a year from the smallest plants and up to 1,000 tons a year from large plants. Moreover, using a blend of ethanol and gasoline in a vehicle causes more pollution than using gasoline alone because ethanol makes gasoline more volatile, resulting in more emission owing to increased evaporation. The scientific explanation is simple. Because biomass has much lower energy density, the carbon oxidation is much higher than fossil energy feedstocks. That is why engine exhaust from gasoline and ethanol mixtures releases more oxides of nitrogen (NO_x), acetaldehyde, and peroxy-acetyl-nitrate than using gasoline alone. Between 2002 and 2007, ethanol refineries in Iowa were cited 394 times for violating health regulations and creating air pollution problems by emitting mercury and other toxins, as well as releasing particulate matter, ethanol vapors, carbon monoxide, volatile organic compounds, and several carcinogenic pollutants.[83]

Soil degradation is another dimension of the environmental impacts of biofuel production. Among crops, corn is the most destructive crop in terms of its overuse of water, synthetic fertilizer, and pesticides. In the 1990s, approximately 9 tons of soil per acre were being eroded each year by wind and rain in corn-growing areas, which was 20 times faster than soil reformation; the replacement cost of the natural soil nutrients lost to erosion was estimated at $20 billion per annum.[84] Traditionally, American farmers practiced important components of agroecology such as crop rotation and fallowing portions of their holdings, to allow the soil to replenish itself with essential agronomic nutrients. For example, corn used to be planted in an annual rotation with soybeans that naturally fix nitrogen, enhancing soil fertility while avoiding the need for costly synthetic nitrogen. Soybean plant roots are naturally equipped to fix nitrogen gas from the atmosphere or extract it from other vegetative sources. It is no surprise that less than 2 percent of reactive nitrogen from commercial fertilizer was used on soybean cultivation in 1997 compared with the 40 percent of reactive nitrogen that was used in corn cultivation. According to one study, 34 pounds more reactive nitrogen is applied to continuous corn-on-corn cultivation than corn/soybean rotation.[85] Under temporal urgency to increase supply of feedstocks to the ever expanding biofuel industry, farmers now practice a corn-on-corn mode of monocultivation in which fields are sown with corn year after year using massive amounts of synthetic fertilizer; corn crop rotation with soybeans, wheat, or fallow is abandoned altogether as commercial fertilizer reigns supreme. For example, the application rate of reactive nitrogen to corn in the Midwest rose from 49 to 129 pounds per acre from 1965 to 1980. On the whole, commercial fertilizer application rates from Indiana to Nebraska were on the order of 40,000 pounds per square mile.[86]

Numerous studies indicate that the absence of crop rotation results in yield drag ranging from 5 to 15 percent for second-year corn compared to first-year corn, depending on soil, location, and weather, while "soybeans will yield 5 to 8 percent higher when they follow two or more years of corn as opposed to just one year."[87] Thus, the overly aggressive intensification of corn production means more application of synthetic agrochemicals, resulting in more loss of these agrochemicals to surface and groundwater. Furthermore, the growing demand for corn feedstock triggers more cultivation of highly erodible and marginally productive land, with concomitant repercussions on erosion, soil carbon oxidation, and wildlife habitat destruction.[88] The fragmentation, degradation, drainage, and conversion of wetlands to farmland in the U.S. corn/soybean heartland in particular have negatively impacted hydroecological ecosystems and coastal waters.

Water contamination is still another consequence of biofuel production. Even though the U.S. federal government spent $150 billion per year on cleaning the nation's water, soil, and air in the 1990s, 50 percent of the country's lakes were deemed unsafe for recreational activity.[89] As the deteriorating state of drinking water in the United States continued, in 2015 the EPA warned Americans that upgrading the nation's deteriorating drinking water infrastructure and waste water treatment facilities would require fresh investment of $633 billion over the next twenty years (in 2007 dollars). In the nation's system of water pipes, key to bringing drinking water to homes and businesses, around 237,600 water main ruptures occur every year; cities and communities also lose over 46 billion gallons of water per day through leaking pipes; this amount of precious water lost through leaks could be enough to supply the ten largest American cities for two weeks. The nation's drinking water quality is also under existential threat from the dilapidation of waste water treatment facilities. For example, up to 3 billion gallons of contaminated sewage water is estimated to pour into the Anacostia River near Washington, D.C., each year.[90] Many of the country's streams and coastal waters are found not meeting water-quality standards. According to data submitted by the states to the EPA in 2004, 51 percent of the waters they surveyed were too contaminated for basic uses, such as fishing and swimming, due to unacceptable levels of nutrient overloading.[91] All told, 98 percent of the 5.2 million kilometers of streams in the coterminous United States had been found anthropogenically altered in such ways that they were not meeting stringent requirements for protection. As a result, more than 100 freshwater fish species were added to the threatened or endangered list and more than 250 freshwater fish species were in danger of disappearing.[92]

Since the transformation of American agriculture into a food manufacturing system during the era of the green revolution, much of the pollution in U.S. water is due to agriculture's overuse of fertilizers and pesticides. The annual use of reactive nitrogen in agriculture progressively increased from less than 1 million tons in 1950 to 10 million tons in the early 1980s, and that of phosphorus rose from less than 500,000 tons to 2 million tons during the same period. The effects of this magnitude of reactive nitrogen has been matched by the annual excretion of 6 million tons of nitrogen and nearly 2 million tons of phosphorus as manure. While nitrogen and phosphorus inputs into the watershed originates from commercial fertilizer, 25 percent of nitrogen and 40 percent of phosphorus inputs are deposited from manure. In contrast, a mere 2.5 million tons of nitrogen are deposited from the atmosphere on the whole United States each year.

Citizens who rely on water withdrawn from wells or reservoirs near corn farms are most affected by lower-quality drinking water. There are 43 million Americans who rely on private wells whose quality and safety are not publicly regulated; it is up to the owners to maintain and monitor the wells, which is, in most cases, beyond their financial and technical capacity. Fifteen million Americans fetch water from shallow wells where the maximum contaminant level is above the national safe drinking-water standard. Findings from a water-quality study based on 500 streams and over 5,000 wells in 51 major hydrologic systems across the United States, carried out from 1992 to 2001, indicate that concentration and distribution of nitrogen and phosphorus in streams and wells were 2 to 10 times greater than regional nutrient criteria recommended by the EPA. Concentrations of nitrate, ammonia, total nitrogen, orthophosphate, and total phosphorus were found to have been above background levels at more than 90 percent of 190 streams draining agricultural watersheds, and nitrate concentrations were above background levels in 64 percent of 86 shallow aquifers in agricultural areas.[93] Moreover, of the 241 water facilities surveyed for nutrient contamination, 82 percent showed odor and taste issues due to eutrophication (overfertilization of water bodies) associated with agricultural runoff. Indeed, the annual cost of coping with the eutrophication of freshwater sources was estimated in 2007 at $2.2 billion.[94]

For example, the level of nitrate concentration in the Des Moines and Raccoon rivers in Iowa, on which 500,000 citizens depend for drinking water, has put the health of those citizens at risk for many years. Indeed, the nitrate pollution levels reach epic proportions during the summer months when the rivers transport a heavy nitrogen load; the water becomes so unsafe for human consumption that officials have to deploy workers to the waterworks to clean up the nitrate. For three months in the summer of 2013 huge machines were kept running around the clock to remove the nitrate, and local authorities pleaded with citizens to use less water in order to help with the difficult job of cleaning the waterworks—this is the price for Iowa being number one in corn and ethanol production.[95] In Nebraska, authorities routinely post health alerts to warn residents when algal toxins, due to reactive nitrogen-driven eutrophication, reach levels unfit for recreational activities in specific lakes. Likewise, the overproduction of algae in Lake Erie in August 2014 compelled public authorities to close the local water treatment plant to protect citizens against potential diarrhea, nausea, vomiting, numbness, and liver damage; but this left 500,000 people in Toledo, Ohio, without access to safe drinking water. The source of the algal bloom was nitrogen and phosphorous pollution from the Maumee River that drains agricultural lands in Ohio and Indiana, regularly discharged into Lake Erie.

Water is vital in all stages of biofuels production, ranging from monocultivation of feedstocks through their conversion into biofuels. As a result, runoff and leaching from cornfields and dumping of waste water from plants unavoidably result in immense water contamination. Once applied to farm fields, nitrates can leak into natural water systems, including underground waters, streams, rivers, and lakes where the nitrates do most damage to drinking water and aquatic species. The nitrate pollution results in excessive algae blooms in freshwater bodies and coastal ecosystems that causes seasonal eutrophication, becoming a major threat to aquatic life including important fisheries.

The connectivity of the Mississippi-Atchafalaya River basin and the Gulf of Mexico illustrates this problem. What makes the Mississippi/Atchafalaya watershed unique is not only its geographic extent but also the fact that 80 percent of corn and soybean production, as well as significant livestock operations, take place here. Another crucial geographic dimension is its connectivity with the Gulf of Mexico, which is bordered by five U.S. states. Because the Mississippi and Atchafalaya rivers receive agricultural runoff from 31 U.S. states and two Canadian provinces, it is not difficult to imagine how the magnitude of nitrogen, phosphorus, other chemicals, and sediment loads would be damaging to freshwater and marine life. The Mississippi/Atchafalaya River basin is the third-largest watershed in the world, covering 41 percent of coterminous U.S. territory with over 1.2 million square miles, with 1.18 million farms in the basin, covering about 843,000 square miles.[96] The hydroecological connectivity of these giant natural systems, the Mississippi/Atchafalaya River basin and the Gulf of Mexico, has had far-reaching implications. Historically, hypoxia formation was rare and small well into the twentieth century until the green revolution was ushered in in the 1950s. Since then, nitrogen and phosphorus deposition exponentially increased owing to widespread application of synthetic fertilizer, navigation channelization, deforestation and fragmentation, wetland draining for cropland, and extensive loss of riparian zones. Of the total nitrogen and phosphorus delivered to the Gulf of Mexico, more than 70 percent comes from agricultural sources in the Mississippi/Atchafalaya basin, with corn and soybean production being the predominant source. Nonrecoverable animal manure from pasture/rangelands accounts for around 39 percent of the total phosphorus transported to the Gulf of Mexico.[97] Since more than 11.6 million metric tons of nitrogen is added to the Mississippi and Atchafalaya rivers each year, the extent of the hypoxic zone formed every summer in the Gulf of Mexico is the size of New Jersey, and it is the largest in the United States and the second-largest in the world.[98] Accounting for 80 percent of the annual freshwater discharge to the Gulf of Mexico, the Mississippi and the Atchafalaya rivers are the principal sources of freshwater and nutrients discharged to the Gulf of Mexico.

Hypoxia occurs when oxygen becomes too low for many aquatic and marine species to survive, much less thrive. The noteworthy biogeochemical reality is that, since the nutrient-laden freshwater flowing to the Gulf of Mexico from the Mississippi/Atchafalaya basin is warmer and less dense than the deep ocean water, this warmer water floats at the top, severely restricting the mixing of oxygen-rich surface water with oxygen-poor deep water. In addition, the excess nutrient flow triggers algal overproduction; these algae eventually die off and sink to bottom water and decompose. During decomposition, the dissolved oxygen becomes depleted by bacteria, reinforcing the hypoxic conditions. Exposure to hypoxic events severely affects the health, growth, and reproduction of less mobile marine species such as crabs, shrimp, clams, and worms that are the critical food sources for fish. That is why hypoxia formation in the Gulf of Mexico is damaging to the $2.8 billion seafood industry on which the livelihoods and income of some 24,000 workers hinge.[99]

Between 1980 and 2012, the spatial extent of the hypoxic zone in the Gulf of Mexico was in the range of 15,000 to 20,000 km^2. This was the result of the integration of agriculture into the petroleum and agrochemical industries and an exponential increase in the use of nitrogen and phosphorus fertilizers in the Mississippi/Atchafalaya basin. Of the 11.6 million metric tons of nitrogen added to the Mississippi and Atchafalaya rivers each year, about 51 percent is from commercial fertilizer, and 30 percent is from livestock manure. Between 1980 and 1996, the annual average nitrogen loading from the Mississippi to the Gulf of Mexico was 1.5 million metric tons compared with the annual load of less than 300,000 metric tons in the 1960s, with the Corn Belt states of Iowa, Illinois, Indiana, Ohio, and southern Minnesota being the primary sources of nitrogen discharges. Overall, even though the annual nutrient loads vary from year to year, the pattern has been consistent. For example, in the 1980s and 1990s (even before biofuel production witnessed spectacular growth), the annual nutrient loads ending up in the Gulf of Mexico ranged from lows of 810,000 to highs of 2.3 million metric tons of total nitrogen, and from lows of 73,100 to highs of 213,000 metric tons of total phosphorus. It is instructive to note that the annual nitrate yields in the Corn Belt states between 1980 and 1996 were more than 1000 kg per km^2, while the annual nitrate yields outside the Corn Belt were on the order of 50 to 300 kg per km^2, attesting to the reality that the increasing conversion of farmland to corn production is hydrologically and environmentally more harmful than any other.[100]

As the nutrient load discharge to the Gulf of Mexico continued to grow to alarmingly epic proportions, numerous task forces were assigned to explore ways of reducing nutrient-rich runoff from non-point sources, agriculture being the primary source, accounting for over 70 percent of the nutrient pollution. Today, there are twelve state task forces, set up to monitor nutrient pollution through the development of quantitatively verifiable conservation strategies and practices. These efforts are supported by various federal bureaucracies, the Departments of Agriculture and the Interior and the EPA being the main ones. For example, the USDA formed the Mississippi River Basin Healthy Watershed Initiative, which provided over $341 million in technical and financial assistance across 123 projects and 640 small watersheds in the Mississippi basin in fiscal year 2013.[101] Even though studies and initiatives continued to be manufactured, all efforts have so far failed to arrest the nutrient pollution in the Mississippi River and the hypoxic zone in the Gulf of Mexico. Several redundant action plans had specified quantitative steps to reduce the hypoxic zone in the Gulf of Mexico from 17,000 km^2 to less than 5,000 km^2 by 2015 through the curtailment of nutrient runoff into the Gulf from the Mississippi/Atchafalaya watershed. However, to the consternation of the federal and state task forces, the hypoxic zone has continued to remain at above 15,000 km^2. When the 2013 hypoxic zone in the Gulf was still 15,126 km^2, the task forces were compelled to postpone realization of the target reduction of the hypoxic zone by two-thirds to the year 2035, not 2015 as expected before. The anticipated quantification of progress in the reduction of the hypoxic zone failed because the various task forces failed to seriously grapple with the real roots of the problem, which is anti-agroecology agriculture, defined by its hyperdependency on synthetic external inputs and by its incompatibility with the requirements of hydroecology. The Corn Belt states are entrapped in self-contradiction between continuing the expansion of corn production by bringing more and more land into corn mono-cultivation, attended by the continuous application of synthetic fertilizer, on the one hand, and the hydroecological imperative to protect terrestrial and aquatic resources and life, on the other. But it is virtually impossible to capture the agricultural runoff flowing from 31 U.S. states and two Canadian provinces; farms are spread over tens of millions of acres, all integrated into the fertilizer and agrochemical industries—and this is what makes agriculture the main widely distributed source of nutrient pollution. One 2008 study projected that meeting the U.S. objective of 15–36 billion gallons of biofuels by 2022 through the expansion of corn and soybean monocultivation would inevitably increase the dissolved inorganic nitrogen load to the Mississippi/Atchafalaya rivers by between 10 and 34 percent.

If the United States is serious about reducing the hypoxic zone in the Gulf of Mexico to less than 5,000 km^2, then the nitrogen load must be reduced by 55 percent, which means that the 97 million acres that farmers planted to corn in 2012 will have to be reduced to 44 million acres. However, if the United States holds to its goal of producing 36 billion gallons of biofuels by 2022, then the acreage put under corn production will reach 130 million acres, raising the current level of nitrogen deposition exponentially because of increased fertilizer use by corn growers.

In order to reduce such pollution, it is necessary to reduce both the extent of productionist capitalist agriculture and the application of artificial nutrients. But this requires reversion to agroecology and crop rotation, which will allow soils to rely more on natural fertilization than on the petroleum and chemical industries. This general observation was supported by the EPA's own inspector general in 2014. He indicted both the EPA and the state task forces for lack of rigor, coherence, and commitment to adequately carry out their expected obligations to reduce the nitrogen and phosphorus loads in the Mississippi/Atchafalaya watershed by at least 45 percent, as recommended by EPA's own scientists, in order to meaningfully reduce the hypoxic zone in the Gulf. According to the Inspector General:

> The OIG [Office of Inspector General] found that states had not been motivated to create these standards because implementing them is costly and often unpopular with various constituencies. Additionally, the EPA has not held the states accountable for milestone commitments nor had the agency adequately, until recently, used its CWA [Clean Water Act] authority to promulgate water quality standards for states. . . . As of February 2014 most of the Task Force states had not completed their strategies. Further, our review of draft and completed strategies indicates that few states are committing to specific nutrient reduction targets or timelines.[102]

Of the 12 Corn Belt states, only Iowa and Wisconsin had established nitrogen and phosphorus reduction goals without a specific time line for achieving those goals. The EPA blamed its inadequacy to carry out its obligation on the corn states for not providing the agency with data and the required quantification of measures taken to address the problem. In turn, the corn states blamed their limited financial and technical capacity to monitor nutrient pollution in their respective jurisdictions.[103] For example, the Minnesota state government report made the financial burden of complying with the expected mitigation measures much clearer. According to the report, in order to meaningfully decrease the high levels of nitrate deposition from the state's water systems would require at least $1 billion annually to bring about significant changes in farming practices.

Nitrogen and phosphorus pollution of water is compounded by pesticide contamination, which has been growing since the dawn of the agrochemical-driven green revolution, with U.S. farmers applying nearly one billion pounds of pesticides each year. Monsanto's glyphosate herbicide had been the dominant agrochemical, whose application grew from 85 million pounds in 2001 to 185 million pounds six years later. Most of the approximately 600 active ingredients used in pesticides are carcinogenic, causing multiple health complications. For instance, atrazine, the most heavily used herbicide in corn monocultivation, is the second most common pesticide found in drinking wells. Even though the maximum safe levels of atrazine in drinking water is set by EPA at 3 parts per billion, scientists have found 224 parts per billion in streams and 2,300 parts per billion in Corn Belt irrigation reservoirs.[104] There is no mystery to this reality. As discussed in chapter 1, when raw throughput is converted from useful and available energy to perform work to a useless and unavailable form of energy unable to perform work, the dissipated energy must go back to the environment or to the atmosphere as waste or pollution. In the case of the Corn Belt, cornfields are left bare between harvesting and planting time, which is half of the year when there will be no plants to hold on to the nutrients and protect the soil from erosion. When it rains, the synthetic fertilizer, manure, and pesticides not absorbed by the corn or soybean crops are washed into vital waterways. The disintegration of the wetland ecology in the Corn Belt, where two-thirds of the wetlands are converted to agriculture, as

well as the use of artificial subsurface drainage systems, intended
to protect farms from waterlogging and salinization, have worsened the situation. The artificial subsurface drainage system
facilitates the circulation of nitrogen and phosphorus pollution
from farm fields to waterways. The delinking of agriculture from
the natural conditions of agroecological cultivation and its consequent integration into the petroleum industry to make synthetic
agrochemicals inevitably increases the requirement of artificial
nutrients to make the soil productive, which, in turn, increases
the need to install more subsurface drainage systems to lower the
water table to protect crop roots from waterlogging and excess salt
accumulation. The disappearance of wetlands that once served
as buffers against any residues escaping from agriculture into
freshwaters compounds the problem of nitrogen and phosphorus
pollution and chemical contamination.[105] Nitrates and pesticide
pollution is particularly much evident in shallow groundwater
and streams in rural areas on which millions of Americans rely
for drinking. According to the U.S. Geological Survey, the shallow groundwater in half of America's rural watersheds has shown
highly elevated levels of nitrate. In 20 percent of these watersheds,
the groundwater is found to be unsafe to drink due to high levels
of nitrate; 31 percent of streams in the United States have high
levels of phosphorus contamination and 32 percent of them have
high levels of nitrate contamination; water in 13 percent of these
streams is deemed unsafe for human consumption due to the
nitrate contamination. Corn and soybean crops are responsible
for 51 percent of the nitrogen and 25 percent of the phosphorus
pollution in these streams.[106]

Nitrogen and phosphorus pollution results not only from the
application of the agrochemicals to cornfields but also from biorefineries. Following the conversion of the corn starch into ethanol,
what remains is what is referred to as distillers' grains, composed
of residual synthetic nutrients, protein, and fiber, which is fed to
livestock. Consequently, animal manure becomes rich in nitrogen and phosphorus. When used in cornfields and pastures as

fertilizer, the synthetic nutrients in the manure are released back to the environment, doubling down on polluting the natural water systems, compounded by effluent from ethanol refineries. During the conversion process, the 160 gallons of wastewater that are generated for each gallon of corn ethanol produced are dumped into the hydroecology.[107]

The transformation of agriculture into food manufacturing systems, dependent on synthetic agrochemicals, and the provision of clean healthy water are incompatible. New York City discovered this truth some twenty years ago. The drinking water supplied to the city, coming from the Catskill Mountains, 125 miles north of the city, was so bad, threatening the health of nine million New Yorkers, that the EPA admonished city authorities that they had to build a new water treatment facility at the cost of around $8 billion, coupled with an annual operation cost of some $400 million. The source of the problem was the unregulated capitalist development and failing septic systems around the Catskills responsible for degrading the quality of the drinking water. City officials were placed between a rock and hard place: whether to expend hard-earned taxpayer money in the suggested magnitude on an artificial filtration system or to innovatively invest in natural capital. Eventually, after much back and forth deliberation, they settled on the second course, betting on nature, rather than on an expensive modern facility whose reliability was questionable anyway. The city allocated $1.6 billion to the restoration of the natural ecosystem around the Catskills watershed by buying the properties from private owners so that nature would do the filtration process. This experiment was so successful that about 140 U.S. cities were contemplating in the mid-2000s to emulate the New York model.[108]

In sum, the mounting evidence of the adverse impacts of nitrogen and phosphorus pollution, chiefly emanating from the expansion of capitalist agriculture, shows how terrestrial and aquatic life is under peril. The deleterious conditions include algal blooms, reduced spawning grounds and nursery habitats, massive fish kills, oxygen-starved hypoxic zones where fish and aquatic life can no longer thrive, much less survive, and public health concerns related to impaired drinking water sources and increased exposure to toxic microbes such as cyanobacteria.

The expansion of biofuel production, at both the cultivation and refining stages, entails public health hazards. Air pollution, soil degradation, and water contamination due to excessive use of agrochemicals compromise the health of millions of people, including farm workers, and communities in the vicinity of farms or ethanol refineries. This is what a panel of epidemiologists, toxicologists, and health scientists confirmed in 1993. Based on studies of two hundred people who reported exposure to job-related insecticides and herbicides as well as others exposed to herbicides as a result of industrial accidents, the panel found a strong statistical association between herbicides and three types of cancer: soft-tissue sarcoma, non-Hodgkin's lymphoma, and Hodgkin's disease. In addition, the panel found substantial evidence of a link between herbicide exposure and chloracne (a type of skin disorder), and porphyria cutanea tarda (a liver disorder that causes skin blistering). The panel also found an important association between exposure to herbicides and lung and throat cancers, prostate cancer, multiple myeloma (a cancer of the bone marrow), immune disorders, renal cancer, leukemia, birth defects, and infertility.[109] Other studies have subsequently confirmed previous reports of the link between agrochemicals and a host of maladies. EPA data show that 18 percent of all insecticides and 90 percent of all fungicides are carcinogenic. The types of chronic health effects of pesticides include neurological effects, respiratory and reproductive effects, cancer, sensory disturbances, memory loss, language problems, learning impairment, infertility, asthma, and chronic bronchitis.[110]

Drinking water contaminated by nitrate is a potential risk factor for cancer, reproductive problems, and methemoglobinemia (blue-baby syndrome), which disrupts oxygen transport in the blood of infants.[111] There is a very strong association between health complications and a group of herbicides belonging to the family of chlorotriazine (consisting of atrazine, simazine, and cyanazine); these have been widely used in corn production throughout the United States. These chemicals pose significant health risks because they are highly mobile. It is estimated that up to 3 percent of atrazine applied in corn production is carried by runoff to aquatic environments following heavy rains, posing risk to aquatic life. Surface and groundwater contaminated with atrazine, also pose a great health risk to humans. In Kentucky, where more than one million pounds of these herbicides were used annually over a 35-year period, researchers found significant levels of atrazine and cyanazine in ground and surface water. The researchers found an important link between these herbicides and human breast cancer, the result of reliance on wells as sources of drinking water contaminated with the herbicides.[112] To be sure, the increasing reliance on these carcinogenic chemicals to increase corn and soybean yields can only worsen the injurious effects of the relentless expansion of biofuel production.

The impact of biofuel production on forest ecology is another area of grave concern because of the greater push for lignocellulosic fuel and commercial wood pellet production. Indeed, the development and commercialization of bio-based products in combination with the expansion of biofuel production raises a fundamental question pertaining to the sustainability of biological feedstocks required to sustain the synthetic biological revolution. For instance, the global bioplastics market today is just 300,000 tons compared to the 181 million tons of petroleum-based synthetic plastics produced annually.[113] Let's suppose that it is possible to raise the market share of bioplastics to 90 million tons per annum or nearly 50 percent of the overall global plastics market. What amount of biological feedstocks will have to be removed from the environment without affecting the rates at which the environment regenerates and self-cleanses? Any answer to this question must be placed in the context of the biological feedstock requirements of other bio-based product sectors such as biofuels, pulp and paper, biochemicals, and so forth. After all, the global pulp and paper industry alone consumes over 400 million metric tons of forest resources annually. As the largest producer and consumer of pulp and paper in the world, the United States has already drawn down half of its natural forest resources in the past two hundred years.[114]

Nowhere is the depletion of the country's natural forest resources more apparent than in the 13 southern states of the United States where 60 percent of forest harvests occur, contributing $211 billion to the U.S. economy annually. In this region, the area of native forests declined from 351 million acres, when European settlers began to dispossess Native Americans, to 201 million acres by 2000, still projected to further fall to around 150 million acres by 2040. Between 1962 and 1996, forest harvests in the South more than doubled from 4 billion cubic feet to 10 billion cubic feet annually. Over a period of three years between 1998 and 2000, mills processed 131 million green tons of chips to meet growing demand for biomass energy production.[115] Projecting into the future, nearly all 33 percent of the expected increases in timber production in the United States between 1995 and 2040 will come from the South; the region is expected to increase softwood production by 56 percent and hardwood production by 47 percent. As a result, harvesting levels of wood in the South for bioenergy production will expand by between 54 and 113 percent by 2050 over the 2010 levels.[116] The ferocious decimation of longleaf pine forests ill-portends for other trees species in the Southeast. In the past, there were 90 million acres of longleaf pine forests, but by 2010 reduced to a shadow with only 3.4 million acres still standing.[117]

Today, seen as the "wood basket" of the nation, the southeastern region of the United States has become the prodigious focus of relentless exploitation of priceless natural forests to meet the growing demand for bioenergy feedstocks. The region has already been producing such wood energy products as wood pellets, hog fuel for process heat, and wood chips for electricity generation. In addition, new facilities have been under construction to produce bioethanol and biodiesel from wood chips in order to meet the 36 billion gallons of biofuels mandated by the 2007 legislation. The Obama administration's announcement of the Clean Power Plan in June 2014, calling for a 32 percent reduction of emissions from power plants by 2030 over the 2005 levels while producing 30 percent more renewable energy, enough to power 30 million homes, has placed operators under pressure to shift out of coal-fired plants to the use of wood pellet. The promulgation of the Clean Power Plan extravagantly promises reduction of CO_2 emissions in the power sector by 32 percent in 2030 from the 2005 levels; prevention of more than 310,000 non-fatal heart attacks and 90,000 asthma attacks in children; eliminating 300,000 missed workdays and schooldays; boosting renewable energy generation by 30 percent in 2030 while creating tens of thousands of new jobs; saving enough energy to power 30 million homes in 2030; and saving U.S. consumers $155 billion between 2020 and 2030.[118] Thus, according to the U.S. EIA projection, renewable electricity generation would increase by 72 percent from 2013 to 2040, accounting for more than one-third of new electricity generation capacity, something that would place power plant operators under pressure to descend upon biomass plants.[119] Biomass-based energy generation is projected to increase, on average, by 3.1 percent per year, led by mixing biomass-based fuel with coal at existing coal plants through 2030; thereafter, new dedicated biomass plants are expected to account for the majority of the growth in biomass-based energy generation.

For now, though, U.S. coal-fired plant operators could count on the shale resource boom to slow their migration to wood pellet usage to generate electricity and heating. Today, the existential threat to the biodiversity of the region's forest ecosystems comes from Europe's coal-fired power plant operators, who are ramping up their wood pellet utilization to meet the EU Commission's guidelines to reduce greenhouse gas emissions by 20 percent over the 1990 level by 2020. As a result, the southern U.S. forests have become the wholly owned reserves of the European Union, supplying most particularly wood pellets for electricity and heat generation; exports of U.S. wood pellets increased from 1.6 million short tons in 2012 to 5.7 million short tons in 2015, with 98 percent destined for the EU of which 99 percent originated in the South. The top three importing countries of U.S. wood pellets were the United Kingdom, accounting for 53 percent of U.S. wood pellet export; Belgium with 21 percent; and the Netherlands with 14 percent; Denmark and Italy were major pellet importers as well.[120]

In early 2015, *Forbes* reflected the soaring optimism and excitement of wood pellet manufacturers when it announced to the world: "It's a good time to be in the American wood pellet business," as dozens of wood pellet manufacturers, based in the southeastern United States, began increasing wood pellet production, making the country the largest wood pellet producer in the world.[121] Unsurprisingly, the southeastern region accounted for 62 percent of national wood pellet production in 2013, up from just 12 percent in 2003.[122] No wonder that Enviva's marketing director, Elizabeth Woodworth, was even more exuberant when she reminded North Carolinians of the rosy prospects for wood pellet producers in these glowing terms: "What we consider as biomass is wood. Those pellets are incredible. We use residue from sawmills, chips from other facilities, tree tops, limbs and round [forested] logs to produce our product. You're blessed here in North Carolina with an abundance of forests, about 18 million acres. In the United Kingdom, they have about 6 million acres. The United States has about 750 million acres, about 200 million of that is in the southeastern states. So that gives us an opportunity to supply some of Europe's energy needs."[123]

Enviva is the largest wood pellet manufacturer and exporter in the United States, supplying pellets to British utility Drax Power, which owns and operates the largest British coal-fired power plant, and is converting three of its six units to pellet-fired plants. Enviva operates five wood pellet plants in Virginia, North Carolina, and Mississippi with a combined production capacity of 1.7 million metric tons per annum.[124] In addition, Enviva operates a deep-water terminal at the Port of Chesapeake, capable of receiving and storing three million metric tons of pellets destined for Europe. In 2011, Enviva opened its flagship pellet-manufacturing mill in Ahoskie, North Carolina, capable of converting 850,000 tons of trees into wood pellets to feed European power plants under the guise of generating a renewable form of electricity. In 2013, Enviva also opened another large mill in Northampton County, North Carolina, and by 2017 had opened others in Virginia and Mississippi. Other companies are closely following Enviva's example by prodigiously building wood pellet facilities throughout the Southeast. For instance, in 2012 Biomass Power Louisiana built a wood pellet mill, capable of producing up to 2 million tons of pellets annually. Georgia Biomass, based in Waycross, wholly owned by the German company RWE, is another bioinvader, which has built one of the largest wood pellet mills, capable of processing up to 1.5 million metric tons of log obtained from the virgin forests of Georgia. The Atlanta-based Enova Energy Group is still another biovandalizer, which announced in 2012 its plans to build three new pellet mills in South Carolina and Georgia, with combined production capacity of 1.3 million short tons of pellets annually destined for Europe.[125] For its part, Drax Power Station, determined to whitewash itself as a clean energy producer by converting its dirty coal-fired plants to supposedly clean pellet-fired plants, announced in 2012 that it was going to open four new large pellet mills in Mississippi, South Carolina, and Louisiana.[126]

The impetus for this extraordinarily rapid wood pellet production is driven by the European Commission's classification of pellets as carbon-neutral, prompting coal-fired plant operators to shift to wood pellets in the generation of electricity and heating as fast as they can in order to meet the requirements of the Renewable Energy Directive. This corporate response to the commission's flawed classification of all biomass source of energy as renewable resources is undergirded by the subterfuge that burning any type of biomass resource is carbon neutral because of the regrowth of trees. Thus, European power plants, supported by the European Commission and their home governments, are capitalizing on the traditional conception of wood pellets as carbon-low and thus environmentally friendly because they are made from by-products of sawmill operations such as sawdust and chips that quickly decay and release carbon dioxide if left on the ground unused.[127]

To meet the growing demand for pellets, manufacturers have begun felling whole trees to process them into pellets, making biomass resources a source of CO_2 emissions, rather than an alternative to fossil fuels. Since pellet manufacturers now harvest whole hardwood trees, which take a long time to regrow, the corporate claim that pellets are carbon-neutral is patently bogus. By measuring carbon output, the Natural Resources Defense Council (NRDC) confirmed that burning wood pellets in the generation of electricity can increase emissions compared to using fossil fuels if the pellets are manufactured from whole trees. "When the proportion of whole trees in pellets ranges from 40 percent to 70 percent," the emissions exceed those from fossil fuels by significant margins.

The modeling shows that it will take approximately 55 years for forest regrowth to recapture enough carbon from the atmosphere to reduce the plant's cumulative emissions below those of coal. At levels greater than 40 percent, pellets emit more carbon than coal for most of this period. In addition, as the percentage of whole trees increases above 70 percent, the level of carbon emissions continues to increase. When whole trees make up 20 percent of the wood in pellets, emissions are slightly higher than natural gas and slightly lower than coal for a period of approximately 55 years. Even when whole trees make up as little as 12 percent of pellets, our modeling showed that burning pellets still produces emissions comparable to natural gas trend line for approximately 50 years." After all, "wood is less energy-dense than fossil fuels, so burning biomass generally emits more carbon than fossil fuels to produce the same amount of energy.[128]

Thus, the felling of whole trees for pellet production is threatening the entire forest ecology in the southeastern United States today as pellet manufacturers scramble to increase the bottom line. Most of the wood that Enviva uses in its North Carolina Ahoskie plant is composed of hardwood trees, including wetland forest trees. According to the Southern Environmental Law Center, over 50 percent of the biomass sourcing area for the Ahoskie mill are wetland forests. As a result, over 168,000 acres of wetland forest near the mill appear to be bound for harvesting to produce wood pellets for export to Europe. This presages an ominous development for the forest and and wetland ecologies, not only in the Southeast, but everywhere. According to one projection, if wood pellet manufacturers seek to produce just 6.4 percent of global electricity from burning wood pellets by 2035, then the global commercial tree harvest (excluding trees felled for traditional firewood) must increase by 137 percent, since most fossil fuel-fired power plants in the United States and elsewhere are under pressure to follow the example of European utilities in order to mask their dirty practices.[129] Considering the strong undercurrent fostering the wholesale use of forest and wetland resources, the natural resources in the Southeast are particularly vulnerable to bio-devastation. Because, unlike in the western states, most forests in the Southeast are privately owned, 180 million acres (89 percent) of the forests there are privately held and only 21 million acres are publicly held with the federal government managing a mere 11 million acres. In comparison, the U.S. Departments of Agriculture and the Interior together manage nearly 600 million acres of forests, wetlands, parks, and land in the rest of the country, mostly in western states, benefiting from federal protection. Even though the Energy Independence and Security Act of 2007 sets limits on the types and quantities of trees that could be used as feedstocks in the production of biofuels or solid biomass energy, which means that any woody biomass must come from non-federal lands, from roundwood and mill residue in existing plantations, from pre-commercial thinning operations, and from wildfire hazard reduction materials, yet the forest resources in the Southeast seem to be free for all without a modicum of federal protection. As the law stands now, no protection is accorded to privately held forest resources, which explains why wood pellet manufacturers are concentrated in the Southeast and why wood pellet production there has been projected to rise from 27 million green short tons in 2015 to 49 million green short tons in 2020.[130]

Researchers at the U.S. Forest Service express grave apprehension over the demand for bioenergy futures that can trigger profound structural changes in forest conditions, entailing decreased water availability and degraded water, especially if placed in the context of climate change, urban population growth, spread of invasive plants, droughts, fires, and the increasing intensity of hurricanes and tornados.[131] The increasing frequency of forest fires in recent years is a good illustration of the impending disasters associated with bio-vandalization and fragmentation of forests and weather-related change. The 38 major forest fires that occurred between 1995 and August 2015 classified as weather-related natural disasters, affected more than 108,000 Americans and the economic cost was $11 billion.[132]

Of course, the costs of these consequences are discounted to future generations while accumulators reap the benefits here and now. Indeed, there are numerous sustainability ramifications of the domestic and European bioinvasion of the South. Traditionally, wood pellets have been made from wood waste such as saw-dust, shavings, and wood chips that result from wood-processing activities, or from the by-products of the pulp and paper industry without harm to virgin forests, but now they are produced from logging residues and from unprocessed harvests of whole trees. Historically, it was uncommon to remove logging residues whole-sale for fuels; much of the logs were left to decay into organic matter, replenishing forest soils. It was a common practice to leave at least 35 percent of timber residues in the forests, where they strengthened the forests' capacity to store carbon.[133] Now, however, the growing controversy surrounding the use of grains for biofuel production in the face of growing grain shortages and price hikes, the biofuel industrial complex is emphasizing the importance of cellulosic fuels and solid biomass energy in order to keep accumulation going. Today, the top five largest wood pellet companies have been found to use whole trees for pellet production. This prompts forest owners to resort to fast-growing short rotation industrial tree plantations, composed mostly of pines, non-native poplars, and eucalyptus. Since 5 million private owners control 89 percent of the 201 million acres of forests in the South under the neoliberal deregulation and privatization regime, the temptation to hollow out natural forests by converting them into industrial tree plantations is very much in prospect.

Predictably, the deforestation in the Southeast, spurred by the growing demand for wood pellets, will have far-reaching repercussions on wetland ecology, precisely because of the teleconnection of forests and wetlands. The loss, fragmentation, and degradation of forests are reflected in equal proportion in the fragmentation and destruction of wetlands, which themselves are subjected to conversion to farmland and provision of throughput required by biofuel and wood pellet producers, resulting in significant changes in water flow, increased pollution, increased erosion, and deposition of sediments and habitat devastation.[134] When forests are cut down, the law of gravity forces eroded soils, silts, minerals and all sorts of residues to flow to lower areas, which happen to be wetlands. A noteworthy historical reality is that, prior to European settlement, the extent of riparian land in the floodplains of the lower 48 states was 49 million hectares, reduced to 9.3 million hectares by the 1980s; 22 states had lost more than 50 percent of their wetlands; in the case of California, the loss of wetlands is a staggering 90 percent.[135]

Floods from the upper reaches of the ecology, previously covered by forests, inevitably hollow out the ecological integrity of wetlands, as well as their capacity to provide storm buffers, absorption of pollution, and vital habitat for wildlife. The situation is made worse when wetland forests themselves become targets for exploitation by wood pellet manufacturers for feedstocks. Note that the overall net loss of forested wetlands in the United States between

2004 and 2009 was over 633,000 acres, mostly in the southeastern states, with freshwater wetlands of the Atlantic and Gulf coastal plain and the Lower Mississippi River experiencing the greatest losses. Compared to the 1997–2004 time frame, the net loss of forested wetlands increased by 140 percent between 2004 and 2009. In the Southeast, stretching from North Carolina to Florida on the Atlantic, and from Florida to Texas on the Gulf of Mexico, the forested wetland area declined by approximately 443,780 acres between 2004 and 2009. Even though part of this total was cleared and converted to other wetland types such as fast-growing industrial tree plantations, the alteration of the original wetlands in this manner will have harmful effects on the hydroecological functions of the wetlands.[136]

What has been taking place in the southeastern United States is not out of the ordinary; indeed, it is consistent with the historical patterns of accumulation by alienation of nature. Virtually all ecosystem types in the Midwest and far West had been ruthlessly subjected to the same processes of alienation since the 1930s, with drastic acceleration taking place since the 1950s concomitant with the extraordinary transformation of American agriculture into a food manufacturing system, supported by equally extraordinary amounts of synthetic nutrients and multipurpose super-giant dams. The radical alteration of 5.2 million kilometers of streams in the contiguous 48 states by the development of hydrological structures for irrigation, hydropower generation, and navigation have violated all requirements for protection of wildlife and aquatic species. By the turn of the century, 578 aquatic species had been listed as endangered nationwide under the Federal Endangered Species Act, including 37 percent of freshwater fish, 70 percent of mussels, 64 percent of crayfish, and 29 percent of amphibians; thousands of aquatic species more had also been at risk of being endangered or disappearing. Agriculture had been regarded as the primary source of imperilment for 45 percent of listed fish and 64 percent of mussels, while water pollution had been identified as a source of endangerment for 55 percent of fish and 97 percent of mussels.[137]

In light of the facts and factors, it must be obvious to any clear-eyed analyst that America's biofuel production is not only unsustainable, but also harmful in terms of ecology, hydrology, biodiversity, food ecology, environment, and human welfare. Indeed, the illusionary quest for liquid biological fuels has already worsened the ill-effects of the country's industrial capitalist agriculture and has created new conditions that are anti-nature, anti-people, and pro-corporate wealth accumulation.

Finally, the United States is the largest producer and exporter of corn and soybeans in the world, and the diversion of these crops to biofuel production has significant international implications for the circulation of agricultural commodities. Corn is the staple food for a billion people worldwide, their principal source of nutrients and calories. Furthermore, corn is a key component of animal feed, so any price increase in corn is immediately reflected in increased prices for milk, cheese, eggs, and milk. What makes corn particularly hypersensitive to market price volatility is that the United States historically has been the largest producer and the largest exporter of this critically important crop; so any change resulting from the U.S. diversion of corn to domestic ethanol production will have far-reaching implications for world corn markets. Thus, given the size of U.S. agriculture's influence on international markets, it is inevitable that producers and consumers overseas will react to market conditions or policy-related events in the United States. The international price for corn soared from $50 per ton in 2000 to $350 a ton in 2012.[138]

If we use the past as a guide, a reduction in the delivery of U.S. corn and soybeans to the global market because of biofuel production will continue to send shivers across agricultural commodities as has happened on several occasions. For instance, the U.S. federal mandate privileging biofuel production over grain export between 2006 and 2011 escalated the international price of corn, resulting in the addition of more than $6.5 billion to the food import bills of third world countries. North African countries witnessed $1.4

billion in ethanol-related import costs between 2006 and 2011, with Egypt accounting for $679 million of that cost. The additional cost for the net food-importing countries in Sub-Saharan Africa was $1.6 billion over the same period. Similarly, the ethanol-related cost of corn imports from the United States for Latin American countries between 2006 and 2011 was more than $2.4 billion, with the poor nations of Central America incurring $368 million additional cost of corn import. The poor nation of Guatemala spent $91 million as its corn import from the United States soared from 9 percent in the 1990s to 40 percent by 2011. Between 2004 and 2011, the additional cost of corn import from the United States to Mexico stood at a staggering $1.5 billion due to the diversion of corn to ethanol production. All told, induced by the 2008 food price hikes, the least developed countries in the Global South imported over $26.6 billion in agricultural commodities. In contrast, they exported a mere $9.1 billion, incurring a trade deficit of $17.5 billion.[139]

According to researchers at the New England Complex Systems Institute, expansion of ethanol production was responsible for 27 percent of the 40 percent in global corn prices in 2007–2008; financial speculation was responsible for 13 percent. The financial speculation as a corrosive dynamic in global agricultural commodities was triggered by the perception that price hikes associated with the conversion of corn to ethanol in the United States and the conversion of oilseeds to biodiesel in Europe would make the global commodity market a lucrative source of new profits under the neoliberal deregulation regime.[140] Predictably, the ballooning prices, prompted by the expansion of biofuel production, has had considerable social and political costs. For example, tortilla prices rose by 69 percent, the result of costly corn imports. This created a tortilla crisis in Mexico, prompting tens of thousands of people to take to the streets. By some estimates, more than 5 million Mexican children went hungry as a result.[141] In 2008 alone, there were 60 reported food riots in 30 third world countries.[142] According to a comprehensive study by the Washington-based International Food Policy Research Institute, between 52 and 58 percent of children under age five in Bangladesh, the DRC, Ethiopia, Nigeria, and Pakistan were classified as stunted or wasted. Overall, by the beginning of 2015, 2 billion people worldwide were experiencing micro-nutrient malnutrition and 794 million people were calorie deficient; and 161 million children under age five were stunted and another 51 million were described as wasted; 40 percent of the stunted and 50 percent of the wasted children were in India. The study further notes that such infectious diseases as diarrhea, malaria, acute respiratory infections, and tuberculosis were unmistakably linked to nutrition-related morbidity and mortality, compounded by the lack of clean water and sanitation. No wonder that 45 percent of deaths of children under five are linked to malnutrition.[143]

Another crucial dimension of the expansion of biofuel production in the Global North has been the initiation of a new cycle of struggle for land resources in the Global South. When U.S. corn began to be diverted from food to ethanol fuel production, the resulting price increase for corn prompted farmers to convert their soybean fields to cornfields. This, in turn, triggered higher international prices for soybeans in response to the decline of soybean production in the United States. When American farmers increased the area dedicated to corn production by 25 percent during the 2007–2008 season, for example, the land devoted to soybean production fell by 16 percent, resulting in the reduction of soybean reserves by 75 percent and in the consequent increase of soybean prices by 80 percent.[144] This new dynamic triggered an unprecedented rush to convert forests in the Global South to soybean fields as farmers sought to take advantage of the rising international price for this flexible commodity. Here, a far-reaching dialectic became operational. A diversion of just an acre of traditional field cropland in the United States to grow feedstocks for biofuel production has had to be compensated for somewhere in the Global South in such countries as Brazil, Argentina, Bolivia, and Paraguay by destroying virgin forests. It is this reality that has made Brazil the largest soybean producer and exporter in Latin America. In 2013, Brazil produced 86.8 million metric tons of soybeans, of which 46.8 million metric tons were available for export. In 2014, Brazil's soybean production reached 96 million metric tons, of which 45.3 million metric tons were projected to be exported.[145] The further expansion of Brazil's soybean fields into virgin forests continues unabated. The country's soy fields already cover over 42 million hectares, representing 21 percent of the nation's cultivated area; plans are underway to bring another 60 million hectares under soy cultivation. When all plans are fully implemented, Brazil will have 100 million hectares under soy production, mostly sown in Monsanto's transgenic soybeans, accompanied by some 65 million hectares of sugarcane plantations, all taking the place of virgin forests.[146]

The conversion of Brazil's forests to soybean fields is a lucid illustration of how the logic of outsourcing operates. If and when the biofuel industrial complex encounters or senses domestic supply constraints, transnational corporations will outsource the required feedstocks to the Global South. When President Bush led a biofuel mission to Latin America in March 2007, the sole aim was to calibrate the business climate for bioenergy crop and biofuel production. The mission was accomplished as Brazil turned out to be the green goose that lays golden eggs for corporate transnationals and venture capitalists. U.S. transnationals, including giant financial service corporations such as the Carlyle Group and Goldman Sachs, began to pour their capital into Brazil's bioenergy sector following President Bush's mission to the region. Even the International Finance Corporation invested $200 million in Brazil's bioenergy sector, and the InterAmerican Development Bank invested $500 million in Brazil's bioenergy sector. The financial role of the InterAmerican Development Bank was expected to reach $3 billion, as it was involved in four projects to triple ethanol production in Brazil by 2020, including the extension of $500 million in credits to boost milling capacity in São Paolo, and $2 billion for new ethanol plants in two other states.[147]

Oil oligopolies were not far behind in moving to Brazil's booming ethanol sector. In 2008, BP became the first oil oligopoly to invest in Brazil's biofuel sector and as of 2012 it was operating three ethanol plants. In 2012, BP announced $350 million of investment in one of these ethanol plants to double the plant's sugarcane processing capacity to five million tons to generate 450 million liters of ethanol a year.[148] Determined not to be left out from Brazil's hyped ethanol bonanza, Shell jumped full steam on the bandwagon of Brazil's biofuel production. In 2011, Shell joined Cosan (Brazil's giant sugar company) to create a $12-billion sugar and ethanol joint venture, named Raizen, intent on producing 2 billion liters of ethanol and 20 billion liters of other industrial and transport fuels per year for domestic and international markets. The 24 sugar mills at Raizen's disposal were equipped to process 62 million tons of sugarcane per annum into ethanol and sugar.[149]

The grain transnational trading corporations have also been betting on Brazil's biofuels sector to expand their portfolio. By 2014, ADM was operating Brazil's largest biodiesel plant, and had majority control in one of Brazil's largest ethanol plants; in November 2008, ADM poured $370 million into Grupo Cabrera, a sugar bioethanol company, headed by Brazilian former agriculture minister Antonio Cabrera. With this fresh injection of cash, the joint venture was projected to generate up to 90 million gallons of sugar bioethanol annually. By 2008, in addition to having a majority stake in one of Brazil's ethanol distilleries, Cargill had become the largest exporter of Brazilian raw sugar and soy for purposes of biofuels and animal feed production; by then, Cargill was processing and exporting half of the soybeans produced in Brazil's Cerrado. The corporation had 13 soybean silos and four illegal ports in the Amazon, while Bunge and ADM have six and four silos, respectively.[150] Moreover, Cargill had the largest soybean processing plant in Paraguay and the largest maize processing plant in Argentina; Cargill also acquired a 63 percent stake in Cevas, one of the biggest corporations in São Paolo. America's Global Foods and Brazil's Santa Elis formed a partnership to create the National Sugar and Alcohol (CNAA) company, investing R$2 bn ($500 million in 2018 United States dollars) in four sugar mills with funding coming from IDB.[151] Not to be outdone, Monsanto took its biotech prowess to Brazil by acquiring two Brazilian companies in November 2008, known for their sugarcane expertise.

The immediate casualty of these biovandalizations has been Brazil's virgin forest resources. As Brazil is poised to become the premier model of biofuel production in the Global South, the forests are rented out to domestic and foreign biofuel producers and timber extractors. Between 2006 and 2007, for example, the rate of deforestation in several Brazilian states had been over 84 percent. As a result, the annual rate of deforestation in Brazil had been responsible for releasing 150 million metric tons of greenhouse gases, accounting for 70 percent of that country's ghg emissions. The scope of deforestation had been so massive that many analysts have suggested that half of the Amazon's forests might be completely gone by 2030, since the annual average rate of deforestation in the region between 2000 and 2005 was already 2.2 million hectares.[152] The new wave of bioinvasion of Brazil by metropolitan transnationals has been a vivid demonstration of accumulation by occupation and dispossession. Outsourcing the acquisition of the required biological feedstocks to the Global South is the necessary default option for biofuel producers. If the United States were to convert 500 million acres of farmland to feedstock production, biofuels could possibly supply 55 percent of liquid fuels that the country consumes.[153] But if this option is chosen, the United States will become a net food importer, to the tune of $80 billion per annum, by 2050 instead of the net food exporter it is today. It is safe to assume that the United States is likely to fall back on its default option to outsource biofuel production and import the fuels rather than importing food, most likely because of domestic pressure spurred by the livestock and poultry sectors. Moreover, even if the country uses its total arable land of 500 million acres to produce biofuels, it will not be nearly enough to meet the energy needs of the country since the dedication of the total farmland can produce only 25 EJ of ethanol compared to the 100 EJ used in 2000 and 120–170 EJ per year in 2050.[154] Thus, if the economy completes its transition to a post-petroleum bioeconomy through the synthetic biological revolution, the United States will have to heighten its geoeconomic agent role to aggressively promote and defend disciplinary neoliberalism in the Global South on behalf of the global corporate dinosaurs. In other words, the United States will deepen the processes of neocolonization and dispossession of tens of millions of people in the Global South.

At this juncture, the United States is prepared to fulfill its geoeconomic agent role to keep wealth accumulation going by outsourcing the required biological feedstocks to the Global South in general and to Latin America in particular. All the pretensions of the state as a free agent having melted away, it will be the corporate oligopolies that determine, shape, and guide the trajectory of U.S. foreign economic relations. To be sure, the rapidity with which the integration and consolidation has taken place among grain-trading oligopolies, biofuel producers, biotech companies, commercial proprietary seed and agrochemical manufacturers has crystallized almost beyond comprehension, making the collective power of oligopolies formidable. One does not have to travel any further to find a validation for this sorry conclusion than the U.S. Supreme Court, which bestowed personhood upon corporations by its 2010 majority decision in *Citizens United v. FEC*. With the elevation of corporations to this new status, the corporate minions now have unlimited power to spend as much financial resources as they wish to influence the outcomes of elections.

---- 4 ----

The Three Deceptions: Abundance, Green Environment, and Blue Skies

Global oligopolies and their supporters have manufactured a series of myths and falsehoods to promote GE crops and biofuels as the long-awaited answers to the world's problems of hunger, climate change, and energy shortages. Petroleum price hikes and the diversion of food crops to biofuel production during the 2007–2008 financial crisis triggered global food price surges, thereby throwing at least 100 million people into destitution, hunger, and malnutrition. In 2007 alone, consumers living in developing countries were subjected to an increase in the international prices of maize, rice, and wheat, which led to a record spending of $400 billion on food imports by developing countries.[1] According to the World Bank, the prices for crops that are used to produce biofuels rose faster than other foods between 2006 and 2007, with the prices for grains going up 144 percent and for oilseeds 157 percent, while the prices for other food prices went up only 11 percent. These price hikes were in response to the fact that three-quarters of the increase in global maize production between 2006 and 2008 went to ethanol production; the five million hectares of cropland that could have been used to grow wheat were devoted to rapeseed and sunflowers feedstock for bio-diesel production.[2]

The integration of industrial agriculture into the petroleum industry has made matters worse. Even though inorganic nitrogen is abundant in the atmosphere, it must be transformed into assimilable reactive nitrogen for plants to use it as fertilizer. The conversion process requires massive amounts of fossil resources, particularly natural gas and coal. So, as the price for fossil energy goes up, so does the price for fertilizer, raising the production costs of all crops. Because of the correlation between synthetic fertilizer prices and fossil price fluctuations, the global food market becomes volatile. Between 2006 and 2008, in response to soaring energy prices, the international price of synthetic fertilizer increased by 170 percent.[3] The unprecedented global oil price increase raised the price of synthetic fertilizers and agrochemicals, and conse-quently the prices of agricultural commodities. In the United States, the price of synthetic fertilizers skyrocketed 160 percent in the first two months of 2008 compared with the same period in the previous year. The soaring oil price increase was made even worse when the biofuel companies diverted 93 million metric tons of American corn, wheat, and soybeans to biofuel production in 2007, twice the 2005 amounts. This represented more than half of the growth in American corn production during that period.[4] Similar developments had taken place in the EU countries, Brazil, Japan, and China. In all, between 2000 and 2007, global ethanol production increased by threefold and biodiesel production by tenfold, reaching 62 billion liters and 10 billion liters, respectively. Worldwide, 295 million tons of grain were diverted to biofuel pro-duction in 2006 alone, representing 17 percent of world total grain production.[5] The cumulative result of the conversion of grains to biofuels was that developing countries had to pay more for cereal imports, without necessarily increasing the volume of basic grains they imported. On average, prices for vegetable oil, cereals, dairy products, and rice, increased by 97 percent, 87 percent, 57 percent, and 46 percent, respectively, during the first half of 2008, compounded by speculation by financial institutions, banks, and hedge funds as they saw a new line of lucrative accumulation in global agricultural commodities.[6]

THE DECEPTION OF FOOD ABUNDANCE

The facts above support the conclusion that there is a definite connection between biofuel production and food consumption. In the United States, the diversion of corn to bioethanol production reduced the total volume of grain available to consumers, leading to increased prices for products such as beef, chicken, milk, pork, eggs, cereals, and bread by between 10 and 30 percent.[7] Between January 2005 and February 2008, the international prices for maize and wheat increased by 131 and 177 percent, respectively, while prices for rice went up by 165 percent between April 2007 and April 2008. Between the end of 2005 and the beginning of 2008, the international prices for palm oil and soybeans also went up by 165 and 175 percent, respectively.[8] All current trends point toward unprecedented price hikes in the range of 30 to 50 percent in the coming decades, attended by greater international food price volatility.[9] It goes without saying that poor undeveloped countries will continue to bear the brunt of food price hikes. In 2011, for example, the rise in grain prices cost undeveloped economies a whopping $324 billion.[10]

The preceding observations demonstrate how bio-based energy generation and food production are locked in perpetual competition for the same throughput. The "food versus fuel" debate is not a false one, as the UN Food and Agriculture Organization (FAO) and allied agencies profess. Which is why these agencies, unable to dispute their own statistics, are compelled to change the lyrics of their pro-corporate anthem. Now they grudgingly say that there could be competition between first-generation biofuel production and food consumption. Feedstocks dedicated to biofuel production must of necessity be diverted from direct human food consumption and animal feed to biofuel production, since there is no room for greater grain harvests without further drawing down forests and grasslands or without worsening the plight of the global poor.

In its projection through 2022, the U.S. Department of Agriculture anticipates intense competition between the demands for biofuel expansion and food and feed production. In the United States, EU, Canada, Argentina, China, and Brazil, ethanol and biodiesel production will expand by 40 percent and 30 percent, respectively, cutting deeply into grains available for food and feed consumption. Between 2013 and 2022, within the European Union, biodiesel and ethanol production is projected to expand by 45 percent and 60 percent, respectively; maize and wheat feedstocks are expected to account for over 80 percent of the expansion in ethanol production. To meet the 10 percent road transport biofuel mandate by 2020, member states of the EU will have to dedicate up to 31 million hectares to feedstock production. Since the EU cannot afford to dedicate land resources of this magnitude to feedstock production, up to 19 million hectares of land must be found outside Europe.[11] Even if this happens, biofuel-driven competition for agricultural commodities is projected to push up the prices of vegetable oils by 36 percent, cereals by 22 percent, and oilseeds by 20 percent by 2020.[12]

Similarly, Brazil plans to expand sugar ethanol production by 90 percent and biodiesel production by 50 percent, while Argentina anticipates its biodiesel production to increase by 80 percent and its maize-based ethanol to double by 2022. By then, 40 percent of U.S. corn output will also be going into ethanol production as in 2012. According to the U.S. Department of Agriculture, the major biofuel-producing countries will not have sufficient national feedstocks to sustain mandated biofuel consumption in the future, and grain exporting countries will not be in a position to satisfy global demand for bioenergy feedstocks, considering that future demands for food and animal feed are also expected to significantly rise in parallel with global population growth. For example, Canada plans to increase its ethanol production by 35 percent by 2022 with large amounts of imported corn, while it projects its biodiesel production to increase by 28 percent using canola as its main input, thereby reducing the amount of canola it usually exports. At the same time, Mexico anticipates the quantity of maize it imports to rise from 9 million tons in 2012 to 17 million tons in 2022. It must be borne in mind here that diverting U.S. corn to ethanol production had already made Mexico vulnerable to price gouging, as Mexico's corn import bill from the United States soared from $1.5 billion in 2005 to $3.2 billion in 2011. The country's overall agricultural trade went from a modest surplus in the early 1990s to a deficit of $1.3 billion in 2000, which then grew to $4.5 billion in 2008 as its food imports from the United States steadily soared from $2.6 billion in 1990 to $6.4 billion in 2000 and then to $18.4 billion in 2011. Due to ethanol production-driven price increases in the United States, driven by use of corn for biofuel production, tortilla prices in Mexico rose by 69 percent. The cost of the basic food basket that the typical Mexican family consumed increased by 53 percent as of 2011 when 56 percent of Mexicans were experiencing some form of food insecurity while another 11 percent of the population were suffering from acute food insecurity and 5 million children were going to bed hungry. The number of Mexicans in extreme poverty increased from 14 percent of the population in 2006 to 20 percent in 2010.[13]

There remains the effect of intensified livestock production on the competition between food grains and biofuels. In parallel with the increase in cereal production since the dawn of the green revolution, the shift in the livestock sector's dependency on feed has grown significantly. In 2008, the amount of cereals, protein-rich crops, roots, and tubers fed to livestock was 1.25 billion metric tons. By 2020, the amount of cereals alone fed to livestock will likely be nearly 1 billion metric tons. The demand for other sources of feed will similarly skyrocket. The consumption of soybeans alone had already climbed from 130 million metric tons in 2002 to 307 million metric tons in 2015, which will continue to grow even further in line with the projected increases in population growth and urbanization. For example, global demand for meat is forecast to increase from 229 million in 1999 to 465 million metric tons in 2050, and that of milk from 580 million to 1.5 billion metric tons. This means that 50 percent of world cereals will go to feed livestock to keep up with the rise of global meat consumption from 37.4 kg per person per year in 2000 to more than 52 kg by 2050.[14]

The foregoing analysis makes the future of the global food system extremely precarious when juxtaposed with the FAO's projections. In October 2009, the FAO convened agricultural experts to sound the alarm regarding the bleak prospects of global food distribution. What emerged from the convocation was the realization that global cereal production would have to increase by 1 billion metric tons and meat production by 200 million metric tons by 2050 to feed 2 billion more human beings without increasing hunger, malnutrition, and food insecurity. If the world is to meet these food requirements, $83 billion must be invested annually in agriculture in developing countries, and 125 million hectares of arable farmland must be found, presaging a further drawing down of forest and grassland resources. Unfortunately, even if such investment in agriculture is made, the net cereal imports of developing countries are still projected to increase from 135 million metric tons in 2008–2009 to 300 million metric tons by 2050. The pressure of competition on global food supply must be juxtaposed against the present baseline of world poverty and hunger, as well as against changing demographic conditions.[15] Various statistics amply demonstrate that 1.25 billion people worldwide go to bed hungry; hunger-related health complications kill more people annually than malaria, tuberculosis, and AIDS combined; 25 percent of children in developing countries are underweight; and 6 million children under five years die from malnutrition-related health complications each year. In 2012, for example, the World Food Program distributed food assistance to one million Senegalese, in a country where 20 percent of the population were suffering from acute malnutrition and 30 percent of children were stunted for lack of adequate nutrition. Yet the regime bargained away over 650,000 hectares of farmlands to foreign land grabbers for biofuel production. Meanwhile, the food crops annually converted to biofuels in the G7 countries could have fed 441 million people.[16] The unsavory conclusion is that the food gaps between the overfed Global North and the underfed Global South do not seem likely to close. Meeting the current annual food demand in industrial countries of 550 kg of cereals per person and 78 kg of meat per person, compared with 260 kg of cereals and 30 kg of meat per person in the Global South, will require enormous mobilization of land and water resources that are hard to come by.[17]

The contradictions between food, feed, and biofuels are complicated by the financialization of agricultural commodities and the speculation bubble. The outcome of the liberalization and deregulation of financial markets following the triumph of the Washington consensus has been the emergence of unregulated and largely unscrutinized shadow banks, with combined holdings that had rocketed to $75.2 trillion by 2013.[18] The crowning moment of the financialization of the global economy occurred in 1999 when successive U.S. Treasury secretaries (Robert Rubin and Lawrence Summers, both under President Clinton) effectively shepherded the demolition of the New Deal–era firewall between investment banks and commercial banks that was intended to insulate the former from corrosive speculation. Since then, shadow banks, which proliferated in the form of hedge funds, mutual funds, pension funds, insurance funds. and sovereign wealth funds, have been empowered to create complex financial instruments, the chief ones being derivatives, which function without regulation or accountability. In response to the collapse of the subprime mortgage markets and the concomitant amplification of price movements in agricultural commodities during 2002–2008, the corporate holdings in agricultural commodities grew from $13 billion in 2003 to $400 billion in 2011. Barclays Capital alone injected $60 billion into speculative agricultural commodity markets in 2010.[19] To get a complete historical picture, note that just prior to the financial crisis of 2008, the size of the global financial markets was a staggering nine times the size of global trade, with $200 trillion invested in financial assets compared to $18 trillion in world merchandise trade.[20] These numbers do not even reflect the true size of the global derivatives market, which was estimated at $1.2 quadrillion in 2012, twenty times the global GDP of $60 trillion that same year.[21] These financial instruments had to find new outlets if the vulture fund managers were to continue to make money, and it was in this context that speculating in agricultural commodities was seen as another outlet. Ultimately, speculation in agricultural commodities went beyond the commodities themselves to the land on which the agricultural commodities are produced. Following the financialization of agricultural commodities and the multiplication of biofuel mandates since the beginning of the new century, the shadow banks poured tens of billions of financial assets into dodgy land deals, covering 227 million hectares between 2001 and 2010, mostly grabbed from defenseless rural communities for purposes of bioenergy crop and biofuel production. According to the World Bank, 56.6 million hectares of farmlands were negotiated away to corporate land grabbers in developing countries between October 2008 and August 2009, of which 66 percent were in Africa. Indeed, the scramble for land in Africa in 2009 was equal to the total cropland expansion of the twenty previous years. By some estimates, between August 2008 and April 2010, the amount of land resources acquired in Africa by foreign entities was between 51 million and 63 million hectares. Of the 464 land projects, with a median size of 40,000 hectares, which the World Bank scrutinized between October 2008 and August 2009, the focus of 37 percent of the projects was on food crops, 21 percent on biofuels, and 21 percent on industrial cash crops.[22] There is no mystery about corporate land grabbing; the competition over agricultural commodities necessarily drives the competition for land, water, and nutrients.

The competition of biofuels with food, feed, and fiber and the financialization of agriculture are further compounded by the law of diminishing returns. The green revolution, dependent as it was on intensive use of fertilizers, pesticides, and irrigation waters, has reached its outer limits. Yields have plateaued and the major cereals have long faced yield stagnation. Between 1962 and 2006, during the zenith of the green revolution, the conversion of 500 million hectares (almost all of it in the Global South) into agriculture and pasture, and the tripling of irrigated areas, in combination with the use of synthetic nitrogen, pesticides, fossil fuels, and hybrid seeds, led to an increase in world agricultural production by 70 percent in the 1970s and 1980s. However, despite intensified use of arable land, the growth of world agricultural production sharply declined by 30 percent by the 1990s and 2000s. For example, grain yields in the U.S. increased by 3 percent per annum between 1950 and 1980, but precipitously dropped to 1 percent per year since then.[23] Worldwide, the average yield growth rate for wheat declined from 2.92 percent between 1961 and 1979 to 1.78 percent between 1980 and 1997; and for maize the average yield growth rate slipped from 2.88 percent to 1.29 percent over the same period, while the average yield growth rate for rice remained stagnant at 1.95 percent throughout the entire period.[24] According to another FAO calculation, the growth rates in yields of wheat declined from 5 percent per annum in 1980 to 2 percent in 2005, while yield growth rates in rice and maize dropped from over 3 percent to around 1 percent in the same period. Notwithstanding these facts, the FAO still insists that 80 percent of the required increases in world food production must come from the intensification of agriculture. But even if such gains could be achieved, real price increases for maize, rice, and wheat are projected to increase by 104, 79, and 88 percent, respectively, and the prices for beef, pork, and poultry will rise by 32, 70, and 77 percent, respectively, by 2050. In part, such price increases are correlated with climate change, which is projected to decrease yields for maize, rice, and wheat by 9–18, 7–27, and 18–36 percent, respectively, by 2050. Under the predicted level of global warming, yields for maize will decline by 1,500 kg per hectare, for soybean, by 800 kg per hectare, for sorghum, by 1,000 kg per hectare, and for wheat by 500 kg per hectare.[25]

The ultimate reflection of yield stagnation is that the average world per capita grain output declined to 305 kg in 2006 from a peak of 376 kilograms in 1985. During years when nature unleashed its destructive forces in the form of droughts, excessive rainfall, floods, and cyclones, the global average per capita grain output dropped below 300 kilograms. More important, the global average per capita masks severe variations between regions and among countries within regions. For instance, the output of grain per person in the United States is 1,230 kilograms, most of which is fed to livestock, which translates to the average American eating more than 10,000 calories per day. In comparison, the average per capita output in China is 325 kilograms with average daily caloric intake of 2,700 per person, while Zimbabwe's meager 90 kilograms per capita grain output yields just 670 calories per person per day. Moreover, only three countries (the United States, China, and India) are responsible for 50 percent of world cereal grain production.[26] No wonder that 3.7 billion (56 percent of the human population) were classified as malnourished in 2008 by the World Health Organization.[27]

The looming danger of climate change could make cropland degradation even worse. If global warming increased by 2 degrees Celsius by 2050 as projected, global yields of wheat, maize, and soybeans could fall by 14–25 percent, 19–34 percent, and 15–30 percent, respectively, at a time when world population would have grown to 9.6 billion, requiring 1 billion metric tons of additional cereal grains and 200 million metric tons of additional meat products. It must be restated here that the increased crop yields during the green revolution period were made possible by constantly increasing irrigated areas, which tripled to over 300 million hectares between 1962 and 2006, accounting for 44 percent of world crop production. But here is the inescapable dilemma: there is little cropland left that is suitable for irrigation. The FAO projects that there are fewer than 20 million hectares that can potentially be irrigated in the next four decades, since water is already overdrawn in the world's most productive agricultural areas. In fact, by 2050, wheat production in China is predicted to drop by 40 million tons due to water shortages, and much of the irrigated area on which 175 million Indians depend for livelihoods will be dry by then.[28]

In addition to the growing shrinkage of arable land, water resources remain a key determinant with respect to how much land could be put under cultivation. Today, there are already 888 million people without access to clean drinking water; 2.6 million people do not receive sanitation services; and 1.4 million children under the age of five die every year for lack of clean water and adequate sanitation.[29] Furthermore, 1.6 billion people live in countries that are extremely vulnerable to weather-related food crises, where most grain production is from rainfed cropland. Crop yields from rain-fed agriculture in southern Africa are projected to fall by up to 50 percent by as early as 2020 due to water shortages. The water crisis is thus bound to confound the situation further. By 2020, it is conservatively estimated that up to 250 million people in Africa will experience greater water supply shortages because of climate change; this is a continent whose total population is predicted to more than double to 2 billion by 2050 from 900 million in 2012. Likewise, substantial reduction of water flow from mountain glaciers could affect up to one billion people in Asia in the coming decades; in Central and South Asia, crop yields are predicted to fall by 30 percent by 2050. The net result of climate change could be the addition of 50 million and 132 million people by 2020 and 2050, respectively, to the roster of hungry people.[30]

In light of this, it is impossible to overstate the cumulative effects of competition between biofuels, food, and animal feed—contextualized by the financialization of world agriculture and the scourge of climate change—on the food security of developing countries, where people spend between 50 and 80 percent of their income on basic foods, where 500 million small farmers are responsible for feeding 80 percent of the people, and where 75 percent of the poor live in rural areas. Thus the costs associated with the combined effects of competition of biofuels with food and feed are borne by the more than 5 billion people who live in the Global South. But this festering sore of material deprivation is something that the biofuel-biotechnology industrial complex views simply as a source of accumulation that can and must be tapped. They reassure us that future crop yields will be unprecedented when the transition from the green revolution of yesteryear to the gene revolution of tomorrow reaches its apotheosis. Monsanto vice president Donald Easum put it this way in a letter sent to African leaders:

> In agriculture, many of our needs have an ally in biotechnology and the promising advances it offers for our future: healthier, more abundant food, less expensive crops, reduced reliance on pesticides and fossil fuels, a cleaner environment. With these advances, we prosper; without them, we cannot thrive. As we stand on the edge of a new millennium, we dream of a tomorrow without hunger. To achieve that dream, we must welcome the science that promises hope. We know advances in biotechnology must be tested and safe, but they should not be unduly delayed. Biotechnology is one of tomorrow's tools in our hands today. Slowing its acceptance is a luxury our hungry world cannot afford. To feed the world in the next century, we need food that is more plentiful and more affordable than it is today. With more productivity needed from less tillable land, we need new ways to yield more from what is left—after development and erosion take their toll. To strengthen our economies, we need to grow our own food as independently as we can. Agricultural biotechnology will play a major role in realising the hope we all share. Accepting this science can make a dramatic difference in millions of lives. The seeds of the future are planted. Allow them to grow. Then let the harvest begin.[31]

However, the historical record does not support this hyperbole. Domination of world agriculture by biotech corporations will strip the world's farmers of their ability to control the food crops they grow, while diverting inordinate amounts of engineered food crops to biofuel production in order to grease the machine of global capitalism.

There is an even darker side to the advocacy for the transition from the green revolution to the gene revolution. It totalizes the objectification and neoliberalization of nature and human dispossession. The growing choke-hold of biotech crop breeders on their global commercial seed market has already reached alarming proportions, representing 82 percent of the $34.5 billion global commercial seed market as of 2011. Monsanto, whose biotech crops and traits accounted for 87 percent of the world's area devoted to genetically engineered crops in 2007, is the vanguard player in this gene revolution. By 2007, Monsanto had licensed its biotech crops and gene traits to more than 250 seed companies. In March 2007, Monsanto and BASF (the largest chemical corporation) pooled $1.5 billion for research on how to increase overall yields in GM crops and to manufacture so-called drought-tolerant maize, canola, cotton, and soybeans. Likewise, in September 2007, Monsanto and Dow AgroSciences pooled their resources to jointly develop the first ever engineered maize, loaded with eight different genes.[32]

The domination of biotech oligopolies over the global food manufacturing system is of such magnitude today that there is no shortage of arrogance in expressing their limitless capacity to biologically manipulate the characteristics and behavior of virtually every living species. This means that practically every plant species stands to be patented under the brand name of a corporation regardless of its impacts on human health, farmers' welfare, biodiversity, and the environment. Between 2008 and 2010, 1,663 biotech patent documents were issued; 77 percent of these patents were controlled by just eight gene giants, and only three of them controlled 66 percent of the patents.[33]

To be sure, the drive toward completing the genetic modification of world agriculture, and corporate consolidation and concentration in commercial food, health, drugs, biofuels, and biochemicals are moving in tandem at an accelerated pace under the guise of producing sufficient crops for food, feed, and bio-fuel production. From thousands of seed companies and public breeding institutions in the 1980s, just ten corporations control 76 percent of global proprietary seed sales today. Only three companies, Monsanto, DuPont, and Syngenta, control 53 percent of the total global proprietary seed market; 65 percent of the proprietary maize seed market; and over 50 percent of the proprietary soybeans market. Similarly, just six giant corporations control two-thirds of total global biotech industrial output, while another ten corporations control 90 percent of global agrochemical sales; the top five grain-trading corporations control 75 percent of the global grain trade; the ten biggest corporations control 52 percent of the global animal feed market; and the largest ten animal pharmaceutical companies control 76 percent of animal pharmaceutical sales. The ten biggest forestry corporations control 40 percent of the global forest market. With respect to vegetable seeds, Monsanto by itself controls 30 percent of the seed market for beans, cucumbers, hot peppers, sweet peppers, tomatoes, and onions.[34]

The centralization and concentration of commercial seed and agrochemical production and marketing have continued unabated at dizzying pace. The six giant agrochemical corporations (BASF, Bayer, Dow, DuPont, Monsanto, Syngenta) that dominate commercial proprietary seed, synthetic fertilizer, and pesticide markets globally are looking forward toward completing the neoliberalization of nature under absolute corporate monopoly domination. Their preoccupation now is with how to further accelerate the synthetic biological revolution. This requires the placement of $39 billion of proprietary seeds, $175 billion of fertilizer, $54 billion of pesticides, and $116 billion of farm equipment markets under a single corporate umbrella. They justify this by pointing to the looming dangers of climate change, demographic explosion, food insecurity, and energy supply shortages, which, according to them, could be solved only with continuous deployment of huge financial resources and new scientific innovations, meaning further unhampered centralization and concentration of production and marketing through mergers, acquisitions, strategic alliances, and partnerships.[35] Monsanto collaborates with Deere & Co., CNH Industrial, and AGCO (the world's largest farm machinery corporations); while Deere has been enjoying strategic partnerships with five of the Big Six agrochemical and commercial seed corporations. This reality is further compounded by corporate cross-pollination through vertical and horizontal clustering. Crop producers, grain traders, commercial seed providers, agrochemical manufacturers, and supermarkets are now forged into clusters; and all can be found in one another's backyards. For example, the four grain-trading oligopolies are now major biofuel producers, with the leading ADM producing 1.1 billion liters of ethanol per year. Operating over 250 plants in more than sixty countries, ADM has become an omnipotent global conglomerate. Another privately held TNC, known for its aggressive vertical supply chain integration and conglomeration, is Cargill, which operates in more than seventy countries. The U.S.-based Bunge also operates in nearly seventy countries with 450 plants. The French-based conglomerate Dreyfus, in addition to having a notable presence in international trade in agricultural products, is active in producing biofuels, the refining of petrol, trade in crude oil and gas derivatives, as well as in the real estate sector. Moreover, the grain-trading majors also dominate the fertilizer market in South America, bundling fertilizer sales with the purchase of harvests, holding farmers hostage to source all their inputs from the same oligopolies. In Brazil, for example, ADM, Bunge, Cargill and Dreyfus control 57 percent of the primary processing of soybean; and Bunge, Cargill, and ADM control 68 percent of soybean oil production.[36]

These behemoth corporate entities are linked to agrochemical and commercial seed suppliers like Monsanto, DuPont, BASF, and Syngenta, which themselves have become major biofuel producers as well.[37] Down the chain, all these corporations are connected to multinational supermarkets to distribute whatever they crank out. Fifty-five percent of the global wheat flour processed in mills operated by Cargill, ADM, and ConAgra, and 71 percent of the soybean flour processed by ADM, Bunge, and Cargill are distributed through multinational supermarkets.

With the neoliberalization of nature and the globalization of the food manufacturing system, humans are now involuntarily being placed under compulsion to eat unsafe and environmentally risky GM products. To make matters worse, with the state opting out of its professed social obligations, GM companies now conduct their own bogus testing of the foods they supply to the market. The U.S. FDA, for example, does not independently test GM foods on the market; it simply trusts the providing companies and expects them to voluntarily follow food safety guidelines.[38] In all, at least 7 dangerous effects of the so-called gene revolution on world agriculture have been identified, namely horizontal GM gene flow to non-GM crops and wild relatives; the potential emergence of new forms of resistance and pest problems; the potential of recombination, i.e., the production of second-generation plants containing traits not found in the parent plant, which can produce new pathogens; the potential emergence and propagation of direct and indirect effects from new toxins; the inevitable loss of biodiversity from changes to farm practices; manifestation of allergenic and immune system reactions; and the problem of antibiotic-resistant marker genes.[39]

What makes biotech oligopolies omnipotently dangerous is the reduction of the state to irrelevancy insofar as societal interests are concerned. When private corporations make false representations that GM crops are identical to natural crops and better in terms of nutrition, the burden of challenging them falls on highly fragmented and less coordinated non-governmental groups. If and when their deceitful maneuvers and manipulations are exposed, the oligopolies quickly marshal their resources to hire public relations experts to greenwash their actions, and they buy politicians and legislators through monetary donations to rebuff any challenge to their dominion. In 2013, for example, Monsanto, DuPont, Syngenta, and Cargill together spent $40.4 million on lobbying the U.S. Congress to defeat a bill requiring labeling GMOs.[40]

Bear in mind that commercial enclosure of nature involves transformation of biotic resources, which had been naturally and historically within the public domain. Proprietary ownership of resources under the brand names of corporations establishes monopoly control over the crossbred and genetically manipulated crop, plant, or organism. In other words, any cross-bred and biologically engineered crop genes now fall under the intellectual property rights regime and are off-limits even to indigenous farmers who domesticated the grain or plant in the first place. With the entire public domain of crops and plants surrendered to corporations, farmers have lost control over their crops and food sovereignty. Users of what had been public domain seeds are under compulsion to purchase cross-bred and GM seeds year after year from corporations; farmers will not be able to even save seeds from current harvests for replanting in the next season. Farmers' dependency on commercial seed companies will not be limited to the purchase of seeds alone, as they also have to buy all the agrochemicals needed to support the planting of hybrid and GM seeds. Thus, while the vulnerability of farmers to corporate stranglehold increases, GM seed and agrochemical companies maximize profits from double dipping.

A bizarre aspect of patent legislation in the United States is that obligations are unilateral, borne by farmers. Commercial seed corporations have no liability whatsoever for any nonperformance of the seeds, defects, or incidents of any sorts. For example, if pollen from a field sown with Roundup Ready soybeans is blown onto a field sown with organic soybeans and, as a result, becomes contaminated, the farmer who owns the organic soybean-growing field will be held liable for using Roundup Ready soybeans without Monsanto's permission. Instead of obliging Monsanto to compensate the farmer for the biological contamination, the farmer is identified as a thief under the law, and must pay Monsanto up to 100 times more than the presumed damage. Moreover, Monsanto has the right to visit soybean farms anywhere and anytime without the permission or presence of farmers.[41]

To enforce its power Monsanto has deployed a large army of "seed detectives" throughout rural America to spy on farmers, collecting royalty fees plus hefty fines from thousands of soybean growers on grounds of alleged infringement of its patented GE seed. Monsanto also established a toll-free tip line for farmers to inform on neighbors, pitting farmers against farmers.[42] In the 1990s, Monsanto's 1,800 detectives spied on soybean farmers and GM seed dealers, resulting in placing 475 farmers under criminal investigation, identified as seed "pirates." In 1998, the pro-corporate court found soybean farmers in Kentucky, Iowa, and Illinois guilty of saving GM soybean seeds in contravention of their obligations to the oligopoly, and ordered them to pay Monsanto $35,000 each. Exhilarated by the court's ruling, Monsanto's manager for intellectual property protection, Scott Baucum, boasted in these terms: "We say they can pay (either of) two royalties—$6.50 at the store or $600 in court."[43]

The use of spies and legal proceedings proved costly for corporations, however, so to lower costs, they sought to develop seed sterilization technologies. The design would involve engineering seeds to commit suicide after each harvest. Even if farmers saved the seeds from the first year's harvest and replanted them, they would not germinate, leaving the farmers with no option other than to come back to the seed biomanufacturers for a new supply of seeds year after year. With this objective in mind, in 1983, the U.S. Department of Agriculture in conjunction with the Mississippi-based Delta and Pine Land Company started working on genetic use restriction technology (GURT), commonly called terminator technology. Then, in March 1998, the USDA and the company obtained the license to commercialize the terminator technology, applying for patents in seventy-eight countries. As developed, the terminator patent would indiscriminately cover plants and seeds of all species. Within two months of the announcement of the terminator technology patent, Monsanto entered into direct negotiation with the USDA over the acquisition of an exclusive license, and offered to buy the Delta and Pine Land Company for a whopping $19 billion.[44]

Another version of the terminator technology is what is known as genetic trait control, which would make plant growth or the expression of specific genes responsive only to particular chemicals designed by a company. Accordingly, a company can develop certain traits to produce crops or grow plants that would fail to grow properly unless they are regularly exposed to the company's chemicals. In this situation, if farmers want to turn on the herbicide-resistant seeds acquired from the company or to turn off the sterility traits of the seeds, they would be compelled to apply commercial proprietary chemicals to the crops or plants as they grow or pay the company to have the seeds or plants soaked in catalyst solutions before planting. Thus the terminator and genetic trait control technologies would hold farmers as permanent hostages, bioserfs who must come back to the company year after year for new seeds. The bioserfs would not be able to grow self-pollinating and self-germinating crops such as wheat, rice, oats, sorghum, soybeans, and cotton. In the end, a few biomanufactured seeds would replace the hundreds of thousands of seeds that were developed over millennia, grown and adapted to highly varied and complex geoecological and hydroclimatological conditions, endowing communities with complete sovereignty over their food ecology. However, the bioinvention of terminator and genetic trait control technologies effectively completed the transfer of power from the natural producers of our foods to transnational oligopolies. The biological weaponry of these technologies has been referred to as a "neutron bomb" of agriculture.[45] Until the 1990s, cereals such as wheat, rice, oats, barley, and rye were resistant to hybridization on a grand commercial scale. Now however, their biological fate changed, extending corporate monopoly over all life-sustaining food sources to a level beyond even the influence of producers. In particular, control over wheat and rice represents a catastrophic risk for poor farmers in the

Global South. Note that, in 2015, the combined global production of maize, rice and wheat was nearly 2.3 trillion metric tons, accounting for three-fourths of the sources for human nutrition.[46] Thus control of these three major cereal grains through the application of terminator technology would effectively cement corporate domination over our food.

The USDA and the corporations have certainly taken to heart Henry Kissinger's counsel that to control food is to control people. Melvin J. Oliver, the USDA molecular biologist who was the primary inventor of terminator technology, was frank when he stated without a trace of reflection that seed-saving by farmers was tantamount to open theft of intellectual property. In his words: "My main interest is the protection of American technology. Our mission is to protect U.S. agriculture, and to make us competitive in the face of foreign competition. Without this, there is no way of protecting the technology [patented seed]." If Oliver was frank about the bioinvention of the terminator technology, USDA spokesman Willard Phelps was even more blunt when he told the public that the overarching goal of the terminator technology was "to increase the value of proprietary seed owned by US seed companies and to open up new markets in second and third world countries."[47]

The announcement of the terminator technology patent made many eyebrows go up. Almost universally, plant and animal breeding institutions throughout the developing world threatened to boycott sterilized seeds, and other critics raised many issues regarding the numerous threats posed by the novel technology, not only to the food ecology but also to the general environment and public health. Martha Crouch, a molecular biologist at Indiana University, observed that the use of terminator technology poses a grave danger to agrodiversity because the sterility traits of the engineered seed could contaminate not only surrounding organic farms but also wild relatives via the spread of pollen, potentially making all seeds sterile with no liability for the GM seed manufacturers.[48] The horizontal transfer of transgenes from GM crops to wild relatives is a near certainty given the evolutionary process of natural selection. Terminator technology–based transgenes presage the transfer of undesirable traits, resulting in the permanent transformation of food crops and plants, attended by the emergence of novel forms of resistance and/or secondary pests and weeds. Even before the introduction of GM crops into modern agriculture, numerous agrochemical-resistant species had become problematic. By the late 1990s, there were more than 500 species of insects and mites resistant to one or more synthetic compounds, 400 herbicide-resistant weeds, and 150 resistant fungi and bacteria. Greater danger to human health could emerge from the recombination of viruses and bacteria, resulting in the appearance and proliferation of new pathogens if viruses or bacteria incorporate transgenes into their genomes, which could potentially result in the expression of harmful new traits.[49]

Proponents of this perilous technology respond by claiming that, since the engineered seeds or plants are sterile to begin with, the pollen blowing to adjacent fields would also be sterile without the capacity to biologically contaminate. They claim the best way to restrict or eliminate the spread of genes from GE crops or plants to other crops and plants in the natural environment is through terminator or genetic trait control technologies, insulating the natural agrodiversity against any accidental or intentional introduction of GE crops and plants.[50] The truth is that nobody, much less managers of seed companies, can know the long-term effects of the biological interactions between pollen from terminator seeds and organic seeds. However, it is certain that the prevention of cross-pollination of crops or contamination of wild species is virtually impossible.

THE DECEPTION OF A GREEN ENVIRONMENT

In chapter 1, we saw that the economy is a subsystem of the environment to which it is permanently attached. The economy receives continuous inflows of throughput from the environment to carry out production functions, while it continuously sends out inordinate amounts of waste and pollution for assimilation or processing into harmless substances. The conversion of through-put into exchange goods, resource depletion, and environmental exhaustion take place simultaneously. For example, to produce one liter of bioethanol, a typical feedstock plant receives clean water and when its conversion into liquid fuel is complete, dumps thirteen liters of wastewater into the environment.[51] The environment can perform these two requirements of the economy only if the parameters of sustainable scale are observed. If the exactions for throughput exceed the environment's regeneration capacity and if the insertions of waste and pollution into the environment exceed its self-cleansing capacity, the supply of raw materials from the environment progressively diminishes and the quality of the environment steadily decreases, leading to environmental exhaus-tion, degradation, and possibly eventual collapse. These negative conditions are cumulative. The whole environment may not be exhausted or degraded at once; its parts deteriorate at different intervals and different rates until noticed on a macrostructural scale. Biologists use the concept of "punctuated equilibrium" to describe these kinds of situations, where changes occur incremen-tally in ways that are not noticeable until the whole edifice of the system begins to crumble due to the cumulative weight of lon-ger-term changes within it. Forestalling such a scenario requires unconditional observance of the cardinal principle of sustain-able scale in which the throughput taken from the environment must be exactly proportional to its regeneration capacity and the amount of waste returned to the environment must be equal to its waste assimilative capacity.

Blinded by both ignorance and apologetics, many bourgeois analysts offer multiple research scenarios about how biofuels can be obtained from the conversion of living things without resource exhaustion and environmental degradation. For example, the IEA counsels OECD countries that 23 to 27 percent of primary energy, equal to 225 EJ, could be obtained from biomass by 2050. This would require the harvest of 1,500 metric tons of throughput per year, with half of the feedstocks grown on 375–750 million hectares, and the other half coming from forest and crop residues.[52] But bioenergy experts Timothy Searchinger and Ralph Heimlich recently dealt a serious blow to the IEA's projection. They asked: "How much plant material would that require? To get a sense of how much, consider that in 2000 the total amount of energy in all the crops, plant residues, and wood harvested by people for all applications (e.g., food, construction, paper) and in all the biomass grazed by livestock around the world was roughly 225 EJ."[53] Even if we suppose that it is possible to obtain this amount of bioenergy, we run into the following problem. According to OECD projections, global primary energy use in 2050 will reach 900 EJ per year, which means that 675 EJ of global primary energy must still come from fossil resources. To put this insight into historical perspective, in 2000 the total global primary energy use was on the order of 400 to 500 EJ. Thus:

Using all of the world's harvested biomass for energy would provide only 20 percent of the world's energy needs in 2050. Note: a total amount of crops, harvested residues, grass eaten by livestock, and harvested wood contained 225 EJ, but would replace only 180 EJ of fossil fuels because of conversion efficiencies from biomass to useable energy. Put another way, meeting this bioenergy target would require not only all of the world's recent crop harvest, but also all of its crop residues, harvested trees, and grass consumed by livestock. And yet the world would still need food for people, fodder for livestock, residues for replenishing agricultural soils, wood pulp for paper, and timber for construction and other purposes. To meet these needs and at the same time meet a 20 percent bioenergy target, humanity would therefore need to double the world's recent annual harvest of plant material. In fact, it would have to do even more than that because humanity also needs to produce about 70 percent more food by 2050.[54]

The crux of the problem for corporations stems from the fact that subordinating production to the principle of sustainable scale runs counter to the logic of capital accumulation, which recognizes no limitations in nature nor does it respect boundaries. Further accumulation requires continuous flows of throughputs in ever larger quantity; if the home country cannot supply the demanded resources, then accumulators outsource the material, in effect, outsourcing throughput exhaustion and environmental degradation to other countries. In other words, globalizing environmental exhaustion and degradation becomes the net outcome. This is the very definition of contemporary capitalism. In the remainder of this section, I shall explore how the relentless pursuit of GM monocultivation and biofuel production affect four critical areas of the environment, vitiating the corporate promise to create a green environment through the acceleration of the transition to the gene revolution and green transport fuels. These areas are the competition for land with serious implications for forest, savannah, and grassland resources; the relentless expansion of industrial tree plantations; the competition for water resources; and the profusion of agrochemicals.

The literature on the state of global forest ecosystems amply clarifies the darker side of late capitalism. Historically, the central drivers of forest, grassland, and savannah depletion and degradation have been population growth, which necessitated the extension of farmland, livestock grazing, and fuelwood extraction. This development was followed by commercial logging to serve the pulp and paper industry, reflected in the exponential increase in forest vandalization since the 1950s. As a consequence, forest, grassland, and savannah depletion and degradation led to widespread erosion and greenhouse gas emissions. Between 1950 and 1995, for example, deforestation-driven erosion was responsible for the loss of 580 million hectares of fertile land worldwide; this was larger than the geographic area of the whole of Western Europe. By the mid-1990s, a mere 22 percent of the original forest ecosystems was classified as intact frontier forest, while 78 percent was composed of fragmented, secondary growth, and isolated patches of primary forests.[55]

Until the turn of the twentieth century, temperate forests were the most affected forest ecosystems. This is because the temperate regions of the earth are occupied by countries where capitalism first found its hospitable residence. The favorable hydrometeorological conditions and fertile soils in temperate regions led to wholesale clearing of temperate forests. By the 1990s, a mere 3 percent of temperate forests were designated as undisturbed frontier forests. This has led to the outsourcing by transnational corporations of the forest resources they require to the Global South where tropical forest resources are in abundance. Thus, the deepening processes of globalization and the growing appetite of late capitalism for ever larger inputs extended the subjection of tropical frontier forests to the same processes of depletion and deforestation. As a result, between 1960 and 1990, the world lost 450 million hectares, or 20 percent, of the original tropical forest cover.[56] Lurking behind this forest destruction have been commercial logging, mining operations, petroleum and natural gas exploration, construction of hydrodams and transmission lines, and large-scale infrastructure projects. Then since the 1990s, biofuel production and thermochemical-driven electricity generation have added another layer to the mix of drivers of forest depletion and degradation, threatening additional tropical forest ecosystems by clearcutting or replacing them by industrial tree plantations. In 2000, 24,000 hectares of industrial tree plantations in Malaysia and 60,000 hectares in Indonesia were established inside intact frontier forests.[57]

Because tropical forest ecosystems sequester about 600 billion metric tons of carbon dioxide, the progressive reduction in the areal extent of tropical forests results not only in the substantial diminution of their capacity to remove carbon dioxide from the atmosphere, but the forests' destruction or degradation also results in more emissions. The corporate invocation of biofuels and wood pellet production as clean and green, hence environment-friendly, obfuscates this reality. Biofuels and wood pellets cannot be made from nothing. The natural forests, bioenergy crops, and the industrial tree plantations must grow on land and must be watered. As more and more land and water resources are dedicated to the production of feedstocks, encroaching upon land resources needed for food and feed production, more land must be found elsewhere to grow food crops and animal feed consistent with the growing needs of a growing human population.

Since intense competition of biofuels with food and feed production for land resources becomes unavoidable in a full world, the profound contradictions can be contained, if at all, by finding additional land resources—in other words, by drawing down the remaining forest resources. The resulting conversion of more and more forests and wetlands will then substantially reduce the size of the green natural ecology. In turn, this will erode the natural ecology's capacity to sufficiently capture solar radiation as before, to remove carbon dioxide from the atmosphere and sequester it, and to provide other invaluable ecosystem services.

The number of competitors for land resources are manifold. According to the Gallagher Report, the additional land requirement to grow food crops globally by 2020 could be on the order of 144–334 million hectares.[58] Meanwhile, the additional land requirement to produce feedstocks is projected to be in the range of 35–166 million hectares by 2020. If the world is to obtain 10 percent road transport fuels from first-generation biofuels, the additional required land for feedstocks will be on the order of 118 million to 508 million hectares by 2030, amounting to between 8 and 36 percent of existing cropland and permanent pasture. In fact, according to a more recent projection, the additional gross land resources required by 2050 to produce food, feed, and feedstocks will be in the range of 320–850 million hectares, or between the combined sizes of Indonesia, Ethiopia, and Brazil, crossing the threshold of all parameters of sustainable scale. Therefore, "expansion of such magnitude is simply not compatible with the imperative of sustaining the basic life-supporting services that ecosystems provide, such as maintaining soil productivity, regulating water resources, sustaining forest cover or conserving biodiversity."[59]

This projection seems plausible since the scramble for land acquisition by foreign bioinvaders and domestic corporate elites in the Global South is being ratcheted up at the expense of forests, savannahs, and grasslands. The Indonesian elites, for example, have plans to put 20 million hectares of additional peatland under oil palm plantations by 2020, of which two-thirds will take the place of intact peatland rainforests.[60] The fact is that, since the total global cropland had already covered 1.5 billion hectares in 2000, and since the safe operating space of cropland is considered to be around 1,640 billion hectares, the conversion of an additional 320–850 billion hectares of forests, savannahs, and grasslands to cropland will place world agriculture outside a safe operating space by a wide margin. The current capitalist scramble to transition to a bioeconomy, centered on the production and circulation of biobased products such as bioplastics, biochemicals, and biopolymers, is bound to deepen the capitalist contradictions surrounding the competition for steady flows of throughputs. This will drive the conversion of more forests, savannahs, and grasslands to biomaterial production. As of 2008, the cropland dedicated to biomaterial production stood at 100 million hectares, expected to increase by 104–215 million hectares by 2050.

The conclusion is unmistakable. The gene revolution and the transition toward green fuels is not giving us a healthier environment but a planet on the verge of collapse. It must be remembered that what makes the environment green and clean is preservation of what nature has proffered. Global plants capture 75,000 million tons of oil equivalent (Mtoe) or 3,150 EJ a year of the solar radiation that strikes the earth, which is six to seven times the current global energy demand, essential for photosynthetic action, in addition to the sequestration of massive amount of carbon dioxide.[61] In reckless disregard of this reality, the bourgeois world continues to encourage more and more harvesting of these precious natural resources in order to keep accumulation going indefinitely. After having exhausted their own natural resources, industrial countries are encouraging corporations to outsource biopredation and pollution to the tropics and subtropics under the guise of promoting development, eradicating poverty, and improving climate change. And then they turn around and blame third world countries for depleting or degrading their forests. In sum, the repercussions of land competition, land use change, and land use intensification at the expense of forests, savannahs, and grasslands are and will continue to be catastrophic in scale. If the current rates of resource extraction continue, between 104 million and 347 million hectares of additional forests could be gone by 2030, and the areas of savannahs and grasslands could shrink by 37 and 100 percent, respectively, by then.[62]

The second area where the environmental ramifications of biofuel production must be assessed involves the intensified use of corporate-owned tree plantations, particularly in the Global South. It is no accident that industrial monoculture plantations grew from an area of 12 million hectares in 1980 to nearly 300 million hectares today. However, industrial tree plantations cannot replace the ecological functions performed by natural forests. Because single species–based commercial plantations lack biological diversity and biocomplexity, the biological, biochemical, and hydroecological services that they furnish cannot equal the same services provided by natural ecosystems. This inherent deficiency in monoculture tree plantations is compounded by the regular harvesting of the trees to feed the pulp and paper industry, as well as thermochemical-driven electricity production, which severely curtails the capacity of industrial plantations to remove and store carbon, even if we assume that they have the capacity for doing so. In 2013–2014, for example, 65 percent and 45 percent of the forest loss in Malaysia and Indonesia, respectively, occurred within industrial tree plantations due to frequent harvesting.[63] Such rapid harvesting is due to capital's insistence on quick profits. Thus, we need to look at the environmental effects of industrial plantations within the context of the impacts on the health of indigenous vegetation, conservation of indigenous plants, water allocation, water quality, biophysical processes, biodiverse habitat, pollution and contamination, and fire hazards.[64]

To begin with, industrial plantations are very poor nutrient-builders but voracious nutrient consumers. Rich plant growth and wildlife in tropical wetland systems are not indications of high fertility, but of higher consumption and recycling of nutrients, which cumulatively result in nutrient depletion, necessitating human intervention through the use of synthetic fertilizer and pesticides at much higher cost compared to natural forest ecosystems. Natural forests are composed of a rich variety of plant species with different ages that produce a variety of leaf litter containing a complex diversity of organic matter that degrades at different speeds. As a result, soil formation and organic matter recycling in natural forest ecosystems are continuous. In Nigeria, for example, it was found that leaf litter of indigenous trees contains much higher levels of humus because decomposition occurs within 27 months, in interaction with diverse floral and faunal communities. This contrasts with an industrial pine plantation where the decomposition of pine needles takes between 3 and 6 years. Frequent use of heavy machinery in industrial tree plantations during the preparation of the soil and harvest time also results in soil compaction, erosion, and displacement of the nutrients and organic material naturally found in leaf litter and topsoil. Moreover, the cultivation of homogenous fast-growing trees of the same age cannot reach the level of biodiversity and biocomplexity of natural forest ecosystems because they are cut regularly. Genetic contamination of natural ecosystems by commercial short rotation plantations also present a threat to the conservation of biodiverse native plants. Exotic monoculture plantations are known for their ruthless bioaggression against indigenous plants through competition, outgrowth, and suffocation, in addition to making adjacent indigenous vegetation vulnerable to pests, pathogens, and fire risk. In South Africa, for instance, the 1.5 million industrial tree plantations quickly spread to areas of adjacent native vegetation, colonizing or replacing another 1.7 million hectares of biodiverse native plants.[65]

This brings us to issue of water. The scourge of water scarcity is upon us. The number of people subject to water stress will increase from one-third of the human population in 2010 to 50 percent by 2030, which means that 3.9 billion people will be living in water stress regions by 2030. To cope with the ever-diminishing supply of water, governments have been spending around $45 billion per year on upstream water development projects, which are expected to grow to $200 billion per year by 2030. China's determination to transfer 45 billion cubic meters of water per year from the south to the north of the country is a good illustration.[66] There will inevitably be distorting effects from governmental hydrological policies, such as privileging some sectors and wealthy classes over small farmers and poor communities. In this respect, the feedstock and biofuel production sector could be among government priorities insofar as massive water allocation goes. For example, 65 percent of the urban residents of Guayaquil in Ecuador receive a mere 3 percent of potable urban water at prices that are much higher than those paid by the wealthy few who are connected to public water mains. Likewise, 50 percent of Mexico City residents receive only 5 percent of piped water, while 60 percent of the urban drinking water goes to just 3 percent of households.[67] On a national level, 12 million Mexicans have no access to clean and adequate drinking water, and another 25 million live in areas where the water supply is limited to just a few hours a week.[68] This state of hydro-destitution in Mexico is not simply a function of water scarcity but rather a result of gross inequality in power and distribution of national wealth.

As things stand now, projections indicate that global water insecurity is bound to get worse, in no small part due to the rush for the green El Dorado. Biofuel production, pyrolysis-driven electricity generation, and the pulp and paper industry all depend on large-scale agro-commercial plantations, which require massive amounts of water resources. Every hectare of land and every gallon of water used to produce bioenergy crops and biofuels is inevitably subtracted from water resources needed to grow food and feed. For example, in 2007, 45 billion cubic meters of freshwater were dedicated to biofuels production, which was six times the total amounts of water resources that the entire global population used for drinking.[69] Note that it takes 2,900 gallons of water to grow a bushel of corn in Oklahoma and it takes another 4 gallons of water to generate one gallon of ethanol; 3,500 liters of water are required to grow sugarcane to produce 1 liter of sugar bioethanol. With soy, it takes 14,000 liters of water to generate one liter of biodiesel, and it takes a whopping 20,000 liters of water to generate one liter of biodiesel from jatropha.[70]

The competition for water resources looms even larger in light of the projected increase in global warming. Climate models suggest uneven spatial and temporal distribution of rainfall, meaning that the availability of freshwater will be a daunting challenge in many regions of the Global South, where 64 percent of the population is expected to live in water-stressed basins as early as 2025. Due to increased population and urbanization, worldwide municipal and industrial demand is forecast to increase by 200 percent by 2050. Moreover, meeting the environmental flow requirements in important river basins may necessitate more than 50 percent of the mean annual runoff; thus water availability for global agriculture is projected to fall by 18 percent by 2050.[71]

The race to blanket vast areas in the Global South with fast-growing short-rotation trees will have even more significant bearing on the availability and distribution of water in the future. The water requirements of industrial plantations are highly correlated with hydrological scarcity. In contrast, intact natural forests, equipped with vast undergrowth, are crucial to the regulation of the hydrologic cycle. A study of Southeast Asian forests found that undisturbed contiguous forests intercept 35 percent of rainfall, while logged forests capture less than 20 percent, and commercial rubber plantations intercept less than twelve percent of the rainwater.[72] An important aspect that influences the regulation of the hydrologic cycle is the presence of undergrowth in forests, which acts like a sponge, retaining water without evaporation, and slowly releasing it to the soil. In addition, the presence of rich humus and the depth of roots and diversity of biomass in natural forest ecosystems modulate the infiltration and recharge of downstream natural water systems. Industrial tree plantations, devoid of undergrowth and planted in fixed distances in rows, have lower levels of rainwater infiltration, aggravated by compaction of the soil that takes place during soil preparation and harvesting, thereby facilitating rapid evaporation, erosion, and sedimentation of natural water systems. The long-range impact of industrial tree plantations is not limited to water depletion. Industrial tree plantations are notorious for discharging a wide range of toxic chemicals to the environment such as chlorinated pesticides, herbicides, fungicides, timber preservation treatments, and nitrates.[73]

In all, the diversion of water to irrigate bioenergy crops and industrial tree plantations and the production of liquid biofuels means exposing the once green lush components of the environment to desiccation and desertification. At the same time, reducing overall water yield and flow has significant implications for downstream users and aquatic life.

In the final analysis, it all comes to choosing between using massive amounts of water resources to grow bioenergy crops and industrial trees to produce biofuels to meet the demand of the affluent Global Northerners or using the same amounts of water resources to grow enough food to feed the 1.25 billion poor Global Southerners. The present corporate choice entails converting more cropland to bioenergy crop production and industrial tree plantations, accompanied by the diversion of massive quantities of water, and then running the risk of widening and deepening global poverty. Meanwhile, the conversion of more and more forests, savannahs, and grasslands to create cropland for bioenergy crop production and industrial tree plantations runs the risk of exacerbating the rate of global deforestation, desiccation and desertification and, by extension, climate change and global warming.[74]

THE DECEPTION OF BLUE SKIES

Proponents of biofuels have succeeded to some extent in perpetuating the myth that biofuels and pyrolysis-driven electricity production are clean, green, and renewable. They embed the case for biofuels in what has now become a misleading concept of "carbon negative" or "carbon neutral" bioenergy. This is how one research team attempted to make the case: "Bioenergy is a promising tool for achieving a sustainable development. Using bioenergy can help to mitigate greenhouse gas emissions as bioenergy can be a neutral source of energy."[75] Capitalizing on the general faulty perception of biotic resources as renewable and clean, proponents portray them as economically, environmentally, and socially sustainable. Even though the jury is still out as to whether second- and third-generation biofuels are universally cleaner than fossil fuels or even whether they are feasible, we know that first-generation biofuels are hardly cleaner or safer than conventional sources of energy. For example, scientific evidence derived from analysis of biofuel consumption in EU countries indicates that achieving a target of 10 percent of transport biofuels would lead to up to 167 percent more ghg emissions than using fossil fuels to meet the same requirements. At 2011 levels of biofuel consumption, the EU will add 56 million metric tons of carbon dioxide to the atmosphere by 2020, which is equal to putting more than 26 million new cars on the road.[76]

There is no getting around the fact that the emission of harmful pollution begins with cultivation of bioenergy crops and industrial tree plantations. Synthetic fertilizer production and burning fossils during monocultivation emit 41 million tons of CO_2 annually. The use of heavy farm machinery and equipment results in the emission of another 158 million tons of CO_2 to the atmosphere each year, while irrigation pumps spew 369 million tons of CO_2 per year.[77] If all factors involved in growing the feedstocks, processing the feedstocks, and burning the biofuels are taken into account, biofuel consumption could actually be dirtier than the use of conventional fuels by wide margins. For example, the use of maize-based ethanol has been found to release higher greenhouse gases than fossil fuels. Moreover, even if we assume that biofuels are clean and green, the savings made in terms of improved air quality and climate can be eroded by change in land cover especially when using fire to clear land as in Brazil, China, and Indonesia where the quality of air has been reduced as a result of widespread deforestation.[78] Comparative evaluation of all energy sources would place burning biomass below many energy sources in terms of their environmental and climate benefits, with burning coal being the partial exception. For example, the carbon content of recoverable petroleum reserves is estimated at 120 billion tons; that of natural gas reserves is estimated at 75 billion tons; oil shale reserves hold 225 billion tons; and tar sand reserves store 250 billion tons of carbon. In comparison, terrestrial biomass stores 500 billion tons of carbon, surpassed only by recoverable coal reserves which hold 925 billion tons of carbon. So the progressive burning of forests and converting them to farmland release more carbon. Moreover, the basic reason why burning biomass releases more CO_2 than fossil fuels is that one must burn much more biomass to achieve the same energy unit as from burning fossils because of the lower energy density of biomass. In addition, if the preparation of soil to grow biological feedstocks is included in the computation, the negative consequences of large-scale production and consumption of biofuels and wood pellets are even larger. It is estimated that the quantities of plant roots, organic compounds, and other living and nonliving things held together in the top 100 centimeters of global soil sequester 1,555 billion tons of carbon, which is progressively released during the preparation of the land for industrial biomass production.[79]

Today, Indonesia and Brazil rank third and fourth, respectively, on the global emissions index, after China and the United States, not because they are dirty industrializers, but because they are the worst deforesters. The yearly ghg emissions from Indonesia are 562 million tons, most of it related to deforestation, soil degradation, and peat oxidation. The catastrophic 1997 fire in Indonesia, which devastated 11.7 million hectares of vegetation, precipitated by the rush to clear forests for industrial oil palm plantations, ended up releasing over 2.5 billion tons of CO_2 into the atmosphere. Since Indonesia has dedicated 80 percent of its tropical forests and peatlands to agriculture and bioenergy plantations, Indonesia's contribution to the worsening climatic situation cannot be overstated.[80] Thus, if deforestation of the tropics (which currently releases 1.5 billion tons of CO_2 annually) proceeds unabated in the pursuit of biofuels, the consequences will take on epic proportions. As noted by Tim Searchinger and his colleagues, there is an erroneous logic built into the presentation of biofuels as greener and cleaner than fossil fuels.[81] The error stems from the fact that greenhouse gases resulting from the cultivation of feedstocks and production of biofuels are undercounted or not counted at all in the lifecycle analysis. This fallacy inheres in the argument that the crops and plants used in biofuel production have already removed the carbon dioxide from the atmosphere while growing. Therefore, it is not necessary to count the carbon dioxide released during the production and consumption of biofuels since doing so would represent double counting. This contradicts both the first and second laws of thermodynamics. The law of conservation tells us that one cannot make anything out of nothing; the making of anything requires the use of available energy. This means that the life cycle involved in the cultivation, production, processing, and distribution of bioenergy crops requires raw matter/energy, which simultaneously produces both useful and useless energy, which is transformed into unavailable and useless energy in the form of emissions. However, because biofuels are marketed as clean and green, the emissions resulting from the metabolic transformation of matter/energy are discounted. The costs incurred from clearing forests, woodlands, grasslands, wetlands, and peatlands to grow biological feedstocks are also discounted. Forests and their soils store about 1,100 billion tons of carbon, which is released during forest conversion and soil preparation for crops and plantations.[82]

Biofuel and wood pellet production proponents tend to ignore critical ecosystem functions and associated costs in their bookkeeping. The problem of forest and soil exhaustion and degradation is not confined to industrial monocultivation of inputs. As prices for basic foodstuffs soar beyond the purchasing capability of the poor because of the conversion of huge land resources to biofuel production, poor farmers will by necessity clear more and more fragile forests to grow their own food. These actions cumulatively exacerbate greenhouse gas emissions and climate warming. For example, as ubiquitously mentioned in the literature, Brazil boasts having the cleanest energy sources in the world because of its reliance on hydro-energy for 83 percent of national energy consumption, augmented by substantial amounts of biofuels. However, Brazil outranks India on the global emissions index because of the deforestation necessary for soybean cultivation and sugarcane plantations.[83] Additionally, when refining sugarcane or processing soybeans and jatropha, it uses energy that releases waste and pollution. And when we burn up the ethanol or the biodiesel in our vehicles, the result is more emissions. This is how Tim Searchinger and colleagues summarize the issue at hand:

> For most biofuels, growing the feedstocks requires land, so the credit claimed represents the carbon benefit of devoting land to biofuels. Unfortunately, by excluding emissions from land use change, most previous accountings were one-sided because they counted the carbon benefits of using land for biofuels but not the carbon costs, carbon storage and sequestration sacrificed by diverting land from its existing uses. Without biofuels, the extent of cropland reflects the demand for food and fiber. To produce biofuels, farmers can directly plow up more forest or grassland, which releases much of the carbon previously stored in plants and soils through decomposition or fire. The loss of maturing forests and grasslands also forgoes ongoing carbon sequestration as plants grow each year, and this foregone sequestration is the equivalent of additional emissions.[84]

Despite the ceaseless corporate effort to market biofuels as clean and green, the mounting empirical evidence unambiguously runs counter to what the corporations say. The carbon debt from biofuels in terms of CO_2 emissions has empirically been found to be 17 to 420 times greater than the annual ghg reductions that the use of these biofuels provides by displacing fossil fuels. For example, the ghg savings from using maize ethanol is estimated to be 1.8 tons of CO_2 per hectares per year, while the conversion of the grassland to grow the corn has been found to release 300 tons of CO_2 per hectare per year, and the emissions of CO_2 from the conversion of forest land to corn production is on the order of 600 to 1,000 tons per hectare per year.[85] Since natural forests, savannahs, grasslands, and soils hold 2.7 times more carbon than the entire atmosphere, conversion of these resources (entailing burning of forests, grasslands, and decomposition of organic matter contained in soils) to biofuels releases inordinate amounts of ghg, resulting in greater debt than credit.

As frequently stated by many researchers in the field, primary tropical forests are believed to store up to 400 tons of carbon per hectare; so clearing just one hectare of tropical forest for biofuel production means releasing that amount of CO_2 into the atmosphere. Even secondary natural forest growth stores 100 to 200 tons of carbon per hectare compared to 11 to 61 tons of carbon per hectare of industrial monoculture tree plantations. Not only do industrial monoculture tree plantations store less carbon than natural forests, but they are also environmentally costly since they require great amounts of energy inputs in the form of agrochemicals and deep plowing, which accentuate carbon emissions.[86] The consequences of converting peatlands to oil palm plantations for purposes of biodiesel production are unmatched by other feedstock-producing subsectors. By some estimates, biodiesel produced from oil palm plantations grown on land previously occupied by rainforest could release 2,000 percent more carbon than fossil-fuel based diesel.[87] As conservationist Joseph Fargione and colleagues note, the carbon debt from using Indonesian and

Malaysian palm oil as biodiesel stands at 610 Mg of CO_2 emissions per hectare per year that will take 423 years to repay.[88]

Although peatlands represent a mere 3 percent of the earth's land surface and freshwater, they store between 33 and 50 percent of terrestrial carbon, since each hectare of peatland stores between 3,000 and 6,000 tons of carbon, depending on the geochemistry, hydrology, and depth of the peatlands. Worldwide, peatlands cover over 400 million hectares, including 45 million hectares of undeveloped tropical peatlands; around 27 million hectares of the tropical peatlands are found in Indonesia, which have long been targeted for oil palm plantation establishment.[89] Draining peatlands and the conversion of the peatlands to oil palm plantations allow oxygen to penetrate deep and decompose the vast stores of carbon that was accumulated over thousands of years. Once in contact with oxygen, decomposition and oxidation of the organic matter and emissions continue, releasing over 4,300 tons of carbon dioxide equivalent per hectare over fifty years. The peat deposits in Indonesia and Malaysia are estimated to hold carbon that is equivalent to nine years of global emissions from fossil fuel use.

The amount of carbon-saturated peatland in Indonesia and Malaysia presages disaster for the global climate since these two countries are intent on doubling or tripling the area of drained peatland to serve European biodiesel producers. The emissions from these operations are projected to double or triple to between 5 and 7.5 percent of all global emissions, potentially locking in half of the annual emissions of today's total global emissions from land-use change.[90] This would render the proposed 450 ppm scenario as the stabilization point for global emissions a sheer figment of the imagination. Because the amount of carbon removal from the atmosphere largely depends on the rates of primary production and carbon storage, peatlands are critical players in these processes. Indeed, the amount of atmospheric carbon sequestered in peatlands is believed to have reduced global temperatures by up to 2 Celsius degrees (35.6 degrees F) in the past 10,000 years.[91] Since peatlands are accumulations of partially decomposed organic matter, buffered by permanent waterlogging and acidifying, disturbance of peatland ecosystems can have serious impact on climate change. When peatlands are drained for oil palm plantations, horticulture, and wood extraction, oxidation and decomposition of the organic matter accelerate, and when the organic matter is burned, the carbon stored in the peatlands is released into the atmosphere. This entails double jeopardy to the extent that huge amounts of carbon are released, while, at the same time, liquidation of the peatlands represents permanent loss of future carbon absorption.[92] The danger that deforestation of peatlands poses is conveyed by the 2 billion tons of CO_2 emissions a year from Asia. Of this amount, Indonesia accounts for 75 percent, associated with its massive conversion of peatlands to oil palm plantations. Taking the life cycle analysis of palm biodiesel into account, a ton of biodiesel produced on peatlands yields up to 25 tons of CO_2 emissions, which is five times the CO_2 emission from petroleum diesel.[93] In addition to removing aboveground vegetation, draining peatlands in preparation for palm plantations catalyzes oxidation and decomposition of organic matter, thereby increasing CO_2 emissions. For example, the total net emissions from peatlands with average depth of three meters could be as high as 6,000 Mg per hectare, per year, with a repayment period of 840 years.[94] For comparison, the carbon debt from soy biodiesel in Brazil amounts to 280 Mg of CO_2 emissions per hectare, per year, with a lesser repayment period of 320 years, whereas corn ethanol from newly cultivated grassland in the United States will entail a shorter repayment period of ninety-three years.[95]

Furthermore, the ecological debt associated with biofuel production is compounded by the enormous amounts of fossil fuels that biofuel production requires. According to biologist David Pimentel and chemical engineer Tadeusz W. Patzek, corn-based ethanol production takes 29 percent more fossil energy than the ethanol produced; producing ethanol from switchgrass takes 50 percent more fossil energy than the ethanol generated; producing lignocellulosic fuel from woody plants requires 57 percent more fossil energy than the ethanol produced; soybean-based biodiesel takes 27 percent more fossil energy than the biodiesel produced; and generating biodiesel from sunflowers takes 118 percent more fossil energy than the yield of biodiesel.[96]

Regardless of the enormous costs, biofuel producers are determined to oversell the benefits that could be had from the transition from fossil fuels, but they can do so only by hiding or ignoring the debt incurred by clearing forests and peatlands or converting cropland to bioenergy crops and plantations. Biofuels can never displace fossil fuels in such meaningful ways as to improve energy security or climate change. If the world meets its aspirational target of just 10 percent of global transportation biofuels by 2050, it will generate less than 2 percent of the world's net delivered energy. However, this pitifully insignificant level of biofuels would require 32 percent of the energy contained in all global crops produced in 2010 while, at the same time, widening the food gap between the haves and have-nots from 70 percent to 100 percent. If the world takes to heart the IEA's recommendation to secure 20 percent of global transportation fuels from bioenergy by 2050, it would require the conversion of not only the equivalent of all 2000's global crop production but also the total harvest of crops, grasses, crop residues, and trees.[97]

--- 5 ---

In Place of Conclusion: Can We Overcome the Planetary Emergency?

Can contemporary societies collectively halt late capitalism from slouching into ultimate self-destruction? Can we reverse the damages that have been done to our planet? Can resistance from below at least provide breathing room for the development of alternative ways of living? An interregnum, if you will, similar to that which helped prevent or slow down earlier capitalist depredations.

A previous such interregnum began during the progressive era in the United States and the anarchist, Marxist, and other social movements in Europe. In the end, these gave rise to three world-views: fascism, state welfarism, and communism. Fascism sought to resolve the deepening internal contradictions of capitalism through external aggression and acquisition of new territories, the object being access to natural resources and markets as the panacea for profound internal structural contradictions. State welfarism sought to resolve the same contradictions through an internal restructuring of capitalism, crafting a partial compromise between labor and capital: the New Deal in the United States and, later, the installation of the Keynesian welfare state in Western Europe.

The compromise between labor and capital through the triumph of Keynesian economics over neoclassical economics was made possible by four converging forces. First, the contradiction between the territorial logic of the state and the functional integration of the market acted as a brake on the drive toward widening and deepening globalization. Capital still had a sufficient degree of national character to make the bourgeoisie internally differentiated, as reflected in the conflict between domestic producers and marketers and those invested in multinational production and trade. The latter had not as yet acquired sufficient power to fully capture state institutions to serve their accumulation goals. Second, the sustained struggles waged in the West by revolutionary reformists and radical revolutionaries kept the pressure on the bourgeois state in ways that made elites worry about their own legitimacy if state institutions were to drift toward the right in defense of capital and at the expense of labor. The necessary precondition of the bourgeois state for the preservation of its legitimacy was to steer a middle course, so as not to be overtly associated with either capital or labor. By presenting itself as exterior to accumulation and, instead, as partner to both capital and labor in equal proportions, the state saw itself as a compromise-builder in the market between the excesses of capital and the demands of labor for a living wage; in Europe, they called this compromise the "social market." Third, the crystallization of unequal exchange, grounded in the historically constructed international division of labor between the industrial West and the colonial/neocolonial South, continued to moderate the capitalist contradictions by steering wealth creation and accumulation toward the Global North while, at the same time, subjecting billions of people in the Global South to further dispossession and immiseration. Fourth, the installation of Eurasian communism in the Soviet Union, and later in China, added another external dimension to the struggle against capital in the West, strengthening the pressure against the rise and consolidation of monopoly capital. By presenting capitalism as the root cause of all societal ills, communism saw the answer to the contradictions between capital and labor in total liquidation on a global scale, a paradigm of possibility that terrified the bourgeois state and forced it to extend some concessions to labor.

What happened subsequently is too obvious to rehash here, and the capitalism that had been forged with something of a human face in the form of Keynesian welfarism is gone. Now, the promoters and defenders of the most reactionary form of neoclassical orthodoxy orchestrate the domination and perpetuation of neoliberal globalism by transforming the bourgeois state into the key geoeconomic agent of accumulation by destruction and dispossession. This is the harsh landscape of the struggles that progressive forces face today.

To put it differently, the much-needed radical macrostructural transformation of capitalism requires a thoroughgoing reconstruction of counterhegemonic ideology, revolutionary politics, and dedication to the agitation, mobilization, and organization of the toiling masses to effectively confront what Stephen Gill termed the "new constitutionalism," which is imposed on human societies to ensure the domination of monopoly capital from above and thwart potential resistance from below:

> The new constitutionalism is the political/juridical counterpart to disciplinary neoliberalism. The latter is a discourse that promotes the power of capital through extension and deepening of market values and discipline under the regime of free a market to serve the interest of big capital. The central aim of new constitutionalism is to prevent future governments through precommitments from undoing constitutions, laws, and various institutional arrangements supportive of disciplinary neoliberalism. New constitutionalism redefines political limits of the possible now and the future. This is to contain challenges to neoliberalism through co-optation, domestication, neutralization and depoliticization of opposition. In sum, new constitutionalism is the political-juridical form specific to neoliberal processes of accumulation and to market civilization.[1]

Gill sees hopeful signs of resurgence of a "double moments" trajectory where the resistance to disciplinary neoliberalism from below is in the making. These hopeful signs are entailed by the spread of "countervailing political agency in the form of environmental, ethnic, feminist, and social movements challenging neoliberalism."[2] I share Gill's optimism to the degree that continuous accumulation through ecological destruction and human dispossession and exploitation cannot go on indefinitely under the bogus guise of poverty eradication, climate mitigation, and energy security without provoking contestation and resistance by those who bear the social costs of accumulation and domination. But the greatest challenge facing progressive forces today is how to refuel the resistance from below in such ways as to make it robust and cohesive enough to effect the radical macrostructural transformation of contemporary civilization.

The challenge of developing, executing, and refining robust modes of struggle against disciplinary neoliberalism would certainly require enormous coordination of efforts, extraordinary synchronization of actions, and unprecedented coherence of purposes on a global scale. These modes of struggle involve ideological, political, economic, and technical undertakings. When Barack Obama assumed the mantle of presidential power in 2009, armed with the "audacity of hope," millions of people nationally and internationally grew hopeful that the terms of the debate over the general state of our civilization were finally reframed in favor of poverty eradication, geoecological restoration, and climate change mitigation. The expected results failed to materialize, however, in part due to the powerful entrenchment of the corporate oligarchy and the temporary moderation of the contradictions of late capitalism in the Global North. This sobering reality suggests that the primary terrain of the struggle is in countries of the Global South where the untold material dispossession, social degradation, political suffocation, and ecological evisceration are occurring. Of the 1.3 billion agricultural workers worldwide who can supply the much-needed force for radical transformation, 1.28 billion, or 98 percent, are in the Global South. In Sub-Saharan Africa, 62 percent of the total workforce is engaged in agriculture. In South Asia, 51 percent of the population is engaged in agriculture, including about 129 million child laborers.[3] To be more explicit, if meaningful, durable, and sustainable macrostructural transformations are to occur, they must first occur in the Global South for the reasons that follow.

First, beginning with the imposition of the slave mode of production on Africa during the sixteenth century, the Global South was placed on a trajectory of accumulation by ecological destruction and human dispossession. Notwithstanding the manifold promises from decolonization, the green revolution, disciplinary neoliberal globalization, and the platitudinal pledges of Global North assistance, the Global South is stuck in permanent underdevelopment and abject poverty. Today, 70 percent of developing countries are net food importers, compared to the 1960s when they were net food exporters, enjoying a yearly average surplus of more than $7 billion. Today, Egypt and Brazil alone import 7.7 million and 7.3 million metric tons of wheat annually. This distorted relationship is a result of the imposition of structural adjustments on poor nations, accompanied by trade liberalization. Haiti, which used to be self-sufficient in rice production, offers a paradigm case. In 1994, the IMF forced the country, which consumes 200,000 metric tons of flour and 320,000 metric tons of rice annually, to open its market for food imports. Soon, subsidized U.S. rice flooded the Haitian market, driving out domestic rice farmers. Since the imposition of IMF conditionality, Haiti has imported 100 percent of its flour and 75 percent of its rice, all tied to secular international price fluctuations. Between January 2007 and January 2008, for example, the price for flour and rice went up by 83 and 69 percent, respectively.[4]

This Haitian experience is replicated throughout the Global South. Various studies indicate that 1.4 billion people, over 95 percent of them in the Global South, struggle to survive on less than $1.25 a day; in addition, another another 3 billion live on $1.26 to

$2 a day for a total of 4.4 billion people living on $2 or less a day. As a result, more than half of children under 15 years of age in undeveloped and emerging market countries live in poverty.[5] To put it differently, around 90 percent of the rural population in undeveloped countries struggle on less than $2 a day. The bottom 30 percent of the human population receive a mere 2 percent of global wealth.[6] This overwhelming material deprivation could foment the rejection of disciplinary neoliberalism in favor of radical macrostructural transformation. The scourge of hunger in the Global South that has been looming ever larger year after year is itself a sufficient condition to reject the offer of food assistance from the Global North or the eradication of poverty through biofuel production. In 1996, the UN family of organizations and governments promised to halve the number of hungry people by 2015; instead, the number of people in poverty has increased by a third since this declaration was made. This is not because of shortages in the availability of food, but because of the unequal distributon of resources or the lack of purchasing capability to access the food by the poor. Indeed, the food presently available in the world could feed the current human population one-and-a-half times over if purchasing capabilities were evenly distributed across nations and classes within nations.

In 1996, the Committee on World Food Security named four pillars of food security, considered foundational to promoting global equity in food consumption. The first pillar pertains to the availability of adequate amounts of food that must be produced and placed at people's disposal. The second pillar points to the necessity of access, to ensure that all households, and all individuals within those households, have sufficient resources to obtain appropriate foods for a balanced diet. The third pillar points to the indispensability of proper food utilization that allows the human body to ingest and metabolize food in ways that enhance healthy living and a comfortable social environment. The fourth pillar invokes the paramount importance of food stability to ensure the long-run maintenance of the other three pillars. Since these pillars were identified as critical, many writers have added environmental sustainability as a fifth pillar. True global food security requires that food production and consumption patterns do not deplete and degrade natural resources or the ability of the agricultural system to provide sufficient food for present and future generations. In order to have food stability, food crops and plants must receive sufficient rainwater or irrigation during growing seasons; soil degradation and pollution must be avoided; all natural ecosystems that are critical to the provision of pollination, wild foods, and natural pest controls must be protected and conserved; and meaningful climate adaptation and mitigation options must be explored in order to avoid or reduce the impact of climate change on food production.[7] Since the promised eradication of hunger has fizzled, the UN has again pushed back the goal date for ending global food insecurity to 2030. According to the International Labour Organization (ILO), this would require expenditures of $10 trillion between 2015 and 2030, supposedly flowing from the Global North to the Global South.[8]

The explanation for the prevalence of stagnant poverty and the lack of purchasing capabilities of the global poor is found in how capital accumulation in the Global South has steadily continued to refuel uneven development and uneven wealth accumulation in favor of the Global North. It thus should not come as a surprise that, in 2008, the average GDP per person in the twenty richest countries (all of them in the Global North) was $40,000 compared to a mere $1,000 per person in the 20 poorest countries (all of them in the Global South), a 40-to-1 ratio.[9] The only way out of this perpetual quagmire is through permanent or semipermanent divorce of the political economy of the Global South from that of the Global North.

What emerges is that the future survival of the 5 billion people who live in the Global South hinges on how nations and peoples respond to the wrenching levels of ecological destruction, human dispossession, and poverty, as well as to ecological disasters. There are no avenues to confronting these collective dangers other than robust and outright repudiation of disciplinary neoliberalism foisted by Global North corporations on the peoples in the Global South.

The starting point is agriculture, and for several reasons. Agriculture is still the basis of many economies in the Global South. Almost all agricultural workers are in the Global South. In most undeveloped countries, agriculture is responsible for between 30 and 60 percent of GDP and employs 65 percent of the labor force.[10] Additionally, 3.1 billion or 55 percent of the total population in the Global South, still live in rural areas where agriculture is the mainstay of their existence. Of this rural population, around 2.5 billion are in households directly or indirectly engaged in farming, including 1.5 billion in smallholder households. In other words, 2.6 billion people in the Global South derive their livelihoods from farming, representing 40 percent of the 2010 total world population.[11]

However, agriculture, as practiced today, is fraught with severe problems of hydroecological degradation and emissions. The sector is the largest cause of global biodiversity loss and ghg emissions: responsible for 9 percent of global carbon dioxide, 37 percent of methane, 65 percent of nitrous oxide, and 64 percent of ammonium emissions. The nitrogen pollution from agriculture is four times greater than the capacity of Earth's ecosystems to capture and sequester the nitrous oxide and ammonium pollution. Emissions of methane and nitrous oxide, which are 23 and 296 times more potent than CO_2, respectively, are particularly dangerous in their potency to thicken the atmosphere. Yearly methane and nitrous oxide emissions between 1997 and 2005 were 3.3 billion and 2.8 billion CO_2-equivalent metric tons, respectively, when their combined emissions increased by 17 percent with a projected further increase of 35 to 60 percent by 2030, largely driven by the intensification of livestock production and the increased use of synthetic nitrogen. It must be borne in mind here that, of the total global methane emissions, 60 percent comes from enteric fermentation. In fact, due to the rapid escalation of the shift to a Euro-American-style meat diet in the Global South, increases of emissions from enteric fermentation and manure management are projected to rise by 153 and 86 percent, respectively. In Latin America and the Caribbean, the cattle population increased from 176 million in 1961 to 379 million head by 2004, while the increases in the other livestock categories were in the range of 30 to 600 percent. So, the clearing of more and more native forests to make way for pasture and feedcrop production for biofuels in combination with enteric fermentation from ever growing livestock population present a clear and present danger.[12]

In the long run, the people who bear the brunt of the consequences of atmospheric degradation are in the Global South. The billions of people who live in the poor countries are most particularly vulnerable to a combination of weather-driven changes, dissipation of livelihoods, natural resource degradation, deprivation of access to land, commodification of common resources, and the growing food deficit and volatile international food prices. Taking into full consideration the foregoing description of modern agriculture-related problems, it stands to reason that only the complete restoration of agroecology can solve the appalling poverty, hunger, malnutrition, climate change-driven disasters, social degradation, poor health, and environmental spoliation. The arduous struggle facing the billions of people in undeveloped countries is how to reclaim the title to and knowledge about agroecology that was once thriving and sustainably managed before colonization and the dispossession and commodification of their natural resources. Farmers today can get out from under the yoke of the agribusiness-controlled global food manufacturing system, from the alienation of their natural entitlement, by repossessing what they have lost, and rediscovering their local knowledge and practices, enriched by harnessing scientific knowledge.[13] Fossil-dependent industrial agriculture, which uses ten times more energy than agroecology, is impracticable, unsustainable, and unsuitable for farmers who possess very limited land resources. Of the 525 million smallholders in the world, 404 million farmers grow their food crops on less than two hectares of land, usually under unfavorable biophysical properties and hydroecological conditions. The only way that these small farms can be sustainably operated is through the reconstitution of agroecological practices, preceded by repossession of the means of production. A broad range of surveys of 286 development intervention projects across 12.6 million hectares in fifty-seven poor countries, mostly in Asia and Latin America, showed that integration of natural pest management, natural nutrient management, agroforestry, aquaculture, water harvesting, and livestock increased average yields by 79 percent while, at the same time, increasing efficient water use and carbon sequestration, and reducing pesticide use, as well as protecting ecosystems and improving the provision of critical environmental services. A quarter of these projects reported yield increases of 100 percent. Additionally, pesticide use in 77 percent of the projects declined by 71 percent, while yields increased by 42 percent.[14]

Applying similar approaches to orphan crops such as sorghum, millet, barley, roots, and tubers, forty intervention projects in twenty African countries remarkably benefited 10.39 million families farming 12.75 million hectares with average harvest yields that more than doubled over a period of three to ten years, for a total achieved aggregate food production of 5.79 million metric tons per year. The trick was reliance on crop improvements through participatory plant breeding on hitherto ignored orphan crops, integrated pest management, soil conservation, and agroforestry and livestock integration.[15] Similarly, the application of agroecological farming practices in remote districts of Bangladesh showed impressive results, with benefits flowing especially to marginalized women. Vegetable and fruit production increased by 25–40 percent, rice harvest increased by 5–10 percent, livestock production rose by 30–40 percent, and fish production increased by 20–30 percent—and all these gains were achieved without reliance on synthetic agrochemicals.[16]

These agroecological farming practices openly militate against the global food manufacturing system that has hollowed out the livelihoods of billions of people. During the twentieth century, in parallel with the rapid expansion of capitalism, around 75 percent of plant genetic resources are believed to have disappeared, and one-third of currently existing genetic plants are projected to be gone in the next forty years. Indian farmers who used to grow 42,000 rice varieties were reduced to growing a few hundred varieties after the green revolution.[17] The disappearance of the treasure house of genetic plant diversity has, of course, been the result of the spread of the green revolution to the Global South. By narrowly focusing on hybrid wheat, rice, and maize, all dependent on large quantities of synthetic inputs, agribusiness accelerated the process of the homogenization of cereals. The promotion of genetic uniformity of crops was found amenable to centralization and concentration of production, and a source of quick profits. Synthetic fertilizers soon replaced natural organic matter, and pesticides replaced natural enemies of insect pests and weeds.

Today, a mere ten annual cereals, legumes, and oilseeds constitute 80 percent of the global food manufacturing system. Over 50 percent of world cropland is dedicated to just three cereal grains: rice, maize, and wheat, which account for 50 percent of daily calorie intake globally. Of the 80,000 plant species that have been historically identified as edible and nutritious, only about fifty are used as food sources; of these, just fifteen account for 90 percent of global food supply, with wheat, rice, and maize accounting for 60 percent of the total.[18]

The dominance of the capitalist global food manufacturing system has also orphaned many of the essential crops on which billions of people historically depended, because of the grossly distorted focus on a handful of crops that are deemed amenable to commercial centralization and concentration. As a result, orphan crops in the Global South receive no research attention, much less budget, even though twenty-five orphan crops in developing countries were in 2004 occupying more than 240 million hectares. In 2011, for instance, in Sub-Saharan Africa sorghum and millet (known to be climate-resilient and supporting tens of millions of people) occupied almost the same area as maize and wheat; yet UN institutions and a slew of philanthrocapitalist foundations poured tens of millions of dollars into the expansion of maize production, a grain that is known to be vulnerable to drought conditions.[19]

The narrowing of food grain species is compounded by the hollowing out of what environmental researchers Zareen Bharucha and Jules Pretty call the "hidden harvest" of wild plants, which never figure in official statistics. Wild plants and animal species constitute significant proportions of food for more than 1 billion people worldwide; 350 million people, including 60 million marginalized indigenous people, are dependent on these food sources for most of their dietary intake. At some point in human history, tens of thousands of wild plant species were used as food, and more than 1,000 consumable insects and nearly 1,100 edible wild fungi were important sources of food, protein, and income for millions of people. But these "hidden harvests" have been vitiated by the evisceration of forest ecosystems that provide habitat and forage to wild plants and animals. Forest ecosystems are seen in many localities as natural repositories of plant germplasm that can be directly used as food, medicine, or fodder, or that can be transplanted to family farms. In India, more than 600 wild plants are identified as having important nutritional value. In northeastern Thailand, one-fourth of the 159 wild food species that rice farmers have integrated into their food basket are collected from outside cultivated field boundaries, irrigation canals, swamps, and roadsides. Moreover, in the same region, 88 percent of the home gardens that communities nurture hold up to 200 wild species, in effect becoming conservation harbors for threatened wild species. Similarly, in Tanzania, communities recognize eighty-two wild plants as having multiple uses.[20]

The challenge facing farmers in the Global South today is how to bring back the crops and plant species that are being erased from the memory of farmers. The only way to build food security for billions of people against future ecological, hydrological, and meteorological change is through the reintroduction of the rich variety of crop and plant species that were a part of traditional cultivation.

Thanks to the emergence of intellectuals committed to public service in the last few decades, particularly in Latin America, agroecology as both a discipline and an advocacy has begun to challenge the global food manufacturing complex. As a discipline, agroecology seeks to integrate ecology and cultivation as compatible systems in accord with the laws of evolutionary biology and thermodynamics. In what follows, my purpose is not to rehash, but rather to make a solid case for agroecology as the only beacon of hope to overcome the specter of food insecurity that haunts billions of people.

First, traditional knowledge is the basis of agroecology. Even though organic agriculture (OA) and agroecology are complementary—some use the term interchangeably—the two concepts are not always identical. Agro-ecologist Steve Gliessman categorizes organic farming and agroecology into level 2 and level 3, respectively, with level 1 being conventional agriculture.[21] OA farms rely largely on an input substitution strategy. Using alternative inputs and practices for those used in industrial agriculture, OA incrementally seeks to replace external synthetic input-intensive and ecologically harmful practices and products with those that are derived from natural resources.[22] Even though OA farmers use biologically nitrogen-fixing cover crops, green manure, crop rotations, organic composts to replenish soil organic matter, large numbers of organic farmers are linked to the prevailing commercial market to purchase organic compounds. These conditions make OA food products expensive, accessible mostly to those who can afford to pay premium prices, which is why most of the market for organic farm products is in developed countries. Thus, OA is an adjunct to the global food manufacturing system. Agroecologists Peter Rosset and Miguel Altieri summarized the limitations of OA in these terms: "Organic farming, commonly viewed as a holistic concept, is now heavily commodified and embraced by capital. Publications directed at organic farmers are filled with advertisements for expensive biological pesticides, commercial compost, insectary-produced natural enemies, botanical extracts, microbial and other soil amendments, and the like. Natural food stores are now filled with almost as much processed food as ordinary supermarkets, except that the ingredients are "natural" or "organic," and less fiber has been discarded during their processing."[23]

Over the decades, the extent of organic farming has slowly but steadily moved up from 11 million hectares in 1999 to 43.1 million hectares in 2013, worked by 2 million producers, of whom two-thirds are in the Global South. The 2013 global market value of organic products was $72 billion, up from $15.2 billion in 1999. However, there are unreported areas of organic production that are not included in the above figures, such as wild food source collection areas—for native beekeeping, aquaculture, forest food gathering, and grazing areas. These areas occupy more than 35.1 million hectares. Thus, while OA areas represent 55 percent, non-agricultural organic areas for wild collection account for 43 percent of the nonconventional food production areas worldwide.[24] The weak link in OA is that organic farm operators do not directly challenge the neoliberal global food manufacturing complex. They seek separation, carving out a market niche for organic products within the existing structure.[25] Moreover, surrounded by giant agrochemical-dependent conventional farms, organic farms are vulnerable to pesticide spray drift and genetic contamination by pollen carried by wind.

In contrast to OA, agroecology is a peasant-based mode of cultivation without the use of input substitution, relying instead on ecological processes and natural resources, entirely betting on natural processes to furnish the required renewable nutrients. Steve Gliessman put it best: "Agroecology is more than a way to practice agriculture, such as organic or ecological production. Agroecology is also a social movement with a strong ecological grounding that fosters justice, relationship, access, resilience, resistance, and sustainability. Agroecology seeks to join together the ecological and social cultures that helped human society create agriculture in the first place."[26]

Agroecology seeks a holistic understanding of the dynamic interactions and relationships among all living things, including humans. To put it differently, agroecology seeks to integrate the fundamental ecological principles of sustainable scale, efficient allocation of natural resources, and social justice holistically. Through the application of ecological principles to the design, practice, and management of agriculture, agroecology seeks to mimic natural ecological conditions and processes in holistic manners. Even more important is that agroecology is a farmer-driven, bottom-up approach to diverse natural conditions in which agroecological farms are designed and managed to perform multifunctional needs, including the production of food, feed, fibers, biomass, and medicinal products, while also providing protection to biodiversity, landscape, and hydrogeological structures.

These natural conditions, internally generated inputs, and ecological processes are the essential conditions that make agroecology consistent with the principles of sustainable scale, allocative efficiency, and social justice, however they are measured. Studies indicate that organically nurtured agroecological farms sequester more than 8 metric tons of carbon per hectare compared with synthetic fertilizer-dependent conventional farms. Depending on regional variances and harvesting rates, agroforestry can sequester between 9 and 63 metric tons of carbon per hectare. Furthermore, agroecological farms use 30–70 percent less energy per unit of land compared with industrial agriculture, are more resilient to drought as they have better water holding capacity resulting from increased soil organic matter accumulation, and are more resistant to erosion and runoff during extreme rainfall.[27]

Contrary to corporate propaganda that agroecology is an anti-modern way of farming, agroecology seeks to simultaneously promote collective human welfare and the protection of the natural world through the full utilization of modern science. As a discipline, agroecology celebrates cumulatively received knowledge and seeks to enhance its social and ecological utility with insights from modern science in ways that are adapted to different local ecosystems and cultures. Agroecology is also essentially anti-monoculture, and as such, it is the cornerstone of in-situ conservation of diverse genetic materials and the preservation and circulation of indigenous knowledge. The degree of agroecological diversification is fundamentally what sets it apart from OA. In other words, agroecology puts the premium on ecologically-based intercropping of a diverse range of crop and plant varieties adapted to different local conditions, crop rotations, biological nitrogen-fixing legumes, a diverse range of pest-resistant crop varieties, integrated pest and weed management, agroforestry, and the integration of livestock with crops that supply nutrient-rich manure. By combining traditional local knowledge with modern science, the agroecological mode of production thus seeks to optimize water, nutrients, energy, and land use in conjunction with the management of natural biodiversity and water and nutrient conservation techniques in ways that build system resilience to extreme weather events and other abiotic stressors. Moreover, the manifold agroecological practices provide critical ecosystem services such as the provision of habitat and forage for myriads of pollinators, pest predators, clean water, biodiversity, carbon sequestration in soils and vegetation, groundwater recharge, erosion prevention, and flood protection.[28]

More important, agroecology directly challenges the green revolution and its new companion, the gene revolution, on economic, social, ecological, and political grounds. The negative externalities associated with the industrialization of agriculture are manifested in a cascade of deforestation, human dispossession, land degradation, soil salinization and acidification, overextraction of water resources, erosion of biodiversity, and air and water pollution from the overuse of agrotoxins. In this sense, agroecology has an ambiguous social and political context. It seeks to fight and replace the hegemony of the green/gene revolution, or at least seeks a divorce from it through the development of local and national food self-sufficiency.

While peasant communities are in the trenches to reclaim what naturally and historically belonged to them, intellectuals dedicated to public service are placing the power of their pen at the disposal of the oppressed. For the agroecologist scholar, this is a matter of social patriotism and solemn responsibility, something that invites the wrath of the biofuel-biotechnology industrial peddlers and the constellation of their satellites. The extolling of the productivity gains from the oversimplified monocrop green revolution, on the one hand, and the belittlement of the value of agroecology as romantic primitivism, on the other, are the weapons at their disposal. Proponents of the neoliberal global food manufacturing system are prompted to tell us that irrigated industrial agriculture produces 40 percent of world food grown on only 20 percent of arable land, while the rest of the food, produced on 80 percent of all arable land, represents a mere 60 percent of the total. What they do not tell us about are the differential costs associated with industrial monocultures vis-à-vis organic/agroecological production. To perpetuate their socially constructed myth, biofuel-biotechnology proponents rely on the fetishism of agricultural GDP, which measures only the benefits gained while utterly ignoring the costs externalized to nature and society, such as the cost of soil degradation, salinization, nutrient pollution, agrochemical contamination, biodiversity loss, eutrophication, and ghg emissions, all of which are associated with the green revolution. For example, the global use of synthetic fertilizer, responsible for 40 percent of the food increases during the period of the green revolution, rose by 350 percent between 1961 and 2002, from 33 million to 146 million metric tons.[29] What agricultural GDP does not count is how the use and overuse of synthetic fertilizer has resulted in unacceptable levels of environmental pollution and atmospheric degradation, expressed in soil and water acidification, contamination of surface and groundwater resources, eutrophication of coastal water bodies, devastation of coral reefs, and the exponential release of greenhouse gases emissions. As noted earlier, most of the reactive nitrogen used in industrial agriculture is lost to the biosphere, hydrosphere, and atmosphere. For example, it is estimated that rice and wheat take up a mere 18 to 49 percent of the synthetic nitrogen fertilizer applied, while the rest is lost to surrounding environments, with the concomitant pollution of rivers, aquifers, and coastal waters.[30] In China, less than 28 percent of the synthetic fertilizer used in industrial rice, wheat, and maize production is used up by the crops while the rest of the reactive nitrogen is lost to the environment.[31]

If we add the human cost from industrial agriculture, the cascading effects of industrial monocultures take on even more disturbing dimensions, which are not measured by GDP. Today, there are 162 million stunted or wasted children under five years old, 1.25 billion people live in absolute poverty, and 2 billion more people suffer from acute micronutrient deficiencies. Even in the United States, the largest food producer and exporter in the world, more than 31 million people are food insecure and hungry, relying on local and regional food banks to make it to the next day.[32] But to proponents of industrial monocultures, these human sufferings are simply the collateral damage of doing business.

There is also another important aspect of agroecological farms not captured by the fetishism of the GDP: traditional farmers frequently grow food crops within what is regarded as the main cash crop. In Latin America, farmers grow maize, cassava, and vegetables on small plots among banana trees, the products of which are consumed at home or circulated locally without being counted in GDP. As Brazil's former minister of the environment, Jose Lutzenberger, put it: "It is argued that the Indian peasants in Chiapas, Mexico, are backward, they produce only two tons of maize per hectare as against six on modern Mexican plantations. But this is only part of the picture. The modern plantation produces six tons per hectare and that's it. But the Indian grows a mixed crop. Among his corn stalks, that also serve as support for climbing beans, he grows squash and pumpkins, sweet potatoes, tomatoes and all sorts of vegetables, fruit and medicinal herbs. From the same hectare he also feeds his cattle and chickens. He easily produces more than 15 tons of food per hectare and all without commercial fertilizers or pesticides and no assistance from banks or governments or transnational corporations."[33]

Second, agroecology is the only alternative promising a trajectory of food security, pairing food sovereignty and ecological integrity. According to environmental researcher Jules Pretty and colleagues, small farmers in many developing countries have been able not only to increase quality food production but also to decrease the harmful effects of cultivation on the environment while improving the delivery of important environmental goods and services by adopting a resource-conserving mode of cultivation. Moreover, through agroecological farming that relies on the use of local resources, local control of production and distribution processes, and stewardship of local environment, farmers have been found to insure the multidimensionality of food security, including food availability, accessibility, dietary adequacy, and stability. Furthermore, the reliance on such local inputs as manure, compost, and organic fertilizers, rainwater harvesting, biological control, and the use of leguminous trees could guarantee farmers access to these local resources without the desperate need to beg for (but not likely receive) credit and/or state support.[34]

In a pathbreaking comprehensive evaluation of the benefits of an agroecological mode of production, biologist Catherine Badgley and colleagues show how the world could produce food from agroecological farms on existing cropland without the use of fossil-derived external inputs at a rate at least equal to or even greater than conventional food production, enough to feed more than 9 billion people. In an even more compelling vein, the researchers reckon that the world has more than enough renewable natural inputs to infinitely sustain agroecological production; even if legumes alone are used as green manures, they can furnish enough biologically fixed nitrogen to replace the entire quantity of synthetic nitrogen fertilizer in use today. After examining voluminous data, they reached the conclusion that the average yields from ecological farming could produce 30 percent more food per hectare than conventional agriculture, or 80 percent more food per hectare in developing countries than conventional agriculture.[35]

Moreover, numerous benefits could be derived from the adoption and expansion of the agroecological mode of production without causing environmental and atmospheric damages. To begin with, organic/agroecological farms are energy-efficient because they are not dependent on fossil fuels. Studies indicate that agroecological farms require between 21 and 32 percent less energy compared with industrial farms. Moreover, the use of manure and organic inputs make soils in agroecological farms more stable, whereupon erosion by water and wind is avoided. In eastern Washington State, researchers found that soil erosion by water and wind under OA farms was less than 75 percent compared with conventional agriculture where the loss of soil was three times higher. Moreover, because of the increased accumulation of soil organic matter content, agroecological farms were found to enhance soil structure and the consequent increases in water-holding capacity of the soil. Because agroecological farms do not rely on synthetic fertilizers, nitrous oxide emissions and nitrogen leaching are nonexistent or far lower than in conventional agriculture. Furthermore, soil microfauna populations, microbial biomass, and species richness and abundance are found to thrive more robustly on agroecological farms than in industrial agriculture.[36]

The development of national food security through the scaling out of the agroecological mode of production also has important macro effects on the national economy through the elimination or reduction of "food miles," defined as the distance between the origin of food production and the destination of its consumption. When Ethiopia imports wheat from North America or Europe, most of the money is paid to shippers and insurers. Once in ports, Ethiopia would have to use fossil fuel–guzzling heavy trucks to transport the wheat to different regions and localities of the country at enormous additional cost. Political economist Jennifer Clapp brought home this point when she analyzed the ultimate value of U.S. food aid reaching the intended recipients. According to her analysis, of the $100 million the United States extends to Ethiopia in food aid, only $35 million actually reaches the target population, while $65 million was paid to farmers, shipping and insurance companies. This applies to all imports. In effect, Ethiopia involuntarily subsidizes wealth accumulation in the Global North. By scaling up and scaling out national agroecological food production, Ethiopia could save tremendous resources that could be plowed back into the national economy in ways that would strengthen national food security, in the process contributing to climate change mitigation since the fossil fuel burned by the behemoth transport ships and tracks would be avoided.[37]

Cuba today stands out as a premier model of an agroecological mode of production, showing the pathway to food security and food sovereignty. Following the consolidation of the peasant revolution in the early 1960s, the development of fossil-based industrial agriculture, largely subsidized with Soviet aid, was central to the construction of Cuba's command economy. Before long, 30 percent of arable land in the island nation was dedicated to the monocultivation of sugarcane, which was responsible for 75 percent of foreign exchange earnings. Meanwhile Cuba was importing 57 percent of food and, with industrial agriculture in ascendance, importing 48 percent of fertilizers and 82 percent of its pesticides annually. However, Cuba's chemical-dependent monocultivation reached its outer limits by the 1980s, manifested in widespread soil degradation and acidification, propagation of pesticide-resistant pests, environmental pollution, and, eventually, the decline of yields of important crops such as rice.[38] Then, with the demise of the Soviet Union, and with it the Cold War, all chickens came home to roost as Cuba lost 85 percent of its trade relation, and became unable to import enough food to feed itself, or enough of the synthetic inputs, petroleum, and modern machinery to keep its industrial monoculture going. This presaged an erosion of the social legitimacy of the Cuban system.

However, as necessity is the mother of innovation, Cuba suddenly rediscovered first organic farming, relying on input substitution, such as biocide and biofertilizer, followed by agro-ecological integration as the answer to its chronic food shortages. The government encouraged and permitted its citizens to seek national food security through decentralization of agricultural production and the restoration of local autonomy and authenticity, although still within a system of national planning directed by the state. Cut off from subsidized synthetic fertilizer, pesticide, and petroleum inputs, Cuba's farmers embarked upon a massive conversion to agroecological farms. By 2011, the regime had returned 100,000 farms, covering nearly 1 million hectares, to peasant cooperatives and farmers.[39] With the partial restoration of localization of food production, farmers were prompted to recognize the value of reliance on solar and wind energy, biocontrol of insect pests, biological fixation of nitrogen, ecologically based crop rotations, and the use of crop residues, animal manures, legumes, green manures, and compost. By 2010, 64 percent of peasant farms used organic soil amendments, and 82 percent of the farms were practicing integrated ecological pest management.[40] As a consequence, between 1996 and 2005, Cuba's agricultural per capita growth was an impressive 4.2 percent compared with the regional average of 0.0 percent. Even though the peasant sector occupied a mere 25 percent of agricultural land in 2006, it nonetheless produced 65 percent of Cuba's food. Vegetable production increased by 145 percent by 2007 compared with the 1988 production level, notwithstanding the reduction of chemical use by 72 percent in 2007. Similarly, bean production increased by 351 percent with 55 percent less chemical application, and production of roots and tubers increased by 145 percent with 85 percent less agrochemical use over the same period. Even more impressive was the role of urban agriculture in the reassertion of food sovereignty in Cuba. In 2011, there were 383,000 urban farms, covering 50,000 hectares of previously unused land, which produced over 1.5 million tons of vegetables without the use of synthetic chemicals. These urban farms were supplying 70 percent of the fresh vegetables consumed in Cuba's major cities.[41]

The Cuban experience clearly demonstrates that the agrochemical-dependent green revolution is not the answer to national food security. Today there are no more areas suitable for large-scale irrigation and chemical-dependent farming systems left in the Global South. The best land and water resources are already monopolized by domestic and foreign accumulators in the global food manufacturing system. What is left are the fragmented and isolated small-scale peasant farms that are rain-fed, which are responsible for 60 percent of world food production, feeding 80 percent of people in the Global South. Thus, the relocation and re-nationalization of food security hinges on scaling up these rain-fed farms on the basis of agroecological redesign, research, and public support. The corporate supposition to eradicate poverty through biofuel production or the universalization of GM foods is smoke and mirrors.

Third, the agroecological mode of production is resistant to many climate biotic and abiotic changes. A combination of a diverse range of agroecological methods, including the adoption of multiple inter- and intra-specific crops and plants species, crop rotation, intercrop cultivation with biological nitrogen-fixing leguminous crops and plants, the use of manure, composts, and recycling of crop residues, is what makes agroecology climate sustainable in the long run. Even if some components of the system give in, others can withstand adverse ecological and climatological conditions. In other words, reliance on food crop and edible plant diversification allows farmers a wide latitude to grow a large variety of crops that respond differently to external changes and can thus be harvested at different times. This explains why farmers in the Andes used to plant up to fifty different varieties of potato on their fields, an approach also used by rice farmers in South and Southeast Asia. In Peru, farmers used to plant twenty-seven local varieties of maize from eleven different landraces, known for their distinguished boiling or parching qualities.[42]

The region where agroecology has been witnessing a strong revival is Latin America; of the 9 million hectares of agroecological farms found worldwide, 3 million hectares are located in Latin America, augmented by 6 million hectares of organic farms. Traditional farmers in the region had long ago discovered the integration of farms and the natural ecology as the cornerstone of good husbandry. Preservation of the forests adjacent to farms provides both food and suitable habitat to pollinators and natural enemies of insect pests, essential to farm productivity, and the continuous supply of organic nutrients in the form of litter, as well as protection against storms and extreme winds. In addition, conservation of the forests positively influences the microclimate of an area where farms are located. More important, maintenance of this integration of traditional farms with natural systems ensures preservation of crop and wild plant genetic resources, as well as local food self-sufficiency. In parts of Guatemala, for instance, farmers collect leaf litter from nearby forests and spread it on their farms regularly, which enhances accumulation of organic matter and improves water retention and soil aeration.[43] Falling back on the paramount importance of the multifunctionality of agroforestry, coffee growers in Latin America are using agroforests that commonly contain both annual and perennial plant species to protect the coffee trees against the elements. The agroforests also produce livestock feed, fuel, food, timber, fruit and compost material, and reduce soil erosion, while providing pollinators, insect predators, birds and other beneficial animals with suitable habitat and essential nutrients. Agroforestry around shade-grown coffee has been found to reduce microclimate and soil moisture variability. Shade-grown coffee farms, well protected by such complex agroforestry systems, are found to be higher in yields and superior in quality compared with yields of sun-grown coffee.[44]

Another invaluable lesson we derive from traditional farming systems is the way that traditional farmers manage weeds. In parts of Mexico, indigenous communities developed a very sophisticated classification of non-crop plants into bad and good ones. While the bad weeds are removed manually, the good weeds are preserved as essential nutrition providers and protection against insect pests, thereby improving organic matter accumulation and soil productivity while simultaneously providing invaluable items that are used as supplementary food, medicine, teas, and ceremonial resources. These edible weeds are invaluable, especially in times when bad weather and other extreme events affect harvest of crops.[45] In rural southern Africa, indigenous fruits contribute approximately 42 percent of the natural food-basket. In addition to providing essential vitamins and other much needed micronutrients, rural households rely on these sources of food during lean years as well.[46]

The agroecological mode of production in Latin America has also shown remarkable resilience and resistance to adverse weather events. In the aftermath of Hurricane Mitch, which hit Central America with ferocity, a comparative study was carried out in Nicaragua, Honduras, and Guatemala on 1,804 agroecological and conventional farms occupying the same geoecology, with the purpose of assessing the difference in the effect of the hurricane on the diversified agroecological farms in relation to conventional monocropping farms. The finding pleasantly confirmed the superiority of diversified traditional farms in their capacity to withstand adverse weather-related events, and other biotic and abiotic stressors. This was due to diversification practices that involve the judicious use of agroforestry, intercropping, and cover crops. The result was that the agroecological farms suffered much less damage from the hurricane than their neighboring conventional monocropping farms. Moreover, the diversified agroecological farms were found to have up to 40 percent more topsoil, 69 percent less gully erosion, and greater soil moisture, and experienced much lower economic losses compared to the adjacent conventional farms. The difference lay in creative traditional knowledge about the value of using rock bunds, green manure, crop rotation, ditches, terraces, barriers, organic mulch, legumes, polycultures, agroforestry, and reduced tillage. This unambiguously demonstrates that agroecological practices strongly correlate with higher resistance of diversified farms to extreme events.[47] In addition to the provision of dependable food production, agroecology also substantially reduces ghg emissions because it does not rely on fossil inputs.

Fourth, agroecology is compatible with soil biology, chemistry, and physiology. Reliant on biochemical and biophysical processes, organic material-rich soil is the basis of sustainable agroecology. In two successive publications, University of Illinois scientists established the adverse relationship that exists between soil health and the use of synthetic nitrogen. Indeed, twenty years before the University of Illinois findings, the renowned soil specialist John Reganold and his colleagues had demonstrated the superiority of agroecological farms over conventional agriculture in their research in the Palouse region of eastern Washington State. Like most American farmers, farmers in this region were excited by the quick results they saw in the petroleum industry's entry into American agriculture. They were prompted to purchase synthetic chemicals, tractors, and fossil fuels and converted their organic farms into industrial farms in the 1950s. Three decades later, the farmers found themselves disillusioned with industrial agriculture. To begin with, the tractor-driven tillage exposed the fertile soil of the region to unprecedented rates of erosion by water and wind. By the late 1970s, 10 percent of the cropland in the Palouse region witnessed 100 percent removal of the topsoil, while another 60 percent of the cropland lost 25 to 75 percent of the topsoil to erosion. In addition, along with the topsoil, synthetic fertilizer and pesticides were washed down into rivers, lakes, and ocean.[48]

The Palouse region is one of the most fertile regions in the country in terms of soil productivity, but the topographic conditions are not conducive to industrial agriculture because the rolling hills and loose soil make the area vulnerable to erosion. The average erosion rate in Palouse is 14.1 tons per acre per year compared to the national average of 8.1 tons. Without understanding this essential feature of the landscape, farmers converted their holdings to conventional farms, dependent on synthetic fertilizer. After three decades of experience with conventional farming, farmers discovered that their holdings were less productive, and researchers confirmed that synthetic nitrogen-dependent conventional farming and tractor-based deep plowing were implicated in the growing soil impoverishment. The study also revealed that the annual erosion rate from organic farms was 3.3 tons per acre, well below the tolerance level of 5 tons set by the Department of Agriculture, not to mention the annual average erosion rate from conventional farms of 13 tons per acre. Moreover, the thickness of the rich topsoil on organic farms was 2 feet deep, whereas it was up to 10 inches thinner on conventional farms. The difference lay in the fact that organic farmers relied on natural conditions to conserve soil with the use as green manure. Green plants or legumes are grown and then plowed back into the soil, simultaneously providing biological fixed nitrogen and protection against erosion by water and wind. As a result, the organic farms were found to have higher organic matter content, thicker topsoil depth, and higher polysaccharide, or complex sugar content, and thus higher moisture retention capacity and less soil erosion compared with conventional farms.[49]

The Palouse situation negates the one-size-fits-all recipe of the green revolution. To be sure, food security resides in the compatibility between local ecological context and the food system, one that integrates ecological resilience, social equity, preservation of agrobiodiversity, less soil disturbance, diverse crop rotation, and a locally focused mode of existence. The health of soil is measured by the richness of the diversity and abundance of its biological life and organic matter, and by its resilience and resistance to outbreaks of soil-borne pests.[50] What distinguishes agroecology from industrial agriculture is its reliance on having nutrient-enriching plants, a wide range of pest-resistant crop varieties, routinely practicing crop rotations, intercropping, biological control of pests, insect predators, pollinators, nitrogen-decomposing bacteria, soil-aerating and soil-fertilizing earthworms, and myriad biological soil-activating microbes.[51] As a consequence, agroecology maintains and enriches soil health by relying on natural sources of plant nutrition and organic matter from manure and nitrogen-fixing crops, shrubs, and trees without polluting soil, air, and natural water systems while avoiding salinization and acidification of soil and nitrate contamination of water that are imminent consequences of synthetic agrochemical use. Agroecological farmers boost crop yields by restoring soil health and by controlling insect pests by protecting their natural enemies rather than destroying them through the indiscriminate spraying of crops with toxic pesticides. Pesticides kill not only insect pests, but also their natural enemies, not to mention the harm they cause to farmers themselves and to the environment. Under agroecological conditions, insect pests are kept at bay through the suppression of pathogens through crop rotation, through inter- and intra-specific crop cultivation and enhancing crop and plant diversity, and by managing the types and quality of nutrients in ways that thwart pathogen reproduction.[52] In East Africa, up to $10 billion worth of maize production was often eaten by the tenacious pest known as a stem borer, threatening the livelihoods of 100 million Africans. But now farmers are benefiting from the discovery of a local weed, called napier grass; by planting the grass in rows between the maize and along the edges of their maize fields, farmers lure the stem borer to the grass where it becomes trapped by a sticky substance produced by the grass and dies. As a result, maize yields on such farms increased by 70 percent. Moreover, farmers could harvest the napier grass and sell it as animal fodder, generating additional income.[53]

Although practicing conservation tillage, crop diversification, legume intensification, crop rotation, intercropping, and biological pest control enhance the productivity, resilience, and resistance of agroecological farms, industrial agriculture suffers from continual degradation, salinization, and pollution of soils because of toxic agrochemical use. It is true that synthetic fertilizer increases yields in the short run, but in the long run the continual application of the fertilizer in increasing magnitudes degrades the soil. In contrast, organic nitrogen sources not only take on stable form under agroecology but also enhance the building of soil organic matter, which obviates the need to add new nitrogen sources each year in order to maintain yields.[54]

Another farming method compatible with agroecology is "no-till." Smallholder farmers can optimize the health and productivity of soil by retaining sufficient quantity of vegetation on their farms. In addition to providing soil protection, retaining sufficient crop residues along with sufficient natural vegetation on the soil surface increases water infiltration, promotes water conservation through evaporation prevention and reduction of runoff. Additionally, no-till farming has been found to increase soil carbon sequestration as non-harvested residues and roots are converted to soil organic matter. No-till farming also requires 50 to 80 percent less fuel compared to industrial agriculture.[55]

In Tanzania, for example, after small farmers started growing mixed crops of maize, beans, and pigeon peas by directly depositing the seeds into holes without plowing the land, retaining surface mulch, removing weeds manually without the use of herbicide, and using livestock manure as soil amendment, the average yields of maize increased from 1 metric ton to 6 metric tons per hectare.[56] Similarly, in the highlands of central Mexico, farmers increased maize yields by 30 percent under no-till, with rotation of crops and use of residues as soil cover. Similarly, in the Indo-Gangetic Plain, 620,000 farmers on 1.8 million hectares increased their average income by $180 to $340 per farm after adopting no-till; the gains resulted from avoiding the cost of fossil fuels and agrochemicals.[57] Latin American farmers have begun to increasingly use reduced tillage to increase both crop productivity and ecological protection. In Brazil, the areal extent of farms under minimum-till systems covered 15 million hectares as of 2001; in Argentina, the farms under no-till increased from 100,000 hectares in 1990 to 11 million hectares in 2001.[58]

The fifth reason the agroecological mode of cultivation succeeds in the Global South is that there is a built-in buffer against hydrological variability. Water is a determinant factor in crop productivity in any form of farming. In Asia, the yields of rice grown on irrigated paddies were found to average 5 metric tons per hectare compared to only 2.3 metric tons per hectares grown on rain-fed lowland rice fields.[59] As noted earlier, the great challenge facing farmers today is that, of the approximately 1.4 billion hectares under cultivation worldwide, around 80 percent (or 60 percent of total agricultural output) is rain-fed and thus vulnerable to weather variability. Only 35 to 50 percent of the precipitation falling on farms is taken up by the crops, with the rest lost to runoff or evaporation.[60] Since areas of irrigation are hard to come by, the challenge facing small farmers, particularly in arid and semi-arid regions, is how to grow crops that are adapted to hydrological fluctuations. In many regions of Asia and Africa, indigenous cultivators have, over the centuries, identified and domesticated crop varieties that are adapted to diverse climatic conditions. Most of these crops, such as barley, millet, and sorghum, are orphan crops, neglected by agribusiness, governments, and philanthrocapitalist donors because they do not readily lend themselves to centralization and concentration, and hence to accumulation. However, the future hope to feed the world, especially in the Global South, hinges on the rearticulation of efforts and research funds to strengthen orphan crops through the promotion of agroecology. Crops of the orphan varieties grown in rain-fed environments are known for their capacity to exploit moisture stored in the root zone, something that suggests that rain-fed agroecological farms can perform well by adopting and expanding deep-rooting crops in rotation, increasing the water storage capacity of soil, facilitating water infiltration, and lessening evaporation through organic mulching—functions that take on paramount importance in the context of a changing climate and growing water scarcity.[61]

One exciting area of research is the possibility of integrating perennial grain crops into modern agriculture. Using both direct domestication of wild plants and hybridization of existing annual crop plants with their wild relatives, plant breeders have in recent years initiated research to develop wheat, sorghum,

sunflower, intermediate wheatgrass, and other species as perennial grain crops. In fact, of the 13 grain and oilseed crops widely
grown today, 10 are considered capable of hybridization with their
perennial relatives.[62] Were this to materialize, the food security of
billions of people, most particularly in the Global South, could be
securely placed on a promising trajectory. In contradistinction to
annuals, which must be sown or planted every season, perennials
live for many years once sown or planted. Indeed, before human
intervention transformed the landscape of food production in
favor of annuals, mixtures of perennial plants used to dominate
the earth's landscapes. Even today, over 85 percent of the native
plant species found in North America are perennials.

There are more than 220,000 species of seed-bearing plants on
the planet, occupying every habitat type across wide spectra of
plant morphologies and sizes, all with the potential to transform
global agriculture in revolutionary ways.[63] Because annuals like
wheat, rice, maize, and soybeans have shallow roots and live only
until harvest time and are productive only with the continual addition of synthetic inputs, the landscapes they occupy are susceptible
to erosion, loss of soil fertility, degradation, and desiccation. To
make up for inherent problems stemming from the conversion of
the natural conditions to industrial farming, farmers rely on synthetic inputs and irrigation in ever greater quantities, which in
turn result in more nitrogen leaching, water contamination, and
ghg emissions. The incorporation of perennials into the contemporary food production system can solve many of these problems,
reducing erosion, improving water infiltration, building soil
carbon, promoting resiliency to drought, and resistance to insect
pests and diseases. Because most perennials have roots that exceed
two meters of depth, they are naturally equipped with the capacity
to regulate water flow, retain moisture, and regulate carbon and
nitrogen cycling. Studies indicate a fivefold reduction in water loss
and a 35-fold reduction in nitrate loss from soil planted with alfalfa
and mixed perennial grasses compared with soil under corn and
soybean production. Moreover, because of deeper roots, coupled

with a longer growing season, perennials are efficient carbon stor-
ers, a function that lends itself to increasing soil organic matter by
no less than 50 percent compared with annual-cropped fields. In
addition, since perennials are not replanted every year, there is less
tillage, soil disturbance, and use of heavy machinery, and little or
no synthetic inputs, and therefore little or no compaction, fewer
emissions, and fewer contaminations. Furthermore, perennials
are said to be more adaptable to long-term cultivation on erodible landscapes where annuals cannot become productive without
heavy doses of agrochemicals and huge quantities of water. In
China, India, and Malawi, for example, farmers who grow perennial pigeon peas on steep slopes consider them important food
crops and sources of biologically fixed nitrogen. Simply put, deep-
rooted perennials capture, store, and use more rainwater more
efficiently, whereas the short-lived and short-rooted annual crops
lose more water along with soil nutrients. Moreover, the role of
perennials in climate mitigation appears significant. It is estimated
that the magnitude of soil carbon sequestered under perennial
crops is on the order of 320 to 1,100 kilograms per hectare per year
compared with 0 to 450 kilograms under annual crops.[64]

The new research front on perennials is certainly promising.
However, domestication and hybridization of perennials requires
patience and persistence, and the flow of research funding is
currently wanting. Global North governments and agribusiness
corporations have hitherto shied away from dedicating resources
to this promising sector because they do not see the potential for
commercial concentration of production of perennials in ways that
would allow them to establish monopoly control. Furthermore, the
potential food security and independence of nations in the Global
South through the expansion of perennials is seen as contrary to
accumulation by dispossession. So the pioneering researchers are
attached to small citizen-supported research organizations such as
the Kansas-based Land Institute. It is no accident that agribusiness corporations annually pour tens of billions into feedstock
and biofuel research and production, while the aggregate global

investment in agroecology is less than 2 percent.The fraction of research resources dedicated to perennial grain crops is even more minuscule, barely reaching $1.5 billion. On the other hand, governments everywhere squander hundreds of billions on subsidizing conventional agriculture, courtesy of taxpayers. In 2012, the agricultural subsidies of the top 21 food-producing countries in the world stood at a whopping $486 billion, representing 80 percent of the global agricultural value-added; OECD countries alone spent $258.6 billion subsidizing their conventional farms.[65]

Agroecological farmers can also mitigate the effect of climate change through rainwater harvesting, flood diversion approaches, and supplemental irrigation in ways that contribute to groundwater recharge and reduce losses of soil and plant nutrients through erosion. In arid and semi-arid parts of West Africa, farmers build barriers around their farm fields using stones that help capture and retain rainwater, thereby replenishing water tables, improving soil moisture, and decreasing soil erosion. As a result, soil water retention capacity has increased by up to tenfold, and biomass production up to twentyfold, while livestock also benefits from grazing on grass grown between the stones.[66] Similarly, in Kenya, communities significantly improved their livelihoods through the construction of double-dug beds in their gardens to grow vegetables. These double-dug beds are regularly treated with animal manures and organic composts, improving their water-holding capacity, making them productive even during periods of lower precipitation. The vegetables and pulses grown in these beds include kale, onion, tomato, cabbage, passion fruit, pigeon peas, spinach, pepper, green bean, and soya. More than 75 percent of the households engaged in this practice were found to be free from hunger throughout the year, and the number of households that previously had to buy vegetables from the local market declined from 85 percent to 11 percent. Kenyan women particularly turned out to be the principal beneficiaries of these practice. After constructing twelve double-dug beds on her farm, Joyce Odari found her farm to be so productive that she hired four young men, thus creating jobs for others. She expressed her exhilaration in these terms: "If you could do your whole farm with organic approaches, then I'd be a millionaire. The money now comes looking for me. My aim is to conserve the forest, because the forest gives us rain. When we work our farms, we don't need to go to the forest. This farming will protect me and my community, as people now know they can feed themselves."[67]

Rainwater harvesting involves water conservation in ways that capture and store the rainwater in the root zone of the soil structure for subsequent uptake. For instance, in semi-arid parts of Niger, peasants and agropastoralists grow sorghum and millet on sandy and loamy soils by ingeniously harvesting rainwater and rehabilitating degraded lands. The technique involves digging holes that are shaped like small ridges with soils to capture rainwater. At the start of the rainy season, seeds are directly deposited into the peats, which are fertilized from time to time with manure that enriches the soil and improves water infiltration.[68] In Burkina Faso, a contingent of youth travel from village to village to show farmers land rehabilitation techniques through planting pits and build rock walls and half-moon structures. These techniques have become so successful that farmers can buy degraded lands knowing full well that they can rehabilitate them. In central Burkina Faso, rainfall is so precarious that cereal yields scarcely exceed 300 kg per hectare; but farmers who use the rainwater harvest technique can now produce 700–1,000 kg per hectare, transitioning from a net food deficit of 650 kg to a 150 kg grain surplus. It is no coincidence that over 3 million hectares of previously degraded land in these countries were productively rehabilitated as of 2010.[69]

Another creative form of managing the impact of rainfall fluctuation involves irrigation through harvesting surface runoff. The rainwater stored in ponds, tanks, and contained spaces is used in the critical stages of crop and plant growth, such as during the early grain development or flowering period. Supplemental irrigation does not replace rainfall; it simply augments it in the event of sudden cessation or delay of rainfall. Farmers in Ethiopia harvest runoff and floodwater from seasonal rivers and streams by using temporary stone and earth embankments; then they use hand-dug canals to distribute the water to their vegetables and fruits. In other regions of the Global South, farmers create large ponds to capture rainwater and runoff. This way, they can control the timing of water application, especially during the critical stages of crop or plant growth. In Iran, farmers increased yields of barley from 2.2 to 3.4 metric tons per hectare with just a single application of supplemental irrigation. Similarly, Syrian farmers have been able to double the size of their wheat fields and to increase total production by one-third through the ingenious use of supplemental irrigation.[70]

The growing popularity of agroecology, the spread of peasant-based social movements, and pro-farmer scholarship have begun to unnerve agribusiness and their sponsors and defenders. From a corporate perspective, the farmer-driven scaling-out of agroecology presents the long-term potential of delinking agriculture in the Global South from the corporate-controlled global manufacturing system. This could happen in two crucial ways. First, the anti-synthetic input and anti-GM nature of agroecology could potentially dry out the market for synthetic fertilizers, pesticides, and genetically engineered seeds, depriving TNCs of access to lucrative sources of profit. Second, relocalization of food production and national food security could potentially wean countries in the Global South from dependency on food imports from the Global North, a condition that could deepen the crisis of grain surplus that has long haunted the global grain-trading corporations. The course corporations have chosen is to rely on the age-old adage that the easiest way to capture a fortress is from within. Thus, bilateral and multilateral institutions as well as philanthrocapitalist foundations, including the USAID, the Canadian International Development Agency, the FAO, the World Bank, the Global Forum on Agricultural Research, the European Conservation Agriculture Federation, and the Rockefeller, Ford, Gates, and Clinton Foundations have joined the platform of agroecology, though always under the guise of promoting food security, water and bio-diversity conservation, soil carbon sequestration, reduction in soil ghg emissions, and climate adaptation and mitigation. To do so, agribusiness adroitly mixes organic farming, conventional agriculture, and GM monocropping into a single package, nourished by high synthetic agrochemicals. These anti-agroecology forces never run out of subterfuges. Their recent stratagems to co-opt agroecology include "sustainable intensification of agriculture," or "global climate-smart agriculture," and no-till farming. To build the road to agroecology, President Barack Obama laid the first stones in July 2009, when he announced at the Rome G8 Summit a commitment of $3.5 billion over a three-year period to supposedly accelerate agricultural productivity and to improve nutrition and food security in undeveloped countries. The creation of the Feed the Future Initiative in 2010 was then marketed as the implementation organ. Soon thereafter, another G8 Summit announced the collection of $22 billion from industrial countries for the purposes outlined by President Obama.[71]

Of course, the international initiatives are embroidered with glossy terms such as the inclusion of smallholder and poor farmers, the promotion of food security, and issues of gender and the environment as the primary focus of the collective efforts. But the devil is in the details: the U.S. Feed the Future Initiative, which focuses on nineteen poor countries, makes it explicit that the final decision regarding policies, strategies, priorities, and allocation of funds rests with the donor country, not the recipient targets. Moreover, according to USAID guidelines, Feed the Future investment priorities must be on agricultural projects that have potential to achieve lasting and large-scale impacts that can be easily expanded beyond any Feed the Future operation; that the United States must work in collaboration with host governments, international and regional development organizations, and philanthrocapitalist foundations in order to maximize its influence; that agricultural policies must be consistent with the need to promote the adoption of innovations in agricultural technology; that there must be strategic coordination at the national, regional, and global levels as well as among donors and private investors in order to improve governance and resource allocation, meaning along the lines of neoliberalism; that the role of multilateral institution must be enhanced in order to strengthen their effectiveness in ensuring the alignment of priorities and approaches with neoliberalism; and that priority must be placed on countries that present strong opportunities to foster regional trade and development corridors, integrate markets, accelerate regional growth, and play a major role in regional market integration. In a nutshell, "sustainable intensification of agriculture" is the expansion of industrial agriculture to agroecology through the use of a combination of technologies, known management practices, and high inputs of fertilizer, pesticides, new seed varieties, irrigation, energy, and access to markets. To achieve these objectives, the USAID claims to have spent $4.7 billion from 2010 to 2014, and other U.S. federal government agencies claim to have spent $6.6 billion under Feed the Future program during the same period.[72]

Similarly, the EU has actively supported the U.S.-driven "sustainable intensification of agriculture" ploy. The EU defines "sustainable intensification" in more frank terms by incorporating the development and diffusion of genomic selection, genetic engineering, precision farming, ecotechnologies, and biotechnologies into a single package.[73] The largest mimicker of the U.S. stratagem has been by the UK, which doubled its agricultural donations for purposes of promoting sustainable intensification in the Global South to 188 million pounds. The favorite ally in subterfuge for governments is the Washington-based Consultative Group for International Agricultural Research (CGIAR), home of fifteen research institutions, the brainchild of the Rockefeller and Ford Foundations, which is tasked to promote agricultural research in the Global South. To strengthen its role in the implementation of the sustainable intensification subterfuge, the amount of funding that the CGIAR was receiving increased from $465 million in 2005 to $696 million in 2010, and is projected to rise to $1.6 billion by 2025. In 2010, the top five contributors to its budget were the United States, the Gates Foundation, the World Bank, the UK, and the EU. In 2010, the CGIAR used some portion of the donations to join the Gates Foundation in launching a $70 million sustainable intensification project in Africa, including virus-resistant wheat, GM rice, new drought-tolerant maize varieties, and stress-tolerant GM legumes. This was an opportune moment for the Gates Foundation, which views Africa as a blank slate for trying out new bio-innovations. Between 2005 and 2011, for example, the Gates Foundation reportedly spent $172 million on farming projects, which included GM technologies like drought-tolerant maize for Africa, other stress-tolerant GM crops, and the promotion of plant-breeding and biotechnology research. Furthermore, in February 2012, the UN International Fund for Agricultural Development (IFAD) and the Gates Foundation announced the formation of a partnership to promote sustainable intensification through the propagation of biotechnologies such as the Water Efficient Maize for Africa project and the Africa Biofortified Sorghum. To these and similar projects, the Gates Foundation and IFAD donated $200 million in partnership with DuPont, Syngenta, Monsanto, Cargill, the International Life Science Institute, and Croplife International, among others.[74]

With such encouragement from officialdom, the Agricultural Biotechnology Council—representing the major biotech corporations including BASF, Bayer CropScience, Dow AgroSciences, Monsanto, DuPont, and Syngenta—welcomed sustainable intensification as another convenient weapon to stultify the surge in the agroecological mode of production. The council states: "Biotechnology is one of the tools which farmers can use to achieve sustainable intensification."[75]

Noticing the momentum of agroecology, the FAO also woke from a sixty-year hibernation in September 2014 to hold the first symposium ever on agroecology, in Rome, attended by 400 participants from thirty countries. Characteristically, the agency steered a middle course, offering both proponents and opponents of agroecology what they wanted to hear. In a booklet etitled *Save and Grow: A policymaker's guide to the sustainable intensification of smallholder crop production*, the UN agency had already favorably rehearsed what proponents of agroecology have been saying for quite some time regarding the benefits of agroecology. On the other hand, it highlights the importance of mixing synthetic fertilizers, pesticides, and biotech innovations with naturally provided nutrients to maximize production through sustainable agriculture. Rehearsing what it had been saying for two decades, the FAO argued that food production in the Global South must double in the future to keep pace with population rise, as well as reduce hunger, malnutrition, and food insecurity, and that this can be done only through the properly balanced combination of fertilizers, pesticides, irrigation, and natural conditions of cultivation, as well as the use of molecular biology, biotechnology, and genetic modification. Once again, the FAO chose to strike the sack for fear of the donkey, as the German proverb goes, by avoiding confronting the roots of the problem, namely, the prevailing mode of primitive accumulation by dispossession and maldistribution of national and global wealth. For example, the FAO bemoans the fact that the world today produces 2,000 more calories per capita per day than the current world population consumes while leaving 1.25 billion people hungry and malnourished and another 2 billion suffering from nutrient deficiencies. Since the 1960s, annual global production of cereals, coarse grains, roots and tubers, pulses, and oil crops has risen from 1.8 billion metric tons to 4.6 billion metric tons; yet the number of hungry and malnourished people kept growing as the world had more people in absolute poverty in 2010 than in the 1960s.[76] Notwithstanding this indictment of the prevailing neoliberal mode of domination, the FAO turned around and warned that food production in the Global South must increase by 100 percent in the future through "sustainable intensification of agriculture" in order to feed everyone. Indeed, two broad fundamental questions leap out from this contradictory FAO lamentation: If the world has abundant food surplus today, why can't the world feed the 1.25 billion indigent people? And even if we assume that food production in the Global South will increase by 100 percent by 2050 because of sustainable intensification of agriculture, how do we know that the food surplus will go to feed the indigent? These are questions of the twenty-first century awaiting answers before co-opting agroecology by another name.

As though the sustainable intensification ruse is not enough, on September 23, 2014, more than twenty governments and thirty-five-plus organizations announced with huge fanfare the formation of the Global Alliance for Climate-Smart Agriculture. The declared intent is the transformation of the 500 million small farmers in the Global South to climate-smart farmers by 2030 through speedy extension of foreign expertise, evidence-based practices, technological innovations, the creation of enabling conditions for foreign private investment, and the promotion of public-private partnerships. From GACSO's (Global Association of Corporate Sustainability Officers) mission statement: "The Global Alliance will enable governments and other stakeholders to make these transformations in ways that bridge traditional sectoral, organizational and public/private boundaries. It will broker, catalyze and help create transformational partnerships to encourage actions that reflect an integrated approach to the three pillars of climate-smart agriculture, as well as synergies between them. The pillars include sustainable improvements in productivity, building resilience, and reducing and removing greenhouse gases. The partnerships will inspire the development and dissemination of innovative, evidence-based options for climate-smart agriculture in different settings, and will involve a broad range of government and other stakeholders."[77]

The document they produced is so burdened by glossy jargon that it requires considerable effort to unravel the hidden agenda, which is the extension of industrial agriculture to the realm of agroecology and the complete dispossession of traditional farmers, who are seen as the remaining obstacles to the totalization of the global food manufacturing system. The composition of membership of this fuzzy ad hoc group gives away its intent: the list of the 124 GACSO members as of January 2016 includes Kellogg's, McDonald's, Yara (the world's largest fertilizer manufacturer), Syngenta, Walmart, Global Biotechnology Transfer Foundation, the Fertilizer Institute, Global Forum for Innovations in Agriculture, International Fertilizer Development Center, Koppert Biological Systems BV, Mosaic Company, University of Missouri, National Center for Soybean Biotechnology, Inter-American Development Bank, the World Bank, Fertilizers Europe, World Business Council for Sustainable Development, International Fertilizer Industry Association, Agricultural Model Intercomparison and Improvement Project, Bioversity International, Canadian Fertilizer Institute, Carbon Drawdown Solution, and the Center for Development & Competitive Strategies Ltd. It comes as no surprise that 107 civil organizations, including ActionAid International, Friends of the Earth International, the International Federation of Organic Agricultural Movements, the South Asia Alliance for Poverty Eradication, the Third World Network, Biofuel Watch, and the National Network on Right to Food, rallied against the formation and aims of GACSA. These organizations correctly argued that "sustainable intensification" and "climate-smart agriculture" are nothing but industrial monoculture systems by other names. At the risk of redundancy, it must be said that agroecology is a multiple cropping agrosystem that completely depends on internal biological components of the homeostatic system, while sustainable intensification and climate-smart agriculture still depend on externally manufactured synthetic agrochemicals.[78]

Another penetration stratagem of those who perceive agroecology as a threat to industrial agriculture is the active promotion of the no-till method of cultivation. The issue is not whether no-till is desirable or not, but whether it is based on in-situ organic inputs and natural processes or on ex-situ synthetic agrochemicals. Under natural no-till methods, seeds are directly sown into untilled soil by opening narrow holes or placing the

seeds in shallow ruts to protect the crops and/or plants against
environmental stressors and predators. The use of cover, mulching, and crop rotation protects the soil against desiccation and
evaporation, while the avoidance of tilling leaves the soil and
the vegetation around the growing crops undisturbed. No-till
also avoids mechanical soil disturbance and compaction and
improves water infiltration because the use of heavy machinery is
eliminated. The central purpose is the prevention of soil erosion
and loss of organic matter and the consequent loss of soil fertility, thereby increasing the accumulation of soil organic matter,
carbon sequestration, and mitigation of climate change. In Brazil,
for example, no-till was initially adopted as a remedy to land degradation loss of soil organic matter, compaction, reduction in
water infiltration, and pollution of natural water systems through
runoff and erosion from modern intensive farming.[79]

In due course, as medium and large-scale farms emerged dominant, farmers increasingly resorted to the use of synthetic inputs.
In 2007, the 107 million hectares under no-till—including nearly
50 million hectares in South America, 40.1 million hectares in
North America, and 12.6 million hectares in Australia and New
Zealand—were wholly or in part dependent on external synthetic
inputs. Lately, philanthrocapitalist foundations as well as bilateral
and multilateral institutions have been pushing hard for the incorporation of no-till into African farming. By 2008, some 100,000
small farmers in eastern and southern Africa were said to have
adopted no-till.[80] This is very good as far as it goes. The concern
arises from the double-edged sword nature of no-till. So long as
the method comports with the imperative of natural conditions of
agroecology, small farmers must be encouraged and assisted to use
the method. However, agribusiness and its supporting agencies and
foundations embroider the no-till method with recommendations
to use synthetic agrochemicals (such as glyphosate herbicide) to kill
or contain weeds, and to use improved seeds, including GM seeds.
In addition to making farmers dependent on agribusiness for the
steady supply of agrochemicals, external inputs will contaminate

soils, water, and the environment. In the end, this version of no-till links agroecology to the chemical-dependent industrial agriculture, preempting the intended divorce and independence of small farmers from the global food manufacturing system. That is why big business and neoliberal institutions see no contradiction between the simultaneous promotion of agroecological agriculture and the global food manufacturing system. Moreover, the agrochemical peddlers and no-till proponents conveniently use the purported benefits of carbon sequestration and ghg mitigation from the promotion of agroecological farming as justification for the inclusion of large-scale no-till monoculture in the global carbon market so as to benefit from the Kyoto CDM (Clean Development Mechanism) because, under no-till, carbon is supposedly stored in organic matter and not released to the atmosphere, thus contributing to reduction or prevention of warming.[81] However, when no-till farms are dependent on synthetic fertilizers and pesticides, the manufacturing and use of these external agrochemicals will inevitably use fossil energy, meaning that pollution and emission cannot be avoided. Moreover, small farmers who cannot afford to purchase agrochemicals will be squeezed out, and even those who can afford them will be permanently dependent on agrochemical companies and commercial seed marketers, locking agroecology perpetually into the global food manufacturing system.

IN SUMMARY, THE MAJOR POINTS I have outlined here show agroecology to be the only pathway for communities and nations to reassert their food sovereignty and ensure food security. Everything else is "biofiction" and corporate concoction. It begins with the re-peasantization of agriculture through full repossession of all land resources by the historic producers and owners of the rural means of production. However, rearticulation of agroecology in practical terms is only half of the equation; the other half pertains to concrete political action, which I shall elaborate upon in the concluding paragraphs, following a few words on the question of energy.

Next to agriculture, the area that takes on the most importance for rural communities and nations is the energy sector. Over the past quarter-century, bureaucrats from the rich and the transnationalized poor states as well as from global institutions like the World Bank and UNEP have been unable to resolve the wretched energy situation of the 2.7 billion people in the Global South. One UN declaration was "Electricity for All," which proposed investment of $756 billion between 2010 and 2030. But nothing has come of it because the bulk of the expected money was supposed to flow from the Global North to the Global South, which had no motivation to do so. Meanwhile, poor countries have remained dependent on fossil fuel imports. Between 2003 and 2007, the sudden upsurges in global oil prices increased the oil import bill of developing countries by $971 billion. African countries still surrender 30 percent of their export earnings to oil imports; Kenya and Senegal spend more than half of their export earnings on energy imports. Notwithstanding such squandering of massive resources on fossil fuel imports, the 110 million poor households on the African continent spend more than $4 billion a year on kerosene-based lighting that drains their already meager resources, is inefficient, and is replete with safety and health hazards.[82]

Notwithstanding the endless lip service paid to the need for rural hydroelectrification, rural populations in undeveloped countries have not benefited from the construction of giant hydrodams. On the contrary, giant hydroelectric projects are used to dispossess peasants and indigenous peoples of water, land, and forest resources. Considering the lack of options for accessing a sustainable energy source, rural people rely on firewood for virtually everything: cooking, heating, and smoking food. Cumulatively, such activity has taken a heavy toll on forests, wetlands, and mangroves. As nearby forest resources are depleted or commercially enclosed by corporations, women must travel ever farther to gather and haul firewood. This situation will get worse unless rural people access alternative energy sources. Reliance on fuelwood is known to have perilous health effects. In most cases, homes in undeveloped countries are built with no windows, and the result is indoor pollution that takes heavy a toll on the health of rural communities. Several million people die each year from indoor pollution, most of them women.

This all suggests that undeveloped countries will never find energy security in fossil energy or biofuels. The only pathway to clean and reliable rural and national energy self-sufficiency is the harnessing of solar radiation in ways that simultaneously meet the energy need and conserve natural resources, while promoting healthy living in the countryside. While biofuels compete with food, feed, and fiber for land and water, solar energy does not. As the International Resource Panel stated:

Solar insolation has the highest energy flows of all renewable energy resources with a global mean energy density of around 170 W/m2 [watt per square meter]. Solar power or solar thermal systems make use of 9 to 24 percent of the radiation input. In contrast, biomass in the open field usually captures about 1 percent of the radiation input with maximum values of up to 5–6 percent. Hence, crops grown for biofuels, at no more than 1 W/m2, can require more than 1,000-fold the land area to produce the same energy output as an oil-field at around 1 kW/ m2 energy density. When biomass is grown for liquid transport fuels, typical land use efficiencies range from 700 l/hectare [liters per hectare] for soybean biodiesel up to 4,900 l/hectare [liters per hectare] for sugarcane ethanol.[83]

This is good news for undeveloped countries because they have a rich endowment of solar radiation due to their proximity to the equator. Moreover, since significant advances in solar technology are being made, the opportunity to capture solar radiation in sufficient quantities to electrify isolated and remote rural areas is very much in prospect. In 2014, the solar photovoltaic sector employed 2.5 million people, and the heating and cooling sector added another 764,000 jobs, with China leading in the number of solar installations and employment.[84] Environmental economists Tim Searchinger and Ralph Heimlich trenchantly demonstrate that the use of solar photovoltaic devices alone could generate 55–70 times more energy per hectare than biofuels even if the solar devices are stationed in America's Corn Belt or in Brazil's heartland of sugarcane plantations. Moreover, solar energy does not compete with food, feed, and livestock for land, water, and conservation needs, since the devices can be placed in dry lands or deserts, or on rooftops.[85]

Bangladesh's experience underscores the potential of solar power in rural areas not served by fossil-generated electricity. By March 2015, the state-owned solar energy company had installed 3.6 million units of solar power, to which non-governmental establishments added another 200,000 units. As a result, more than 20 million people in rural Bangladesh have benefited from these solar installations. In fact, the program proved so successful that 2.2 million additional units were expected to be installed by 2016. The overall employment in the solar power sector was equally impressive, reaching 200,000 by 2014. The downstream spillover of the expansion of solar panel installations added another 50,000 jobs as small businesses and retailers began to tap in to solar power. To improve performance, sales, installation, maintenance, and after-sale services, vocational and management training was given to more than 410,000 people, including significant numbers of rural women.[86]

Here in the United States, environmental engineer Mark Jacobson and his colleagues at Stanford University have empirically demonstrated how the country could wean itself from dependency on oil, coal, and nuclear energy sources by transitioning to solar, wind, and geothermal energy. According to the energy blueprint the researchers submitted to Governor Andrew Cuomo, New York State could meet all of its energy needs by 2030 through renewable energy from water, wind, and solar (WWS), while reducing total energy use by 37 percent. The transition to WWS would provide significant reductions in air pollution, water pollution, and global warming, as well as pollution-related deaths. Were New York State to switch to WWS, air pollution–related deaths would fall by 4,000 per year, saving the state around $33 billion per annum, equal to 3 percent of the state's GDP. The savings in health care alone would pay for the new power infrastructure requirements in fewer than seventeen years. Additionally, New York's reduction of emissions would reduce U.S. climate-related costs by $3.2 billion per annum. According to the blueprint, the state would obtain 40 percent of its energy from local wind power, 38 percent from local solar radiation, and the rest would come from a combination of geothermal, hydroelectric, tidal, and wave energy.[87]

Similarly, according to the renewable energy blueprint Mark Jacobson and his colleagues developed for California, that state could count on, year in and year out, clean, abundant, cheap, and reliable energy from WWS. If California were to switch to WWS, it could derive 85 percent of its energy from WWS by 2030 and 100 percent by 2050, reducing energy demand by 44 percent per year. The state could derive 55.5 percent of its energy from solar, 35 percent from wind, and the rest from a combination of geothermal, hydroelectric, tidal, and wave energy. The switch to WWS would reduce pollution-related premature deaths in California by 12,500 per year, saving the state $103 billion per annum, which is equal to 4.9 percent of the state's 2012 GDP. The annual reduction in emission-driven cost would be $48 billion per annum.[88]

If the potential of solar energy is so great, why are nations and business interests reluctant to tap this inexhaustible energy source? There are two answers to this question, one economic and the other political. In the first case, the countries and peoples who desperately need solar energy are in the Global South, but they do not have the financial resources to harness this freely and abundantly available source of energy. In the second instance, the fossil industry in the Global North countries view solar energy as antithetical to their interests. In the North, accumulation by emission/pollution is the defining feature of economic activity, as opposed to accumulation by dispossession in the Global South.

The adoption of clean solar technology would cut deeply into the accumulation of capital. Thus, externalization of emission/pollution to society and nature still remains the principal means of accumulation. Among sources of renewable energy, nothing panics the fossil industry more than the potential scaling up and scaling out of solar energy development. This is because solar radiation is inexhaustible so long as the sun exists, and that will be for a long, long time. There is no such thing as overuse or underuse with solar energy, something that makes price manipulations virtually impossible once the solar energy infrastructure is put in place. Also, solar energy is amenable to decentralization because it does not require complex infrastructure and long-distance transmission lines. Communities or individual homeowners can easily and cheaply install their own off-grid solar panels, giving them energy sovereignty without interference from alien corporate bodies. In this way homeowners can deny utility companies the chance to continue building new plants to make more profit, or to continue manipulating energy prices as Enron did in California. With solar power in ascendance, generating profits from recurring sales of dirty electric power could become a thing of the past. Moreover, the scaling up and scaling out of solar power could end the logic of accumulation by emission pollution. It is this looming prospect of solar energy providers replacing dirty utilities in the United States that has lately unnerved dirty power plant operators, especially since the price of solar panels has progressively fallen by more than 80 percent since 2009, making solar power economically competitive with natural gas and coal.[89]

It is no coincidence that the Koch brothers, who own the Koch Industries conglomerate, as well as utility companies have begun funding front groups such as American Legislative Exchange Council and Americans for Prosperity to mount assaults on solar power at the state level, hiking up rates and even imposing fees on homeowners who dare to use solar power. Florida, where electricity generation is based on 61 percent natural gas, 23 percent coal, and only 1 percent of solar power, presents a textbook case of obstructionism. Florida's monopoly utility law prohibits any entity or individual save the power companies from buying and selling electricity in the state. Even landlords cannot sell power from solar panels to their tenants. Installation of rooftop solar panels is restricted to the small number of homeowners or establishments that can afford the outrageous up-front fees. This explains why there are fewer than 9,000 homes in the state with rooftop panels. Notwithstanding numerous protestations, Floridians have been unable to change the status quo because utility companies have virtual monopoly control over legislators and politicians. Since 2004, the utility companies spent $30 million on lobbying legislators or lavishing attention on politicians to block any effort to loosen the state's energy monopoly law. The Southern Alliance for Clean Energy launched a $2 million constitutional amendment drive to end private monopoly control over electricity production and distribution, but the utility companies, assisted by outside forces, mounted a counteroffensive, pouring in $8 million to crush the "Solar Choice" initiative, and crush it they did, as the pro–solar energy forces were 300,000 short of the 700,000 signatures needed to qualify for the November 2016 elections.[90] The choke hold of utility companies on Florida's politics is such that the Republican governor of the state even ordered all state officials not to mention "global warming" and "climate change" in their official communications.

The political activity of the Koch brothers in the United States illustrates the reality of Florida's experience. For over two decades now, the Kochs have been using bogus front groups to spread misinformation, disinformation, and deception about climate science. In their attempts to discredit the evidence of global warming they demonize scientists who adduce evidence about the perils of climate change, stiffen their opposition to clean energy and climate legislation, and portray dirty fossil corporations as job creators without whose industrial operations the U.S. economy would collapse. Between 1997 and 2009 alone, Koch foundations distributed $55 million to climate-denial front groups for direct lobbying on oil and energy issues, outspent only by Exxon and Chevron at $87.8 million and $50 million, respectively. The Koch brothers channel money through three nefarious foundations they personally control to forty climate-denial front groups and buy politicians and legislators to block legislation that might affect accumulation by emission/pollution.[91] The recipients of this dirty money include Americans for Prosperity, the Institute for Humane Studies, the Heritage Foundation, the Cato Institute, the Manhattan Institute, and the George Mason University Mercatus Center. The proliferation of falsely labeled nonprofit foundations and think tanks, the obscene magnitude of money dedicated to the dissemination of pernicious corporate propaganda, and the donations to political parties and individual political candidates are what make the Koch brothers the most outspoken enemies of clean energy. Under Koch influence and money, thirty-eight freshman congressmen elected in 2010 to the U.S. House of Representatives signed the "No Climate Tax Pledge" to prevent any legislation and policy for climate action. The two brothers singlehandedly raised over $400 million from ultra-conservative and super-rich billionaires to defeat Obama in 2012; in 2014, they raised almost $300 million for the 2014 midterm elections, most of which was spent on 44,000 political advertisements that enabled Republicans to capture the Senate, which turned out to be the biggest industrial machine of obstructionism. For the 2016 presidential election, the Koch brothers managed to raise $900 million from the plutocratic class, to which the two brothers contributed $150 million.[92]

The Koch brothers have extended their anti-clean energy campaigns to the state level with vigor. To undo California's citizen-driven adoption of clean energy legislation, signed into law in 2006, which committed the state to reducing ghg emissions to the 1990 level by 2029 through 33 percent reliance on clean and renewable energy, the Kochs and their front groups launched a ballot initiative in 2010. Their foundations helped to raise nearly $11 million, with 92 percent coming from oil and energy corporations. In addition, more than a dozen front groups and energy corporations, like Exxon and Chevron, deployed huge financial resources and manpower to combat the law. Even though corporate minions portrayed the clean energy bill as anti-green market, anti-small business, anti-job creation, and pro-tax, California's citizens fought back ferociously to expose the sinister aims behind the ploy. Their fight succeeded, and they defeated this corporate warfare, and this explains why California has become the nation's leading solar energy producer and consumer. Similarly, the Koch front groups spent millions of dollars on regional efforts against climate mitigation. Ten northeastern and Mid-Atlantic states established a regional collaborative framework to collectively reduce ghg emissions from power plants in 2007. In a matter of two years, the states raised $770 million, which was funneled into clean energy development, and home weatherization and conservation-related programs that resulted in lower energy bills and decreased energy consumption. In New Jersey, however, the Koch brothers were successful as Governor Chris Christie unilaterally pulled the state out of the regional multistate pact to combat climate change.[93]

What do the Koch brothers gain from blocking clean energy technology? The answer is protection from assaults on their wealth accumulation. With $115 billion annual sales, the Kansas-based Koch Industries is a conglomerate, dominated by petroleum and chemical interests. It is the second-largest privately held conglomerate, after Cargill, with more than 100,000 workers in sixty countries. Charles and David Koch together own $86 billion of the corporation's assets. The industrial reach of this behemoth is such that the brothers have diversified their holdings into biofuel production by acquiring a biodiesel plant in Beatrice, Nebraska, into which they injected more than $100 million to boost the plant's annual biodiesel production to 50 million gallons. Koch Industries' main source of domestic revenue is the externalization of toxic emissions/pollution to citizens and the environment. Among the top thirty corporations identified as the worst polluters of air, water, and climate, Koch Industries is ranked third, after Exxon and American Electric Power. Its Georgia-Pacific paper mill alone dumps more pollutants into U.S. waterways than General Electric and International Paper combined. Moreover, across its business units, Koch Industries generates more than 20 million metric tons of greenhouse gases annually. In 2012, Koch Industries was singled out to be the number-one producer of toxic waste in the United States, producing 950 million pounds of toxic chemical waste.[94]

Notwithstanding having earned the dubious distinction for holding the largest record of criminal actions, the Koch brothers continue to double down on their violations of the law, in utter disregard of societal welfare and environmental health. In 2000, Koch Industries was indicted by the Department of Justice with ninety-seven charges for deliberately discharging benzine from refineries in flagrant violation of federal laws. However, in accordance with the prevailing dominant culture, the corporation settled out of court, paying just $10 million in fines and another $10 million for environmental improvement. Before that, Koch Industries had paid $35 million for the 11.6 million gallons of petroleum spills from its refineries in Corpus Christi, Texas. The reason why the oil spills occurred was that the facilities required $98 million in repairs to meet industry standards. After causing heavy environmental damages, in 2000 Koch Industries signed a consent decree with the EPA and the Department of Justice to spend $80 million on three petroleum facilities to bring them into compliance with the Clean Air Act. Again, to avoid legal action, the Koch brothers signed another consent decree in March 2014 with the U.S. Department of Justice to spend $40 million on a petrochemical facility in Port Arthur, Texas, to bring it into compliance with the same act. This is a facility that produces 2 billion pounds of petrochemicals per year. Moreover, in 1999, a jury awarded $300 million to parents of two teenagers who were incinerated by the explosion of an antiquated butane pipeline, operated by Koch Industries in Corpus Christi.[95] The corporate behavior of Koch Industries is not an exception, but rather the general rule on which the whole architecture of accumulation via emission/pollution rests.

In the last two chapters I have presented the dangers posed by the advocacy for and diffusion of biofuel production and biotechnology—dangers to society, the environment, and the atmosphere. I have also outlined the pathways toward the reassertion of food sovereignty and energy security in the Global South. The solutions I have proposed are as much ecological and economic as political. Ends cannot be achieved, however noble, without appropriate means, and the proper means at this juncture are political. The recognition of the dark reality of contemporary capitalist civilization, brought about by disciplinary neoliberalism, requires us to go beyond the stale strands of bourgeois reformism. We need open declaration of the mother of all revolutionary struggles against the mother of all counterrevolutionary struggles currently being waged against the human race and nature. The objective conditions for radical macrostructural transformations of our contemporary civilization are very much in evidence in undeveloped countries. The crucial factors still missing are the much-needed subjective conditions in terms of collective leadership, coherent strategies and tactics, political mobilization, and coordinated action. There are existing political templates of struggle in the Global South, being waged not by intellectuals and bureaucrats, but by the dispossessed and oppressed people themselves. The struggle to recover and revitalize the autonomy of communities and the territorial and political independence of the national state is the first precondition for transformations that guarantee sustainable economic development, social justice, and environmental stability in accord with the principles of sustainable scale, allocative efficiency, and social justice. This requires bypassing the transnationalized state and confronting the ruthless forces of globalization personified in the global biofuel and biotechnology industrial complex, the global financial and trade institutions, and the global intergovernmental organizations.

Those who seek the salvation of economic prosperity, energy security, and climate change mitigation through the further commodification and modification of nature will naturally make dreadful miscalculations. The sources of such miscalculations could be either the folly of their understanding of what they are doing or the enormous pressure exerted by global corporations, supported by governments with exceptional impudence, ferocity, deception, manipulation, and outright intervention. These forces must be seized upon by the masses of peasants and workers, who together must then begin to create a sustainable world.

Notes

1. The New Geoeconomics of Biofuels

1. Stefan Bringezu et al., *Towards Sustainable Production and Use of Resources: Assessing Biofuels* (Nairobi: UNEP, 2009).

2. Stefan Bringezu et al., *Assessing Global Land Use: balancing consumption with sustainable supply* (Nairobi: UNEP, 2014); IEA WEO, *World Energy Outlook 2011* (Paris: International Energy Agency, 2011).

3. Kenneth S. Deffeyes, *Hubbert's Peak: The Impending World Oil Shortage* (Oxfordshire, UK: Princeton Univerity Press, 2001); Lester R. Brown, *Plan B/2.0: Mobilizing To Save Civilization* (New York: W. W. Norton, 2008).

4. IEA (International Energy Agency), *World Energy Outlook 2013* (Paris: IEA, 2013).

5. Brown, *Plan B/2.0.*

6. James C. Greenwood, "Update from BIO: Biotechnology—healing, fueling and feeding the world," www.bio.org, January 11, 2011.

7. Cited in Vandana Shiva, *Stolen Harvest: The Highjacking of the Global Food Supply* (Cambridge, MA: South End Press, 2000), 11.

8. ETC Group, "The New Biomasters: Synthetic biology and the next assault on biodiversity and livelihoods," *Communiqué* No. 104 (October 2010).

9. David Harvey. *The New Imperialism* (New York: Oxford University Press, 2003).

10. Karl Polanyi, *The Great Transformation: The political and economic origins of our time* (Boston: Beacon Press).

11. Herman Daly, *Beyond Growth: The economics of sustainable development* (Boston: Beacon Press, 1996).

12.   Nicholas Georgescu-Roegen, *The Entropy Law and the Economic Process* (Cambridge, MA: Harvard University Press, 1971).

13.   Herman E. Daly, "Sustainable Development: From concept and theory to operational principles," *Population and Development Review* 16, Supplement (1990): 25–40; Daly, "Steady State Economics: A New Paradigm," *New Literary History* 24/4 (1993): 811–16; Daly, *Beyond Growth*.

14.   Herman E. Daley and Joshua Farley, *Ecological Economics: Principles and Applications* (Washington, D.C.: Island Press, 2003); Georgescu-Roegen, *The Entropy Law and the Economic Process* (Cambridge, MA: Harvard University Press, 1971).

15.   Richard Alexander et al., "Differences in Phosphorus and Nitrogen Delivery to the Gulf of Mexico from the Mississippi River Basin," *Environmental Science and Technology* 42/3 (2008): 822–830.

16.   Charles Perrings, *Economy and Environment* (New York: Cambridge University Press, 1987).

17.   Jeffrey D. Sachs, *Commonwealth: Economics for a crowded planet* (New York: Penguin Group, 2008).

18.   Donald G. Richards, "Contradictions of the 'New Green Revolution': A View from South America's Southern Cone," *Globalizations7/4* (2010), 563–76.

19.   Brown, *Plan B/2.0*.

20.   Lakshman Yapa, "What Are Improved Seeds?: An epistemology of the green revolution," *Economic Geography* 39/3 (1993), 254–73.

21.   Lester R. Brown, *World on the Edge: How to Prevent Environmental and Economic Collapse* (New York: W. W. Norton, 2011).

22.   Herman E. Daly, "Sustainable Development" and "Steady State Economics."

23.   Rachel Smolker et al., *The Real Cost of Agrofuels: Impacts on food, forests, people and the climate*, Global Forest Coalition, Global Justice Ecology Project and Institute for Social Ecology with contributions from Dogwood Alliance and ETC Group; H. Steinfeld et al., *Livestock's Long Shadow: Environmental Issues and Options* (Rome: FAO, 2006).

24.   Hope Shand, "Terminator Seeds: Monsanto moves to tighten its grip on global agriculture, *Multinational Monitor* 19/11 (1998); Miguel Altieri et al., "Peasant Agriculture and the Conservation of Crop and Wild Plant Resources," *Conservation Biology* 1/1 (1987): 49–58; FAO, *Save and Grow: A policymaker's guide to the sustainable intensification of smallholder crop production* (Rome: FAO, 2011).

25.   Nikos Alexandratos and Jelle Bruinsma, *World Agriculture Towards 2030/2050: the 2012 revision* (Rome: FAO, 2012), FAO, *Save and Grow*; Tim Searchinger et al., *Creating a Sustainable Food Future: a menu of*

solutions to sustainably feed more than 9 million people by 2050, World Resources Report 2013–14, Interim Findings, www.wri.org.

26. Searchinger, *Creating a Sustainable Food Future*; H. Steinfeld, *Livestock's Long Shadow.*

27. FAO, *The Global Forest Resources Assessment 2010* (FRA [Global Forest Resources Assessment] 2010) (2011), www.fao.org; Al Gore, *The Future: Six Drivers of Global Change* (New York: Random House, 2013); World Wildlife Fund, *Living Planet Report 2014: Species and Spaces, People and Places* (2014), www.worldwildlife.org.

28. UNISDR, *The Human Cost of Weather-Related Disasters 1995–2015,* UN Office for Disaster Risk Reduction (2015), www.unisdr.org; WWF, *Living Planet Report.*

29. FAO, *The Global Forest Resources Assessment*; Alexandratos and Bruinsma, *World Agriculture Towards 2030/2050.*

30. Gore, *The Future*; H. Steinfeld, *Livestock's Long Shadow.*

31. Ulrich Hoffmann, *Assuring Food Security in Developing Countries under the Challenges of Climate Change: Key trade and development issues of a fundamental transformation of agriculture,* UN Conference on Trade and Development, Discussion paper No. 201 (Geneva: February 2011); Tim Searchinger et al., *Creating a Sustainable Food Future.*

32. Rifkin, *The End of Work*; Searchinger, *Creating a Sustainable Food Future.*

33. Rifkin, T*he End of Work.*

34. Bringezu, *Assessing Biofuels*; Clive James, *Global Status of Commercialized Biotech/GM Crops: 2014,* ISAAA Brief 49–2014 (2014), www.isaaa.org.

35. Rifkin, *The End of Work.*

36. H. Steinfeld, *Livestock's Long Shadow*; Searchinger, *Creating a Sustainable Food Future*; Bringezu, *Assessing Global Land Use.*

37. Nathan Pelletier and Peter Tyedmers, "Forecasting Potential Global Environmental Cost of Livestock Production 2000–2050," *Proceedings of the National Academy of Sciences of the United States of America* 107/43 (2010): 18371–74.

38. H. Steinfeld, *Livestock's Long Shadow*; Searchinger, *Creating a Sustainable Food Future.*

39. Colin Tudge, "It's a Meat Market," *New Scientist* 181/2438 (2004): 9.

40. H. Steinfeld, *Livestock's Long Shadow*; Searchinger, *Creating a Sustainable Food Future,* 2013; Nikos Alexandratos and Jelle Bruinsma, *World Agriculture Towards 2030/2050*; FAO, *World Livestock 2013— Changing Disease Landscapes* (Rome: FAO, 2013).

41. H. Steinfeld, *Livestock's Long Shadow*; WWF, *Living Planet Report 2014.*

42. Bill McKibben, *Deep Economy: The Wealth of Communities and Durable Future* (New York: Times Books, 2007).

43. Smolker, *The Real Cost of Agrofuels*; Nathan Pelletier and Peter Tydmers, "Forecasting Potential Global Environmental Cost"; Searchinger, *Creating a Sustainable Food Future*.

44. H. Steinfeld, *Livestock's Long Shadow*, 2006; Searchinger, *Creating a Sustainable Food Future*, 2013; FAO, *World Livestock 2013*; Pelletier and Tydmers, "Forecasting Poential Global Environmental Cost," 2010; Gowri Koneswaran and Danielle Nierenberg, "Global Farm Animal Production and Global Warming: Impacting and Mitigating," *Environmental Health Perspectives* 116/5 (2008): 578–82; UNEP (United Nations Environment Program), *Environment Outlook of Latin America and the Caribbean* (Nairobi: UNEP, 2010).

45. H. Steinfeld, *Livestock's Long Shadow*.

46. Colin Tudge, "It's a Meat Market"; H. Steinfeld, *Livestock's Long Shadow*.

47. H. Steinfeld, *Livestock's Long Shadow*; WWF, *Living Planet Report 2014*.

48. Andrew W. Mitchell et al., *Forests Now in the Fight against Climate Change* (Oxford, UK: Global Canopy Program, 2008); Norman Meyers, "The World's Forests and their Ecosystem Services," in *Nature's Services: Societal Dependence on Natural Ecosystems*, ed. Gretchen C. Daily (New York: Routledge, 1997), 213–26; Herman Daly and Joshua Farley, *Ecological Economics*, 2003; Robert Nasi et al., "Can They Pay Our Way Out of Deforestation?" Discussion Paper prepared for GEF, www.uneporg.

49. Millennium Ecosystem Assessment, "Ecosystems and Human Well-Being: General Synthesis" (2005), www.maweb.org/; UNEP, *Costs of Inaction on the Sound Management of Chemicals* (Nairobi: United Nations Environment Program, 2013).

50. Marina Fischer-Kowalski et al., "Decoupling Natural Resource Use and Environmental Impacts from Economic Growth," Internationa Resource Panel (Nairobi: UNEP, 2011); Stefan Bringezu, "Assessing Global Land Use"; Stefan Bringezu, "Towards Sustainable Production"; Millennium Ecosystem Assessment, "Ecosystems and Human Well-being."

51. Bringezu, "Assessing Global Land Use."

52. Jay Golden and Robert Handfield, *Why Biobased? Opportunities in the Emerging Bioeconomy*, submitted to: U.S. Department of Agriculture, Office of Procurement and Property Management, BioPreferred 2014, www.biopreferred.gov; Searchinger, *Creating a Sustainable Food Future*.

53. Bringezu, "Assessing Global Land Use"; Lester R. Brown, *Eco-Economy: Building an Economy for the Earth* (New York: W. W. Norton, 2001); H. Steinfeld, *Livestock's Long Shadow*; Smolker, *The Real Cost of Agrofuels*.

54. Smolker, *The Real Cost of Agrofuels*; Searchinger, *Creating a Sustainable Food Future*; Nicola Colbran, "Indigenous Peoples in Indonesia: At risk

of disappearing as distinct people in the rush for biofuel?," *International Journal on Minority and Group Rights* 18 (2011): 63–92.

55. Smolker, *The Real Cost of Agrofuels*; Grant Rosoman, "The Plantation Effect: An ecoforestry review of the environmental effect of exotic monoculture tree plantations in Aotearoa/New Zealand," New Zealand Greenpeace, *REDD Monitor* (1994), www.redd–monitor.org.

56. Fischer-Kowalski, *Decoupling Natural Resource Use*; Bringezu, *Assessing Global Land Use*; WWF, *Living Planet Report 2014*, 2014; Johan Rockstrom et al., "A Safe Operating Space for Humanity," *Nature* 461 (2009): 472–76.

57. Andrew W. Mitchell, *Forests Now in the Fight*.

58. ETC Group, "The New Biomasters: Synthetic biology and the next assault on biodiversity and livelihoods," *Communique* No. 104 (October 2010); Norman Meyers, "The World's Forests and Their Ecosystem Services," in Daily, *Nature's Services: Societal Dependence on Natural Ecosystems*, 213–26.

59. Daly, *Beyond Growth*; Daly and Farley, *Ecological Economics*; Robert Costanza and Herman Daly, "Natural Capital and Sustainable Development," *Conservation Biology* 6/1 (1992): 37–46; Perrings, *Econo and Environment*, 1987.

60. Daly, *Beyond Growth*; Costanza and Daly, "Natural Capital and Sustainable Development."

61. Costanza and Daly, "Natural Capital and Sustainable Development."

62. Daly and Farley, *Ecological Economics*.

63. Robert Costanza et al., "Changes in the Global Value of Ecosytem Services," *Global Environmental Change* 26 (2014): 37–46.

64. Naomi Klein, *This Changes Everything; Capitalism versus the Climate* (New York: Simon and Schuster, 2014). Al Gore, *The Future*.

65. UNEP, *Towards a Green Economy: The Pathway to Sustainable Development and Poverty Eradication* (Nairobi: UNEP, 2011), www.unep.org/greeneonomy; UNEP, *Options for Decoupling Economic Growth*, 2016; Fischer-Kowalski, *Decoupling Natural Resource Use*, 2011.

66. William Stanley Jevons, *The Coal Question*, 2nd ed. (London: Macmillan and Co., 1866).

67. UK Energy Research Centre, *The Rebound Effect: An assessment of the evidence for economy-wide energy savings from improved energy efficiency*, report by the Sussex Energy Group for the Technology and Policy Assessment function of the UK Energy Research Centre, 2007.

68. Robert Costanza et al., "Modeling Complex and Ecological Economic Systems," *BioScience* (1993): 545–55; Costanza and Daly, "Natural Capital," 1992; Daly and Farley, *Ecological Economics*, 2003.

69. Jane Mayer, *Dark Money: The Hidden History of the Billionaires Behind the Rise of the Radical Right* (New York: Penguin Random House, 2016); Wenonah Hauter, *Frackopoly: The battle for the future of energy and the environment* (New York: New Press, 2016); Clare Foran, "The Koch Brothers' Next Frontier," *National Journal* (November 22, 2014); "Inside the Koch Brothers' Toxic Empire," *Rolling Stone*, October 9, 2014; Schulman, Daniel, *The Sons of Wichita: How the Koch brothers became America's most powerful private dynasty* (New York: Grand Central Publishing, 2014); George Monbiot, *Heat: How to stop the planet from burning* (Cambridge, MA: South End Press, 2007).

70. Mayer, *Dark Money*; *Rolling Stone*, "Inside the Koch Brothers' Toxic Empire"; Schulman, *The Sons of Wichita*; Hauter, *Frackopoly*; Green Peace USA, "Koch Industries 2011 Update" (2011), www.greepeace. org.

71. Mayer, *Dark Money*; *Rolling Stone*, "Inside the Koch Brothers' Toxic Empire"; Schulman, *The Sons of Wichita*; Hauter, *Frackopoly*.

72. Ibid.

73. Monbiot, *Heat*.

74. Cited in ibid., 30.

75. Cited in ibid., *Heat*, 38.

76. Food and Water Watch, "Issue Briefing: Biotech Industry Spending to Influence Congress" (2010), www.foodandwaterwatch.org.

77. Brown, *Eco-Economy*.

78. Deborah Cowen and Neil Smith, "'After Geopolitics' from Geopolitical Social to Geoeconomics," *Antipode* 41/1): 22–48.

79. Robinson, "Latin America in the Age of Inequality."

80. Vandana Shiva, *Stolen Harvest: The Highjacking of the Global Food Supply* (Cambridge, MA: South End Press, 2000).

81. Harvey, *The New Imperialism*; Harvey, *A Brief History of Neoliberalism*.

82. Ibid.

83. R. Arezki et al., "What Drives the Global Land Rush?," CESifo Working Paper Series, No. 3666 (2011), www.ssrn.com; S. Borras and J. Franco, *Political Dynamics of Land Grabbing in Southeast Asia: Understanding Europe's Role* (Amsterdam: Transnational Institute, 2011); Almuth Ernsting and Deepak Rughani, "Climate Geo-Engineering with Carbon Negative Bioenergy: Climate Savior or Climate Endangering?," 2008, www.globalbioenergy.org; Tim Searchinger et al., "Use of U.S. croplands for biofuels increases greenhouse gases through emissions from land-use change," *Science* 319/5867 (2008): 1238–40; IEA, *IEA World Energy Outlook 2012* (Paris: International Energy Agency, 2012); T. Searchinger and R. Heimlich, "Avoiding Bioenergy Competition for Food Crops and Land," Working Paper, Installment 9 of Creating a

Sustainable Food Future (Washington, DC: World Resources Institute, 2015); Bringezu, "Towards Sustainable Production."

84. Arezki, "What Drives the Global Land Rush?"; Kate Geary, "Our Land, Our Lives: Time Out on the Global Land Rush," Oxfam International (2012); Bringezu, "Towards Sustainable Production"; HLPE (High Level Panel of Experts), *Biofuels and Food Security and Nutrition* (Rome: Committee of World Food Security, 2013).

85. Oxfam, "Climate Wrongs and Human Rights," Oxfam Briefing Paper 117, www.oxfam.org; Gore, *Future*.

2. The Biofuels Industrial Complex and Its Migration to the Global South

1. National Energy Development Group, *National Energy Policy*, 2001, www.whitehouse.gov/energy.

2. FAO, *Biofuels: Prospects, Risks and Opportunities* (Rome: FAO, 2008).

3. IEA, *World Energy Outlook: World Energy Balances Overview 2017* (Paris: International Energy Agency, 2017).

4. Miguel Carriquiry et al., "Second-Generation Biofuels: Economics and Policies," World Bank Development Research Group, Working Paper 5406 (Washington, D.C.: World Bank, 2010).

5. HLPE (High Level Panel of Experts), *Biofuels and Food Security and Nutrition* (Rome: Committee of World Food Security, 2013); Dominic Waugray, "Financing Green Growth in a Resource-Constrained World," *World Economic Forum Infrastructure Initiative*, 2012, www.3.weforum.org.

6. IRENA (International Renewable Energy Agency), *Renewable Energy and Jobs: Annual Review 2015*, www.irena.org/Publications.

7. Rachel Smolker et al., *The Real Cost of Agrofuels: Impacts on Food, Forests, People and the Climate*, Global Forest Coalition, Global Justice Ecology Project, and Institute for Social Ecology with contributions from Dogwood Alliance and ETC Group, 2008; Jacques Berthelot, "Agribusiness' Headlong Flight to Agrofuels and Their Impact on Food Security," 2009, www.landaction.org; ETC Group, "The New Biomasters: Synthetic biology and the next assault on biodiversity and livelihoods," *Communiqué* No. 104 (October 2010).

8. L. Peskett et al., *Biofuels, Agriculture and Poverty Reduction* (London: Overseas Development Institute, 2007).

9. M. Hoogwijk et al., "Exploration of the Rages of the Global Potential of Biomass for Energy," *Biomass and Bioenergy* 25 (2003): 119–33; M. Verdonk et al., "Governance of the Emerging Bio-Energy Markets," *Energy Policy*, 35: 3909–24.

10. Jeremy Rifkin, *The End of Work*.

11. David R. Baker, "Oil Giant Chevron Gives Biofuel a Try," *San Francisco Chronicle*, June 1, 2006.

12. Ed Crooks, "BP Gets into Position for a Biofuels Era," *Financial Times*, June 26, 2007.

13. Guy Chazan, "Producers–Big Oil Looks to Biofuels: As low-carbon fuels get pushed, BP, Shell and others invest in alternatives," *Wall Street Journal*, October 19, 2007.

14. Charlie Rose, "Charlie Rose Talks to Exxon-Mobil's Rex Tillerson," *BusinessWeek*, March 7, 2013.

15. Crooks, "BP Gets into Position."

16. Chazan, "Producers." Andrew Morton and Graham Applegate, "Global Market Impacts on Asia-Pacific Forests in 2020," in Robin Leslie, ed. *The Future of Forests in Asia and the Pacific: Outlook for 2020* (RAP Publication, Bangkok: FAO's Regional Office for Asia and the Pacific, 2009).

17. Ibid.

18. Michelle Bryner, "BP Invests $500 Million in Biofuels R&D," *Chemical Week* 168/ 21 (June 21, 2006): 11.

19. ETC Group, *Who Will Control the Green Economy*, December 2011, www.etcgroup.org.

20. Bryner, "BP Invests."

21. Adam Helms, "BP Biofuels and AgriLife Research Sign Agreement," *Southwesterm Press*, August 14, 2012.

22. Bryner, "BP Invests."

23. D. Coady et al., "The Large Global Energy Subsidies?" IMF Working Paper 15/105 (Washington, D.C.: International Monetary Fund, 2015).

24. Naomi Klein, *This Changes Everything: Capitalism versus the Climate* (New York: Simon and Schuster, 2014).

25. Susan Lyon and Daniel Weiss, "Big Oil Continues to See Big Profits Pollution while Americans get Robbed at the Pump," April 29, 2010, www.grist.org.

26. Oil Exchange International, "US Fossil Fuels Subsidies," April 24, 2012: www.priceofoil.org.

27. Lyon and Weiss, "Big Oil Continues."

28. Anu K. Mittal, "Unconventional Oil and Gas Production: Opportunities and challenges of oil shale development," testimony before the Subcommittee on Energy and Environment, Committee on Science, Space and Technology, House of Representatives, May 10, 2012, GAO-12-740T (Washington, D.C.: United States General Accountability Office).

29. MITEI (MIT Energy Initiative), "The Future of Natural Gas" (Boston: Massachusetts Institute of Technology, 2011).

30. U.S. EIA, *Technically Recoverable Shale Oil and Shale Gas Resources: An assessment of 137 shale formations in 41 countries outside the United States* (Washington, D.C.: U.S. Department of Energy, June 2013).
31. U.S. GAO. *Oil and Gas Information on Shale Resource Development and Environmental and Public Health Risks,* Report to Congress (Washington, D.C.: US General Accounting Office, September 2012).
32. Marilyn Radler, "Oil, Liquids-Rich Shales Dominate Capital Spending Budgets for 2012," *Oil and Gas Journal,* March 5, 2012.
33. EIA, *Technically Recoverable Shale Oil.*
34. MITEI, "The Future of Natural Gas"; U.S. EIA, *Technically Recoverable Shale Oil.*
35. Jonathan Pearlman, "Trillions of Dollars Worth of Oil Found in Australian Outback," *Telegraph,* January 24, 2013.
36. David Uren, "Gas Heats Investment to $260bn," *The Australian,* May 25, 2012; Klein, *This Changes Everything.*
37. Uren, "Gas Heats Investment to $260bn."
38. Global Data, "Global Oil and Gas Capital Expenditure Breaks $1 Trillion Barrier," August 23, 2012, www.globaldata.com.
39. IEA, *Medium-Term Coal Market Report* (Paris: International Energy Agency, December 18, 2012).
40. Ibid.; GAO, *Oil and Gas Information.*
41. Ailun Yang and Yiyun Cui, *Global Coal Risk Assessment: Data Analysis and Market Research,* World Resources Institute Working Paper, November 2012.
42. IEA, *World Energy Outlook* (Paris: International Energy Agency, 2012).
43. Ibid.
44. IEA, *Medium-Term Coal Market Report.*
45. Brian Smith, "Chevron Gives Up on Coal-to-Liquid Fuel," *Earth Justice,* January 28, 2011, www.earthjustice.org.
46. GAO. *Oil and Gas Information.*
47. Peter Mantius, "'Frackademia': MIT's Ernest Moniz, Obama's top candidate for energy secretary, oversees pro-industry-funded research," (Washington, D.C.: Natural Resources News Service, February 21, 2013).
48. MITEI, "The Future of Natural Gas."
49. Ibid.
50. Mantius, "'Frackademia.'"
51. Ibid.
52. R. Howarth, R. Santoro, and A. Ingraffea, "Methane and the greenhouse-gas footprint of natural gas from shale formations." *Climatic Change* 106/4 (2011): 679–90.
53. Mantius, "'Frackademia.'"

54. Source Watch, "Shale Gas and Oil Reserves," March 9, 2013, www. sourcewatch.org/index.php/Shale_gas_and_oil_reserves.

55. Mantius, "'Frackademia.'"; Terrence Henry, "Review of UT fracking study finds failure to disclose conflict of interest," NPR, December 6, 2012.

56. Jay Rey, "UB Shutting Down Controversial Shale Institute," *Buffalo News,* November 19, 2012.

57. "Worldwide Number of Battery Electric Vehicles," June 2017, www. statista.com.

58. Smolker, *The Real Cost of Agrofuels.*

59. Ausilio Bauen et al., "A Harmonized Auto-fuel Biofuel Roadmap for the EUP to 2030, Final Report," E4tech, November 2013, www.e4tech.com.

60. Clive James, *Global Status of Commercialized Biotech/GM Crops: 2014,* ISAAA Brief 49-2014, www.isaaa.org.

61. ETC Group, "Who Owns Nature," 2008, www.etcgroup.org; ETC Group, "Gene Giants Seek 'Philanthrogopoly,'" *Communiqué,* No. 110, March 3, 2013; Eric Holt-Gimenez and Isabella Kenfield, "When Renewable Isn't Sustainable: Agrofuels and the Inconvenient Truths Behind the 2007 U.S. Energy Independence and Security Act," in *Agrofuels in the Americas,* ed. Richard Jonasse (Oakland, CA: Food First: Institute for Food and Development Policy, 2009), 25–39; Smolker, *The Real Cost of Agrofuels.*

62. World Bank, "Double Jeopardy: Responding to High Food and Fuel Prices" (Washington, D.C.: World Bank, 2008); Holt-Giménez and Kenfield, "When Renewable Isn't Sustainable"; Jacques Berthelot, "Agribusiness' Headlong Flight"; M. Lagi, *The Food Crises: A quantitative model of food prices including speculators and ethanol conversion* (Cambridge, MA: New England Complex Systems Institute, 2011).

63. William F. Engdahl, "World Bank Secret Report Confirms Biofuel Cause of World Food Crisis," *Global Research,* July 10, 2008; World Bank, "Double Jeopardy."

64. FAO, *High-Level Conference on World Food Security: The Challenges of Climate Change and Bioenergy* (Rome: June Food Summit, June 3–5, 2008); World Bank, "Double Jeopardy."

65. FAO, *High-Level Conference on World Food Security.*

66. U.S. Dept. of State, "US Encourages Countries to Lift Barriers to Biotech," June 13, 2008.

67. FAO, *The State of Food and Agriculture 2008.*

68. ETC Group, "The New Biomasters"; Eric Holt-Gimenez and Annie Shattuck, "The Agrofuels Transition: Restructuring places and spaces in the global food system," *Bulletin of Science, Technology and Society* 29/3 (2009), 180–88.

69. World Bank, "Double Jeopardy"; Jacob Chamberlain, "Goldman Sachs's Food Speculation Turns Global Hunger into Wall Street Profit," *Common Dream,* January 22, 2013; Tim Jones, "The Great Hunger Lottery: How Banking Speculation Causes Food Crises," World Development Movement, July 2010, www.globaljustice.org.

70. Lagi, *The Food Crises.*

71. Jones, "The Great Hunger Lottery."

72. Ibid.; World Bank, "Double Jeopardy"; Luca Colombo and Antonio Onorati, "Food, Riots, and Rights" (London: Institute for International Environment and Development. 2013).

73. World Bank, "Double Jeopardy."

74. Holt-Gimenez and Shattuck, "The Agrofuels Transition."

75. ADM, "Understanding ADM and Biofuels," undated brochure, ADM_and_Biofuels_brochure-lores.pdf.

76. Sasha Lilley, "Green Fuels' Dirty Secret," *CorpWatch,* June 1, 2006.

77. Katie Fehrenbacher, "Ten of Cargill's Next-Gen Biofuel Bets." *Gigaon,* August 19, 2010.

78. Louis Dreyfus website, www.louisdreyfus.com.

79. Bunge website, www.bunge.com.

80. Jones, "The Great Hunger Lottery."

81. Action Aid International, *Fuel for Thought: Addressing the Social Impacts of EU Biofuels Policies,* April 2012, www.actionaid.org; M. Lagi,, *The Food Crises.*

82. Lagi, *The Food Crises;* Action Aid International, *Fuel for Thought;* HLPE, *Biofuels and Food Security and Nutrition.*

83. Action Aid International, *Fuel for Thought;* Al Gore, *The Future;* Oxfam, *Land and Power: The Growing Scandal Surrounding the New Wave of Investments in Land,* Briefing Paper 22, September 2011, www.oxfam.org.

84. Timothy Searchinger et al., *Creating a Sustainable Food Future: A menu of solutions to sustainably feed more than 9 billion people by 2050,* World Resources Report 2013-14, Interim Fundings, 2013, www.wri.org.

85. Charles H. Weston, Jr., "The Political Legacy of Lazaro Cardenas," *The Americas,* 39/3 (1983): 383–405.

86. Harry M. Cleaver, Jr., "The Contradictions of the Green Revolution," *U.S. Economic Review* 62/1–2 (1972): 177–86.

87. EIU Viewswire. "World Commodities: EIU's Monthly Wheat Outlook," June 1, 2013.

88. International Maize and Wheat Improvement Center, www.cimmyt.org.

89. Cleaver, Jr., "The Contradictions of the Green Revolution."

90. B. O. Juliano, *Rice and Human Nutrition* (Rome: FAO, 1993).

91. Nikos Alexandratos and Jelle Bruinsma, *World Agriculture Towards 2030/2050: The 2012 Revision* (Rome: FAO, 2012); Beverly McIntyre et al., eds., *Crossroads Agriculture International Assessment of Agricultural Knowledge, Science and Technology for Development* (IAASTD) (Washington, D.C.: Island Press, 2009).

92. Alexandratos and Bruinsma, *World Agriculture Towards 2030/2050.*

93. Philip McMichael, "Rethinking Globalization: The Agrarian Question Revisited," *Review of International Political Economy* 4/4 (1997): 630–62.

94. Fred Pearce, *When the Rivers Run Dry Water: The Defining Crisis for the Twenty-First Century* (Boston: Beacon Press, 2006).

95. Alexandratos and Bruinsma, *World Agriculture Towards 2030/2050*; Searchinger, *Creating a Sustainable Food Future.*

96. Nikos Alexandratos and Jelle Bruinsma, *World Agriculture Towards 2030/2050*; Beverly McIntyre, *Crossroads Agriculture.*

97. Brian D. Richter et al., "Lost in Development's Shadow: The Downstream Human Consequences of Dams," *Water Alternatives* 3/2 (2010): 14–42; World Commission on Dams, *Dams and Development: A New Framework for Decision-Making* (London: Earthscan, 2000).

98. Carolyn Dimitri et al., "The Twentieth-Century Transformation of U.S. Agriculture and Farm Policy," *Economic Information Bulletin* 3 (June 2005).

99. Alexandratos and Bruinsma, *World Agriculture Towards 2030/2050.*

100. Cleaver, Jr., "The Contradictions of the Green Revolution."

101. Engdahl, *Seed of Destruction: The Hidden Genetic Manipulation.*

102. Jennifer Clap, *Hunger in the Balance: The New Politics of International Food Aid* (Ithaca, Ny: Cornell University Press, 2012).

103. Cleaver, Jr., "The Contradictions of the Green Revolution."

104. Joseph Stiglitz, *The Price of Inequality* (New York: W. W. Norton, 2012).

105. Mark Drabenstott, "The 1980s: A Turning Point for U.S. Agricultural Exports?," *Economic Review* (April 1983).

106. Ibid.

107. Ibid.

108. Jeffrey St. Clair, "The Looting of Iraqi Agriculture," *Counterpunch*, July 3, 2003.

109. GRAIN, "Iraq's New Patent Law: A Declaration of War Against Farmers," October 15, 2004, www.grain.org.

110. St. Clair, "The Looting of Iraqi Agriculture."

111. FAO, *Save and Grow: A Policymaker's Guide to the Sustainable Intensification of Smallholder Crop Production* (Rome: FAO, 2011); Jonathan Bloom, *U.S. Wasteland: How America Throws Away Nearly*

Half of Its Food (Boston: Da Capo Press, 2010).

112. H. Steinfeld et al., *Livestock's Long Shadow: Environmental Issues and Options* (Rome: FAO, 2006).

113. Alexandratos and Bruinsma, *World Agriculture Towards 2030/2050;* Vandana Shiva, *Stolen Harvest: The Highjacking of the Global Food Supply* (Cambridge, MA: South End Press, 2000); Searchinger, *Creating a Sustainable Food Future.*

114. Claire Parfitt et al., "Golden Rice Is No Silver Bullet: Hunger Needs a Political Solution," *The Conversation,* February 20, 2013.

115. James Bovard, "Archer Daniels Midland: A Case Study in Corporate Welfare," *The Cato Analysis* 241 (Sept. 26, 1995).

116. Engdahl, *Seed of Destruction.*

117. ETC Group, *Who Will Control the Green Economy.*

118. Carriquiry, "Second-Generation Biofuels."

119. McIntyre, *Crossroads Agriculture International Assessment.*

120. J. C. O'Toole et al., "The Rockefeller Foundation's Program on Rice Biotechnology," in *Rice Genetics IV*, ed. G. S. Khush et al., Proceedings of the Fourth International Rice Genetics Symposium, October 22–27, 2000, Los Banos, Philippines; Engdahl, *Seed of Destruction.*

121. William Engdahl, *Seed of Destruction;* Shiva, *Stolen Harvest.*

122. Engdahl, *Seed of Destruction.*

123. James, *Global Status.*

124. The White House, "National Bioeconomy Blueprint," Office of Science and Technology, April 2012, www.whitehouse.gov.

125. RT News, "No More GMO: Monsanto drops to approve new crops in Europe," July 19, 2013, http://rt.com.

126. James, *Global Status.*

127. Holt-Gimenez and Shattuck, "The Agrofuels Transition."

128. Martin Mittelstaedt, "Jet Fuel from a Forest," *Globe and Mail* (Canada), August 17, 2013; "Rentech Drops Woody Jet Fuel for Wood Pellets," *Northern Ontario Business,* June 10, 2013, www.northernontariobusiness.com.

129. FAO, *The State of Food and Agriculture 2008.*

130. USDA, *Biobased Products Market Potential and Projections through 2025,* February 2008, www.usda.gov.

131. ETC Group, "The New Biomasters."

132. FAO, *The State of Food and Agriculture, Agricultural Biotechnology: Meeting the needs of the Poor?* (Rome: FAO, 2004); C. Walter and M. Menzies, *Forests and Genetically Modified Trees* (Rome: FAO, 2010).

133. James, *Global Status.*

3. Biofuels and the Transformation of the Metropolitan State

1.   Garten Rothkopf, *A Blueprint for Green Energy in the Americas* (Washington, D.C.: InterAmerican Development Bank, 2007).
2.   Doug Koplow, *Biofuels—At What Cost? Government support for ethanol and biodiesel in the United States* (Geneva: Global Subsidies Initiative of the International Institute for Sustainable Development, 2006).
3.   Randy Schnepf and Brent Ycobucci, "Renewable Fuel Standard (RFS): Overview and Issues" (Washington, D.C.: CRS Report for Congress, Congressional Research Service, 2013).
4.   Koplow, *Biofuels*.
5.   Rachel Smolker et al., *The Real Cost of Agrofuels: Impacts on Food, Forests, People and the Climate*, Global Forest Coalition, Global Justice Ecology Project Project and Institute for Social Ecology, with contributions from Dogwood Alliance and ETC Group, 2008.
6.   Ibid.
7.   Koplow, *Biofuels*.
8.   Schnepf and Ycobucci, "Renewable Fuel Standard (RFS)"; Tom Capehart, "Ethanol: Economic and Policy Issues," CRS Report prepared for members and committees of Congress (Washington, D.C.: Congressional Research Service, 2009).
9.   Robert Perlack et al., *Biomass as Feedstock for a Bioenergy and Bioproducts Industry: The Technical Feasibility of a Billion-Ton Annual Supply* (Washington, D.C.: U.S. Department of Energy, Office of Scientific and Technical Information, 2005).
10. David Pimentel et al., "Ecology of Increasing Diseases: Population Growth and Environmental Degradation," *Human Ecology* 35 (2007): 653–68.
11. Liz Marshall and Zachary Sugg, "Corn Stover for Ethanol Production: Potential and Pitfalls," *Energy: Biofuels* 4 (Washington, D.C.: World Resources Institute, 2009).
12. USDA, *RCA Appraisal: Soil and Water Resources Conservation Act*, 2011, www.usda.gov.
13. Pimentel., "Ecology of Increasing Diseases."
14. USDA, *Bio-Based Products Market Potential and Projections through 2025*, February 2008, www.usda.gov; Erin Voegele, "EIA Data Illustrates 2014 Ethanol Production, Consumption Levels," *Ethanol Producer Magazine*, April 3, 2015; Capehart, "Ethanol."
15. IRENA, *Renewable Energy and Jobs: Annual Review 2015*, International Renewable Energy Agency, www.irena.org.
16. J. S. Golden et al., *An Economic Impact Analysis of the U.S. Bio-Based Products Industry: A Report to the Congress of the United States of America*, joint publication of the Duke Center for Sustainability and

Commerce and the Supply Chain Resource Cooperative, North Carolina State University, 2015.

17. Ibid.
18. Capehart, "Ethanol."
19. "Global Biofuels will Struggle to Match Ambitious Objectives," *Oil and Gas Journal,* April 2, 2012.
20. FAO, *The State of Food and Agriculture 2008 (SOFA), Biofuels: Prospects, Risks and Opportunities* (Rome: FAO, 2008); Smolker, *The Real Cost of Agrofuels.*
21. Richard Jonasse, ed., *Agrofuels in the Americas* (Oakland, CA: Food First, Institute for Food and Development Policy, 2009), 15–24.
22. David Pimentel, "Energy and Dollar Costs of Ethanol Prouction with Corn," *Hubbert Center Newsletter,* 98/2 (April 2–6, 1998); David Pimentel et al., "Food versus Biofuels: Environmental and Economic Costs," *Human Ecology* 37/1 (2009): 1-12; Jason Hill et al., "Environmental, Economic, and Energetic Costs and Benefits of Biodiesel and Ethanol Biofuels," *National Academy of Sciences of the USA* 103/30 (2006): 11206–10; Miguel Altieri and Elizabeth Bravo, "The Ecological as Social Tragedy of Crop-based Biofuels Production in the Americas," in *Agrofuels in the Americas,* ed. Richard Jonasse (Oakland, CA: Food First, Institute for Food and Development Policy, 2009), chap. 1.
23. Smolker, *The Real Cost of Agrofuels;* Hill, "Environmental, Economic, and Energetic Costs."
24. "Global Biofuels Will Struggle," *Oil and Gas Journal.* April 2, 2012.
25. Capehart, "Ethanol."
26. Hill, "Environmental, Economic, and Energetic Costs."
27. Pimentel, "Food versus Biofuels."
28. Roberta Rampton, "Retired U.S. Military Brass Wage Political Battle for Biofuels," Reuters, July 12, 2012.
29. Ibid.
30. Peter Schwartz and Doug Randall, "An Abrupt Climate Change Scenario and Its Implications for United States National Security," 2003, www.iatporg.
31. Ibid.
32. IRENA, *Renewable Energy and Jobs.*
33. U.S. Census Bureau, "US International Trade Statistics" (Washington, D.C.:U.S. Department of Commerce, 2016).
34. UNCTAD, *Trade and Development Report* (Geneva: United Nations Conference on Trade and Development, 2015); U.S. Census Bureau, "U.S. International Trade Statistics."
35. Rina Singh, "Bio-Based Chemicals and Products: A New Driver of U.S. Economic Development," in *U.S. Industry Perspective on Assessing*

Sustainability of Bio-based Products, World Congress on Industrial Biotechnology and Bioprocessing, June 2010, www.oecd.org; Jay Golden and Robert Handfield. *Why Bio-Based? Opportunities in the Emerging Bioeconomy,* submitted to U.S. Department of Agriculture, Office of Procurement and Property Management, BioPreferred Program, www.biopreferred.gov.

36. Singh, "Bio-Based Chemicals and Products."
37. James Greenwood, "Update from BIO: Biotechnology—Healing, Fueling and Feeding the World," January 11, 2011, www.bio.org.
38. Ibid.
39. Ibid.
40. BIO, Battelle/BIO State Bioscience Jobs, Investments and Innovation 2014, www.bio.org/Battelle2014.
41. The White House, "National Bioeconomy Blueprint," April 2012, www.whitehouse.gov.
42. Ibid.
43. Koplow, *Biofuels;* David Pimentel et al., "Update on Environmental and Economic Costs Associated with Alien-Invasive Species in the United States," *Ecological Economics* 52 (2005): 273–88; Fred Pearce, *When the Rivers Run Dry: Water: the defining crisis for the twenty-first century* (Boston, MA.: Beacon Press, 2006).
44. Raymond Herrmann et al., *Water Resources Investigation Report* (Washington, D.C.: U.S. Geological Survey, Department of Interior, 1998).
45. Koplow, *Biofuels.*
46. Koplow, *Biofuels;* Pearce, *When the Rivers Run Dry;* Virginia McGuire, *Water Level Changes and Change in Water and Storage in the High Plain Aquifer, Pre-Development to 2013* (Washington, D.C.: U.S. Geological Survey, Department of Interior, 2013).
47. Koplow, *Biofuels;* Pearce, *When the Rivers Run Dry;* Bridget Scanlon et al., "Groundwater Depletion and Sustainability of Irrigation in the US High Plains and Central Valley," *Proceedings of the National Academy of Sciences of the United States of America* 109/24 (2012): 9320–25.
48. McGuire, *Water Level Changes.*
49. Pearce, *When Rivers Run Dry;* Scanlon, "Groundwater Depletion and Sustainability"; Smolker, *The Real Cost of Agrofuels.*
50. Scanlon, "Groundwater Depletion and Sustainability."
51. Michael Cohen et al., *Water to Supply the Land;* Pearce, *When the Rivers Run Dry.*
52. Bureau of Reclamation, "Colorado River Basin Water Supply and Demand Study" (Washington, D.C.: U.S. Department of the Interior, Bureau of Reclamation: 2012).

53. Ibid.
54. Bureau of Reclamation, *Colorado River Basin Water Supply;* Pearce, *When Rivers Run Dry.*
55. Ker Than, "Can California Farmers Save Water and the Dying Salton Sea?" *National Geographic,* February 2, 2014; Michael Cohen, *Hazard's Toll: The Costs of Inaction at the Salton Sea* (Oakland, CA: Pacific Institute, 2014).
56. Bureau of Reclamation, "Restoration of the Salton Sea, Lower Colorado River Region" (Washington, D.C.: U.S. Department of the Interior, Bureau of Reclamation, 2007).
57. Heather Welch et al., *Unintended Consequences of Biofuels Production: The Effects of Large-Scale Crop Conversion on Water Quality and Quantity* (Washington, D.C.: U.S. Department of the Interior, U.S. Geological Survey, 2010); David Pimentel, "Update on Environmental and Economic Costs."
58. Welch, Heather et al., *Unintended Consequences of Biofuels Production: the effects of large-scale crop conversion on water quality and quantity* (Washington, D.C.: U.S. Department of the Interior, U.S. Geological Survey, 2010); Tony Shrader, *Water Levels and Water Quality in the Mississippi River Valley Alluvial Aquifer in Eastern Arkansas,* Scientific Investigation Report 2015-5059 (Washington, D.C.: U.S. Department of the Interior, U.S. Geological Survey, 2012).
59. Raymond Hermann et al., *Water Resources Investigation Report,* US Geological Survey (Washington, D.C.: Department of Interior, 1998).
60. USDA, *RCA Appraisal.*
61. USDA, *RCA Appraisal;* Pimentel, "Update on Environmental Economic Costs."
62. Capehart, "Ethanol."
63. Action Aid, *Fueling the Food Crisis: The Cost to Developing Countries of U.S. Corn Ethanol Expansion,* Action Aid International USA Report, October 2012, www.actionaid.org.
64. M. J. Helmers et al., "Nitrogen Application Rate Under Continuous Corn and Corn-Soybean Rotation Systems," *Canadian Journal of Soil Science* 70/ 9 (2014): 493–99.
65. Clive James, *Global Status of Commercialized Biotech/GM Crops: 2014, Brief 49-2014,* www.isaaa.org; EIU ViewsWire, "World Commodities: EIU's Soybean Monthly Outlook," September 10, 2015.
66. Pimentel, "Update on Environmental and Economic Costs"; USDA, *RCA Appraisal.*
67. Liz Marshall and Zachary Sugg, "Corn Stover for Ethanol Production."
68. Bina Cappiello and Matt Apuzzo, "The Secret Environmental Cost of US Ethanol Policy," Associated Press, November 12, 2013.

69. Schnepf and Ycobucci, "Renewable Fuel Standard"; Cappiello and Apuzzo, "The Secret Environmental Cost of US Ethanol Policy."

70. USDA, *RCA Appraisal.*

71. Cappiello and Apuzzo, "The Secret Environmental Cost of US Ethanol Policy."

72. Ibid.

73. USDA, *RCA Appraisal.*

74. Herrmann, *Water Resources Investigation Report;* Kristen Blann et al., "Effects of Agricultural Drainage on Aquatic Ecosystems: A Review," *Critical Reviews in Environmental Science and Technology* 39/1 (2009): 909–1001.

75. Blann, "Effects of Agricultural Drainage"; Walter K. Dodds et al., "Eutrophication of U.S. Freshwaters: Analysis of Potential Economic Damages," *Environmental Science and Technology* 43/1 (2009): 12–19; N. M. Dubrovsky et al., *The Quality of Our Nation's Waters: Nutrients in the Nation's Streams and Groundwater, 1992–2004,* U.S. Geological Survey circular 1350 (Washington, D.C.: U.S. Geological Survey, 2010); Helmers, "Nitrogen Application Rate"; USDA, *RCA Appraisal.*

76. Herrmann, *Water Resources Investigation Report.*

77. ETC Group, "The New Biomasters: Synthetic biology and the next assault on biodiversity and livelihoods," *Communiqué* No. 4, October 2010.

78. James, *Global Status of Commercialized Biotech.*

79. ETC Group, "The New Biomasters."

80. Rhonda Brooks, "Pioneer Outlines Plan to Protect Intellectual Property," *Farm Journal*, December 2, 2012.

81. Union of Concerned Scientists, "The Corn Belt and Mississippi River Basin," Cambridge, MA, 2011, www.ucsusa.org.

82. Smolker, *The Real Cost of Agrofuels.*

83. Ibid.

84. Pimental, "Energy and Dollar Costs."

85. Dubrovsky, *The Quality of Our Nation's Waters;* Helmers, "Nitrogen Application Rate."

86. Dubrovsky, *The Quality of Our Nation's Waters.*

87. Michael Duffy and David Correl, "The Economics of Corn on Corn," *Integrated Crop Management* 498/1 (2007): 15.

88. Sylvia Secchi et al., "Water Quality Changes Due to Corn Expansion in the Upper Mississippi River Basin," *Ecological Applications* 21/4 (2011): 1068–84.

89. Pimental, "Ecology of Increasing Diseases."

90. The White House, "Fact Sheet: Increasing investment in U.S. roads, ports and drinking water systems through innovative financing," Office of the Press Secretary, January 16, 2015, www.whitehouse.gov.

91. Dubrovsky, *The Quality of Our Nation's Waters.*
92. Herrmann, *Water Resources Investigation Report.*
93. Dubrovsky, *The Quality of Our Nation's Waters.*
94. Dodds, "Eutrophication of U.S. Freshwaters."
95. Cappiello and Apuzzo, "The Secret Environmental Cost."
96. Dan Engelberg et al., *Nutrient Pollution: EPA needs to work with states to develop strategies for monitoring the impact of state activities on the Gulf of Mexico hypoxic zone,* Report No. 14-P-0348 (Washington, D.C.: U.S. Environmental Protection Agency, Office of Inspector General, September 3, 2014).
97. Richard Alexander et al., "Differences in Phosphorus and Nitrogen Delivery to the Gulf of Mexico from the Mississippi River Basin," *Environmental Science and Technology* 42/ 3 (2008): 822–30; Christine Costello et al., "Impact of Biofuel Crop Production on the Formation of Hypoxia in the Gulf of Mexico," *Environmental Science and Technology* 43/20 (2009): 7985–91.
98. Engelberg, *Nutrient Pollution.*
99. Costello, "Impact of Biofuel Crop Production."
100. Donald Goolsby et al., *Sources and Transport of Nitrogen in the Mississippi River Basin,* U.S. Geological Survey, http://co.water.usgs.gov; Simon Donner and Christopher Kucharik "Corn-Based Ethanol Production Compromises Goal of Reducing Nitrogen Export by the Mississippi River," *Proceedings of the National Academy of Sciences of the United States of America* 105/1 (2008): 4513–18; Engelberg, *Nutrient Pollution;* Mississippi River Gulf of Mexico Watershed Nutrient Task Force, *Reassessment 2013: Assessing Progress Made Since 2008* (Washington, D.C.: U.S. Environmental Protection Agency, Office of Wetlands, Oceans, and Watersheds, 2013).
101. Mississippi River Gulf of Mexico Watershed Nutrient Task Force, *Reassessment 2013.*
102. Engelberg, *Nutrient Pollution.*
103. Ibid.
104. Lilley, "Green Fuels Dirty Secret."
105. Dubrovsky, *The Quality of Our Nation's Waters;* Union of Concerned Scientists, "The Corn Belt and Mississippi River Basin"; Cappiello and Apuzzo, "The Secret Environmental Cost."
106. Dubrovsky, *The Quality of Our Nation's Waters;* Union of Concerned Scientists, "The Corn Belt and Mississippi River Basin"; Dodds, "Eutrophication of U.S. Freshwaters"; Alexander, "Differences in Phosphorus and Nitrogen Delivery."
107. Union of Concerned Scientists, "The Corn Belt and Mississippi River Basin"; Pimentel, "Environmental and Economic Costs."

108. Jim Morrison, "How Much Is Clean Water Worth?," National Wildlife Federation, February 1, 2005; Herman E. Daly and Joshua Farley, *Ecological Economics: Principles and Applications* (Washington, D.C.: Island Press, 2003).

109. "Panel Weighs Health Impact of Herbicides," *Science News* 114/5 (July 31, 1993): 70–71.

110. Pimentel, "Environmental and Economic Costs"; Pimental, "Ecology of Increasing Diseases."

111. Dubrovsky, *The Quality of Our Nation's Waters*; Union of Concerned Scientists, "The Corn Belt and Mississippi River Basin."

112. Michele Kettles et al., "Triazine Herbicide Exposure and Breast Cancer Incidence: An Ecologic Study of Kentucky Counties," *Preventive Medicine and Environmental Health Faculty Publications*, Paper 25, 1997.

113. Golden, *An Economic Impact Analysis of the U.S. Bio-Based Products Industry*.

114. USDA, *RCA Appraisal*.

115. David Wear and John Greis, *The Southern Forest Assessment: Summary* (Asheville, NC: USDA Forest Service, Southern Research Station), www.srs.fs.usda.gov, 2001.

116. Ibid.; David Wear and John Greis, *The Southern Forest Futures Project: Summary Report, United States Department of Agriculture Forest Service, Southern Research Station*, General Technical Report SRS-168, 2012, www.srs.fs.usda.gov.

117. NRCS (Natural Resources Conservation Service), Longleaf Pine Range (Washington, D.C.: U.S. Department of Agriculture, , 2012), www.nrcs. usa.

118. The White House, "Climate Change and President Obama's Action Plan," August 3, 2015, www.whitehouse.gov.

119. U.S. EIA, *Annual Energy Outlook 2015 with Projections to 2040* (Washington, D.C.: U.S. Energy Information Administration Office of Integrated and International Energy Analysis, U.S. Department of Energy, April 2015).

120. NRDC (Natural Resources Defense Council), "Think Wood Pellets Are Green? Think Again," Issue Brief, May 2015, www.nrdc.org; Peter Wong and Gwen Bredehoeft, "US Wood Pellet Exports Double in 2013 in Response to Growing European Demand," US Energy Information Administration, 2004; Kaen Abt et al., "Effect of Policy on Pellet Production and Forest in the US South" (Triangle Park, NC: USDA Forest Service, Southern Research Station, 2013).

121. Wong and Bredehoeft, "US Wood Pellet Exports Double in 2013"; *Forbes*, "Wood Pellets Are Big Business (and for some, a big worry)," 2015.

122. Abt, "Effect of Policy on Pellet Production."
123. Dogwood Alliance, "Wood Pellet Manufacturing: Risks for the Economy of the US South," Briefing, 2014, www.dogwoodalliance.org.
124. NRDC, "Think Wood Pellets Are Green?"
125. Ibid.
126. Robert Drouin, "Wood Pellets: Green Energy or New Source of CO_2 Emissions?," E360, Yale School of Forestry and Environment Studies, January 22, 2015.
127. NRDC, "Think Wood Pellets Are Green?"
128. Ibid.
129. Drouin, "Wood Pellets."
130. Abt, "Effect of Policy on Pellet Production."
131. Wear and Greis, *The Southern Forest Futures Project.*
132. UNISDR (UN Office for Disaster Risk Reduction), *The Human Cost of Weather-Related Disasters 1995–2015,* 2015, www.unisdr.org.
133. Abt, "Effect of Policy on Pellet Production"; Dogwood Alliance, "Wood Pellet Manufacturing."
134. T. E. Dahl and S. M. Stedman, *Status and Trends of Wetlands in the Coastal Watersheds of the Coterminous United States 2004 to 2009* (Washington, D.C.: U.S. Department of the Interior, Fish and Wildlife Service and National Oceanic and Atmospheric Administration, National Marine Fisheries Service, 2013).
135. Herrmann, *Water Resources Investigation Report.*
136. Dahl and Stedman, *Status and Trends of Wetlands.*
137. Herrmann, *Water Resources Investigation Report;* USDA, *RCA Appraisal.*
138. Action Aid, *Fueling the Food Crisis.*
139. Ibid.
140. M. Lagi, *The Food Crises: A Quantitative Model of Food Prices Including Speculators and Ethanol Conversion* (Cambridge, MA: New England Complex Systems Institute, 2011).
141. Action Aid, *Fueling the Food Crisis.*
142. Lagi, *The Food Crises.*
143. IFPRI, *Global Nutrition Report 2015: Actions and Accountability to Advance Nutrition and Sustainable Development* (Washington, D.C.: International Food Poicy Research Institute, 2015).
144. Luca Colombo and Antonio Onorati, *Food, Riots and Rights* (London: International Institute for Environment and Development, 2013).
145. EIU Viewswire, "Soybean Monthly Outlook," September 10, 2015; James, *Global Status of Commercialized Biotech.*
146. James, *Global Status of Commericialized Biotech;* Smolker, *The Real Cost of Agrofuels.*

147. Smolker, *The Real Cost of Agrofuels*; FOEI (Friends of the Earth International), "Fueling Destruction in Latin America: The Real Price of the Drive for Agrofuels," Issue 113, September 2008, www. foei.org; Eric Holt-Gimenez and Miguel A. Altieri, "Agroecology, Food Sovereignty, and the New Green Revolution," *Agroecology and Sustainable Food Systems* 377/1 (2013): 90–102.
148. "Global Biofuels Will Struggle to Match Ambitious Objectives," *Oil and Gas Journal*, April 2, 2012.
149. Peter Voser, "Shell, Cosan form Joint Venture in Brazil for Biofuels," *World of Chemicals*, The Hague, June 18, 2011.
150. Eric Holt-Gimenez and Annie Shattuck, "The Agrofuels Transition: Restructuring places and spaces in the global food system," *Bulletin of Science, Technology and Society* 29/3 (2009): 18–188;
151. FOEI, "Fueling Destruction in Latin America."
152. Andrew W. Mitchell et al., *Forests Now in the Fight against Climate Change* (Oxford, UK: Global Canopy Program, 2008); Smolker, *The Real Cost of Agrofuels*; ETC Group, "The New Biomasters."
153. John Reilly and Sergey Paltsev, "Biomass Energy and Competition for Land," Joint Program on the Science and Policy of Global Change, Global Trade Analysis Project, Working Paper No. 46 (Cambridge, MA: Massachusetts Institute of Technology, 2008).
154. Ibid.

4. The Three Deceptions: Abundance, Green Environment, and Blue Skies

1. Luca Colombo and Antonnio Onorati, *Food, Riots and Rights* (London: International Institute for Environment and Development, 2013).
2. Ibid.; FOEI, *Fueling Destruction in Latin America: The Real Price of the Drive for Agrofuels*, Issue 113, September 2008, www.foei.org; World Bank, *Double Jeopardy: Responding to High Food and Fuel Prices* (Washington, D.C.: World Bank, 2008).
3. Colombo and Onorati, *Food, Riots and Rights*.
4. FAO, *The State of Food and Agriculture 2008 (SOFA)*, Part I. "Biofuels: Prospects, Risks and Opportunities" (Rome: FAO, 2008).
5. International Food Policy Research Institute, "Biofuels and Food Prices," 2008, www.ifpri.org.
6. FAO, *The State of Food and Agriculture 2008*; M. Lagi, *The Food Crises: A Quantitative Model of Food Prices Including Speculators and Ethanol Conversion* (Cambridge, MA: New England Complex Systems Institute: 2011).
7. David Pimentel et al., "Ecology of Increasing Diseases: Population Growth and Environmental Degradation," *Human Ecology* 35 (2007): 653–68.

8. Colombo and Onorati, *Food, Riots and Rights.*

9. Ulrich Hoffmann, *Assuring Food Security in Developing Countries under the Challenges of Climate Change: Key Trade and Development Issues of a Fundamental Transformation of Agriculture,* U.N. Conference on Trade and Development Discussion Paper No. 201, February 2011, Geneva, Switzerland.

10. Oxfam, "Climate Wrong and Human Rights," Oxfam Briefing Paper 117, www.oxfam.org.

11. Ed Gallagher, *The Gallagher Review*: "The Indirect Effects of Biofuel Production," 2008, www.unido.org.

12. Action Aid, "Fueling Hunger: New data reinforces why the UK must tackle damaging biofuels policies at the G8 and EU," April 2013, www.actionaid.org.

13. Diana Hernandez Codero, *Biofueling Hunger: How US Corn Ethanol Policy Drives Up Food Prices in Mexico,* Action Aid International, 2012, www.actionaid.org.uk.

14. H. Steinfeld et al., *Livestock's Long Shadow: Environmental Issues and Options* (Rome: FAO, 2006); Olivier de Schutter, "The New Green Revolution: How Twenty-First-Century Science Can Feed the World," *The Solutions Journal* 2/4 (2011): 33–44; Reyes Tirado, *The Seven Principles of a Food System that Has People at Its Heart: Ecological Farming,* Greenpeace International, 2015, www.greenpeace.org; Colombo and Onorati, *Food, Riots and Rights.*

15. Nikos Alexandratos and Jelle Bruinsma, *World Agriculture Towards 2030/2050: The 2012 Revision* (Rome: FAO, 2012).

16. Colombo and Onorati, *Food, Riots and Rights;* Action Aid, "Fuelling Hunger"; UNCTAD (United Nations Conference on Trade and Development), *The Green Economy: Trade and Sustainable Development Implications,* background note prepared by the UNCTAD Secretariat for the Ad Hoc Expert Meeting on the Green Economy: Trade and Sustainable Development Implications, 7–8 October 2010, Geneva, Switzerland.

17. Jules Pretty, "Agroecology in Developing Countries: The Promise of a Sustainable Harvest," *Environment* 45/9 (November 8, 2003).

18. UNCTAD, *Trade and Development Report,* 2015, United Nations Conference on Trade and Development, Geneva. Switzerland.

19. Colombo and Onorati, *Food, Riots and Rights*: Codero, *Biofueling Hunger.*

20. UNCTAD, *Trade and Development Report.*

21. Global Research, "Financial Implosion: Global Derivatives Market at 1200 Trillion Dollars . . . 20 Times the World Economy," Center for Research on Globalization, May 20, 2012.

22. Oxfam, *Land and Power*; Al Gore, *The Future: Six Drivers of Global Change* (New York: Random House, 2013); Stefan Bringezu et al., "Towards Sustainable Production and Use of Resources," *Assessing Biofuels* (Nairobi: International Panel for Sustainable Resource Management, UNEP, 2009).

23. Tim Searchinger et al., *Creating a Sustainable Food Future: A Menu of Solutions to Sustainably Feed More than 9 Billion People by 2050*, World Resources Report 2013–14, Interim Findings, www.wri.org; Lester R. Brown, *Plan B/2.0: Mobilizing to Save Civilization*, 1st ed. (New York: W. W. Norton, 2008); Stefan Bringezu et al., "Assessing Global Land Use: Balancing Consumption with Sustainable Supply" (Nairobi: International Resource Panel, UNEP, 2014); David R. Pimentel, "Food versus Biofuels: Environmental and Economic Costs," *Human Ecology* 37/1 (2009): 1–12.

24. World Resources Institute, "Food Production: Have Yields Stopped Rising?," 1998–99, www.wri.org.

25. Mark Rosegrant et al., *Food Security in a World of Natural Resource Scarcity: The Role of Agricultural Technologies* (Washington, D.C.: International Food Policy Research Institute, 2014); Thomas Cox, "Prospects for Developing Perennial Grain Crops," *BioScience* 56/8 (2006): 649–59.

26. Lester R. Brown, *Plan B/2.0*; International Food Policy Research Institute, "Biofuels and Food Prices," 2008, www.ifpri.org.

27. Pimentel, "Food versus Biofuels."

28. Searchinger, *Creating a Sustainable Food Future*; Nikos Alexandratos and Jelle Bruinsma, *World Agriculture*; Brown, *Plan B/2.0*.

29. UNEP, *Towards a Green Economy: The Pathway to Sustainable Development and Poverty Eradication* (Nairobi: United Nations Environment Program, 2011), www.unep.org.

30. Searchinger, *Creating a Sustainable Food Future*; Lester R. Brown, *World on the Edge: How to Prevent Environmental and Economic Collapse* (New York: W. W. Norton, 2011); Leora Casey and Alex Wijeratna, *On the Brink: Who's Best Prepared for a Climate and Hunger Crisis?* Action Aid, 2011, www.actionaid.org; Oxfam, *Climate Wrongs and Human Rights*.

31. Donald Easum, "Let the Harvest Begin," letter from Global Business Access, Ltd., May 19, 1998, www.ukadc.org.

32. ETC Group, "Putting the Cartel before the Horse," *Communiqué* No. 111, September 2013, www.etcgroup.org; ETC Group, "Gene Giants Seek 'Philanthrogopoly,'" *Communiqué* No. 110, March 6, 2013; ETC Group, "The New Biomasters: Synthetic Biology and the Next Assault on Biodiversity and Livelihoods," *Communiqué* No. 104, October 2010.

33. ETC Group, "The New Biomasters"; ETC Group, "Breaking Bad: Big Ag Mega-Mergers in Play Dow + DuPont in the Pocket? Next: Demonsanto?," *Communiqué* 115, December 2015.

34. ETC Group, "The New Biomasters"; ETC Group, "Putting the Cartel Before the Horse"; ETC Group "Breaking Bad"; Bringezu, "Assessing Global Land Use."

35. ETC Group, "Breaking Bad."

36. Colombo and Onorati, "Food, Riots, and Rights."

37. Ibid.

38. Doug Gurian-Sherman, "Genetic Engineering—A Crop of Hyperbole," *San Diego Union Tribune*, June 10, 2008.

39. Jules Pretty, "The Rapid Emergence."

40. ETC Group, "Gene Giants Seek 'Philanthrogopoly'"; ETC Group, "Putting the Cartel Before the Horse."

41. Isabel McCrea and Sue Mayer, "AstraZeneca and Its Genetic Research"; Vandana Shiva, *Stolen Harvest: The Highjacking of the Global Food Supply* (Cambridge, MA: South End Press, 2000).

42. McCrea and Mayer, "AstraZeneca and Its Genetic Research"; GRAIN, "GMOs: Fooling, er, 'Feeding—the World for 20 Years," May 15, 2015, www.grain.org.

43. Shiva, *Stolen Harvest*.

44. Hope Shand, "Terminator Seeds: Monsanto Moves to Tighten Its Grip on Global Agriculture," *Multinational Monitor* 19/11 (1998); McCrea and Mayer, "AstraZeneca and Its Genetic Research"; Ricarda A. Steinbrecher and Pat Roy Mooney, "Terminator Technologies (GURTs): The Threat to World Food Security," *The Ecologist*, October 1998, www.econexist.info; Pretty, "The Rapid Emergence."

45. McCrea and Mayer, "AstraZeneca and Its Genetic Research"; Steinbrecher and Mooney, "Terminator Technologies (GURTs)"; Pretty, "The Rapid Emergence."

46. "EIU's Maize Monthly Outlook," *EIU Viewswire*, July 1, 2016; "EIU Rice Monthly Outlook," *EIU Viewswire*, June 1, 2016; "EIU's Wheat Monthly Outlook," *EIU Viewswire*, April 1, 2016.

47. Shand, "Terminator Seeds."

48. Ibid.

49. Pretty, "Agroecology in Developing Countries."

50. Steinbrecher and Mooney, "Terminator Technologies (GURTs)"; Five Year Freeze, "Feeding or Fooling the World."

51. David Pimentel and T. W. Patzek, "Ethanol Production Using Corn, Switchgrass, and Wood: Biodiesel Production Using Soybean and Sunflower," *Natural Resources Research Council* 14/1 (2005): 65–76.

52. Bringezu, *Assessing Global Land Use;* IEA WEO, *World Energy Outlook 2011,* International Energy Agency, Paris, France.
53. T. Searchinger and R. Heimlich, "Avoiding Bioenergy Competition for Food Crops and Land," Working Paper, Installment 9 of *Creating a Sustainable Food Future* (Washington, D.C.: World Resources Institute, 2015).
54. Ibid.
55. Dirk Bryant et al., *The Last Frontier Forests: Ecosystems and Economies on the Edge* (Washington, D.C.: World Resources Institute, 1997).
56. Ibid.
57. Rachael Petersen et al., "Mapping Tree Plantations with Multispectral Imagery: Preliminary results for seven tropical countries," *Technical Note* (Washington, D.C.: World Resources Institute, 2016), www.wri.org.
58. Gallagher, "The Indirect Effects of Biofuel Production."
59. Bringezu, "Assessing Global Land Use."
60. Bringezu, "Towards Sustainable Production and Use of Resources."
61. FAO, *The State of Food and Agriculture, 2008.*
62. Bringezu, "Assessing Global Land Use."
63. Petersen, "Mapping Tree Plantations with Multispectral Imagery."
64. Grant Rosoman, "The Plantation Efect: An ecoforestry review of the environmental effect of exotic monoculture tree plantations in Aotearoa/New Zealand," New Zealand Greenpeace, REDD Monitor, 1994, www.red-monitor.org.
65. Ibid.
66. UNEP, *Options for Decoupling Economic Growth from Water Use and Water Pollution* (Nairobi, Kenya: The International Resource Panel, UNEP, 2016).
67. Erik Swyngedow, *Social Power and the Urbanization of Water: Flows of Power* (New York: Oxford University Press, 2004).
68. Maude Barlow, *Blue Covenant: The Global Water Crisis and the Coming Battle for the Right to Water* (New York: New Press, 2007).
69. Brown, *Plan B/2.0.*
70. ETC Group, "The New Biomasters"; Almuth Ernsting and Deepak Rughani, "Climate Geo-Engineering with Carbon Negative Bioenergy: Climate savior or climate endangering?," 2008, www.globalbioenergy.org; Rachel Smolker et al., *Cost of Agrofuels: Impacts on Food, Forests, People and the Climate,* Global Forest Coalition, Global Justice Ecology Project and Institute for Social Ecology with contributions from Dogwood Alliance and ETC Group; Jacques Berthelot, "Agribusiness' Headlong Flight to Agrofuels and Their Impact on Food Security," January 5, 2010, www.landaction.org.

71. Jessica Bellardy, "Cool Farming"; Steinfeld, *Livestock's Long Shadow;* Searchinger, *Creating a Sustainable Food Future.*

72. Norman Meyers, "The World's Forests and Their Ecosystem Services," in *Nature's Services: Societal Dependence on Natural Ecosystems,* ed. Gretchen C. Daily (New York: Routledge, 1997), 213–26.

73. Rosoman, "The Plantation Effect."

74. Harold Liversage, "Managing the Biofuel Boom, Smallholders' Access to Land: Innovative Models in Africa," 2009, www.un.org.

75. M. Verdonk et al., "Governance of the Emerging Bio-Energy Markets," *Energy Policy* 35 (2007): 3909–24.

76. Hoffmann, *Assuring Food Security;* Action Aid International, *Fuel for Thought: Addressing the Social Impacts of EU Biofuels Policies,* April 2012, www.actionaid.org.

77. Kanya D'Almeida, "Climate: at the nexus of agrofuels, land grabs and hunger," *Global Information Network,* December 6, 2011, www.oaklandinstitute.org.

78. L. Peskett et al., "Biofuels, Agriculture and Poverty Reduction" (London: Overseas Development Institute, 2007).

79. ETC Group, "The New Biomasters."

80. Andrew W. Mitchell et al., *Forests Now in the Fight Against Climate Change* (Oxord, UK: Global Canopy Program, 2008); Edward O. Wilson, *The Future of Life* (New York: Knopf, 2002).

81. Timothy Searchinger et al., "The Use of U.S. Croplands for Biofuels Increases Greenhouse Gases through Emissions from Land-Use Change," *Science* 319/5867 (2008): 1238–40.

82. Smolker, *The Real Cost of Agrofuels.*

83. Herman E. Daly and Joshua Farley, *Ecological Economics: Principles and Applications* (Washington, D.C.: Island Press, 2003).

84. Berthelot, "Agribusines' Headlong Flight"; Joseph Fargione et al., "Land Clearing and the Biofuel Carbon Debt," *Science* 319/5867 (February 29, 2008): 1235–38.

85. Berthelot, "Agribusiness' Headlong Flight"; Joseph Fargione et al., "Land Clearing and the Biofuel Carbon Debt," *Science* 319/5867 (February 29, 2008): 1235–38.

86. Ernsting and Rughani, "Climage Geo-Engineering"; Finn Danielson et al., "Biofuel Plantations on Forested Lands: Double Jeopardy for Biodiversity and Climate," *Conservation Biology* 23/2 (2008): 348–58; Mitchell, *Forests Now in the Fight.*

87. Bringezu, *Assessing Global Land Use.*

88. Fargione, "Land Clearing."

89. Danielson, "Biofuel Plantations on Forested Lands"; Joseph Holden, "Peatland Hydrology and Carbon Release: Why Small-Scale Process

Matters," *Philosophical Transactions: Mathematics, Physical and Engineering Sciences* 363/1837 (2005): 2891–2913; S. E. Page et al., "Interdependence of Peat and Vegetation in Tropical Peat Swamps," *Philosophical Transactions: Biological Sciences* 354/1391: 1885–97.

90. Searchinger, *Creating a Sustainable Food Future.*
91. Holden, "Peatland Hydrology."
92. Ibid.; Searchinger, *Creating a Sustainable Food Future;* Paul A. Keddy et al., "Wet and Wonderful: The world's largest wetlands are conservation priority," *Bioscience*59/1 (2009): 39–51.
93. Mitchell, *Forests Now in the Fight.*
94. Danielson, "Biofuel Plantations on Forested Lands"; Fargione, "Land Clearing."
95. Fargione, "Land Clearing."
96. Pimentel and Patzek, "Ethanol Production Using Corn,"
97. Searchinger, *Creating a Sustainable Food Future.*

5. In Place of Conclusion: Can We Overcome the Planetary Emergency?

1. Stephen Gill, "Constitutionalizing Inequality and the Clash of Globalizations," *International Studies Review* 4/2, (2002): 47–65.
2. Ibid.
3. UNCTAD, *Evolution of the International Trading System and Its Trends from a Development Perspective,* Trade and Development Board, 61st session, September 15–26, 2014 (Geneva: UN Conference on Trade and Development, 2015).
4. Luca Colombo and Antonio Onorati, *Food, Riots and Rights* (London: International Institute for Environment and Development, 2013).
5. Tim Searchinger et al., *Creating a Sustainable Food Future: A Menu of Solutions to Sustainably Feed More than 9 Billion People by 2050,* World Resources report 2013–14, www.wri.org; ILO, *World Employment and Social Outlook 2016: Transforming Jobs to End Poverty* (Geneva: International Labor Organization, 2016); IFAD, *Rural Poverty Report 2011, New Realities, New Challenges: New Opportunities for Tomorrow's Generation* (Rome: International Fund for Agricultural Development, 2011); UNCTAD, *The Green Economy: Trade and Sustainable Development Implications,* UN Conference on Trade and Development, prepared by the UNCTAD Secretariat for the Ad Hoc Expert Meeting on the Green Economy (Geneva: Trade and Sustainable Implications, Octoer 7–8, 2010); Francois Bourguignon, *The Globalization of Inequality* (Princeton: Princeton University Press, 2015).
6. ILO, *World Employment and Social Outlook 2016.*
7. FAO, *Rome Declaration on World Food Security and World Food Summit*

Plan of Action (Rome: FAO, 1996), www.fao.org; Searchinger, *Creating a Sustainable Food Future.*

8.   ILO, *World Employment and Social Outlook 2016.*

9.   Bourguignon, *The Globalization of Inequality.*

10. Ulrich Hoffmann, *Assuring Food Security in Developing Countries under the Challenges of Climate Change: key trade and development issues of a fundamental transformation of agriculture,* discussion paper No. 201 (Geneva, Switzerland: U.N. Conference on Trade and Development, February 2011).

11. Hoffmann, *Assuring Food Security in Developing Countries;* UNCTAD, *Evolution of the International Trading System;* IFAD, *Rural Poverty Report.*

12. H. Steinfeld et al., *Livestock's Long Shadow: Environmental Issues and Options* (Rome: FAO, 2006); Jessica Bellard et al., "Cool Farming: Climate Impacts of Agriculture and Mitigation Potential," Greenpeace Internatioinal, 2008, www.greenpeace.org; Andreas Gattinger et al., "No-Till Agriculture—A Climate Smart Solution?" Climate Change and Agriculture, Report No. 2, www.misereor.org.

13. IFAD, *Rural Poverty Report 2011.*

14. Jules Pretty et al., "Resource Conserving Agriculture Increases Yields in Developing Countries," *Environment, Science and Technology* 40/4 (2006): 114–19; UNEP, *Towards a Green Economy: The Pathway to Sustainable Evelopment and Poverty Eradication* (Nairobi: United Nations Environment Program, 2012).

15. Olivier De Schutter, "The New Green Revolution: how twenty-first-century science can feed the world," *The Solutions Journal,* Vol. 2 No. 4 (2011): 33-44.

16. Reyes Tirado, *The Seven Principles of a Food system that has People at its Heart: ecological farming.* Greenpeace International, 2015, www.green-peace.org.

17. Edgar Hertwich et al., *Assessing the Environmental Impacts of Consumption and Production: Priority Products and Materials* (Nairobi: UNEP, International Panel for Sustainable Resource Management, 2010); FAO, *Save and Grow: A Policymaker's Guide to the Sustainable Intensification of Smallholder Crop Production* (Rome: FAO, 2011).

18. Hertwich, *Assessing the Environmental Impacts of Consumption and Production;* Olivier De Schutter, "The New Green Revolution"; Hoffmann, *Assuring Food Security in Developing Countries;* Miguel Altieri and Fernando Funes-Monzote, *Monthly Review,* Vol. 63, No 8 (2012): 23–33.

19. Searchinger, *Creating a Sustainable Food Future.*

20. Zareen Bharucha and Jules Pretty, "The Roles and Values of Wild Foods in Agricultural Systems," *Philosophical Transactions of the Royal Society B* 365 (2010): 2913–26.

21. Stephen Gliessman, "Transforming Food Systems with Agroecology," *Agroecology and Sustainable Food Systems* 40/3 (2013): 187–89.

22. Ibid.; P. M. Rosset and M.A. Altieri, "Agroecology versus Input Substitution: A Fundamental Contradiction of Sustainable Agriculture," *Society and Natural Resources* 10/3 (1997): 283–95.

23. Ibid.

24. Helga Willer and Julia Lernoud, "Organic Agriculture Worldwide: Current Statistics" (Frick, Switzerland: Research Institute of Organic Agriculture, 2015).

25. Rosset and Altieri, "Agroecology versus Input Substitution"; Stephen Gliessman, "Transforming Food Systems with Agroecology."

26. Gliessman, "Transforming Food Systems with Agroecology."

27. De Schutter, "The New Green Revolution"; Miguel Altieri and Victor Manuel Toledo, "The Agroecological Revolution in Latin America: Rescuing Nature, Ensuring Food Sovereignty and Empowering Peasants," *Journal of Peasant Studies* 38/3 (2011): 587–612; Sarah Borron, *Building Resilience for an Unpredictable Future: How Organic Agriculture Can Help Farmers Adapt to Climate Change* (Rome: Food and Agriculture Organization of the United Nations, 2006); Colombo and Onorati, *Food, Riots, and Rights*; Tirado, *The Seven Principles of the Food System*; Pretty, "Resource Conserving Agriculture."

28. Altieri and Toledo, "The Agroecological Revolution in Latin America"; Miguel Altieri and Parviz Koohafkan, *Enduring Farms: climate change, smallholders and traditional farming communities* (Penang, Malaysia: Third World Network, 2008); Tirado, *The Seven Principles of a Food System*; Gliessman, "Transforming Food Systems with Agroecology"; Jules Pretty, "Agroecology in Developing Countries: The Promise of a Sustainable Harvest," *Environment* 45/9 (November 8, 2003); Mark Rosegrant et al., *Food Security in a World of Natural Resource Scarcity: The Role of Agricultural Technologies* (Washington, D.C.: International Food Policy Research Institute, 2014).

29. FAO, *Save and Grow.*

30. Thomas Cox et al., "Prospects for Developing Perennial Grain Crops," *BioScience*, Vol. 56, No. 8 (2006): 649–659.

31. FAO, *Save and Grow.*

32. UNISDR, *The Human Cost of Weather-Related Disasters 1995–2015*, U.N. Office for Disaster Risk Reduction, 2015, www.unisdr.org.

33. Quoted in Five Year Freeze, "Feeding or Fooling the World? Can GM really feed the hungry?," 2002, www.fiveyearfreeze.org.

34. Pretty, "Resource Conserving Agriculture."
35. Catherine Badgley et al., "Organic Agriculture and the Global Food Supply," *Renewable Agriculture and Food Systems* 22/2 (2007): 86–108.
36. John Reganold et al., "Long-Term Effects of Organic and Conventional Farming on Soil Erosion," *Nature* 330 (1987): 370–72; Mark Rosegrant et al., *Food Security in a World of Natural Resource Scarcity: the role of agricultural technologies* (Washington, D.C.: International Food Policy Research Institute, 2014).
37. Jennifer Clapp, *Hunger in the Balance: the new politics of international food aid* (Ithaca, New York: Cornell University Press., 2012).
38. P. M. Rosset et al., "The Campesino-to-Campesino Agroecology Movement of ANAP in Cuba: Social process methodology in the construction of sustainable peasant agriculture and food sovereignty," *Journal of Peasant Studies* 38/1 (2011): 161-191.
39. Miguel Altieri and Fernando Funes-Monzote, "The Paradox of Cuban Agriculture," *Monthly Review* 63/8 (2012): 23–33.
40. Rosset, "The Campesino-to-Campesino Agroecology Movement."
41. Ibid., Altieri and Funes-Monzote, "The Paradox of Cuban Agriculture"; Altieri and Toledo, "The Agroecological Revolution in Latin America."
42. Isabel McCrea and Sue Mayer, "AstraZeneca and Its Genetic Research: feeding the world or fueling public hunger?" Action Aid International, 1999, www.actionaid.org; Miguel A. Altieri et al., "Peasant Agriculture and the Conservation of Crop and Wild Plant Resources," *Conservation Biology* 1, No. 1 (1987): 49–58; Miguel Altieri and Parviz Koohafkan, *Enduring Farms*; Ulrich Hoffmann, *Assuring Food Security*; IFAD, *Rural Poverty Report 2011*; Vandana Shiva, *Stolen Harvest.*"
43. Altieri, "Peasant Agriculture."
44. Ivette Perfecto et al., "Synergies between Agricultural Intensification and Climate Change Could Create Surprising Vulnerabilities for Crops," *BioScience*, Vol. 58, No. 9 (2008).
45. Altieri, "Peasant Agriculture."
46. De Schutter, "The New Green Revolution."
47. Ibid.; Perfecto, "Synergies between Agricultural Intensification and Climate Change"; Eric Holt-Gimenez, "Measuring Farmers' Agroecological Resistance after Hurricane Mitch in Nicaragua: A case study in participatory, sustainable land management impact monitoring," *Agriculture, Ecosystems and Environment* 93/1–3 (2002): 87–105; Altieri and Toledo, "The Agroecological Revolution in Latin America."
48. Reganold, "Long-Term Effects of Organic and Conventional Farming"; David Huggins and John Reganold, "No-Till: The Quiet Revolution," *Scientific American* 299/1 (July 2008).
49. Reganold, "Long-Term Effects of Organic and Conventional Farming."

50. Badgley, "Organic Agriculture"; Altieri, "Peasant Agriculture and the Conservation of Crop and Wild Plant Resources"; FAO, *Save and Grow.*
51. Altieri and Koohafkan, *Enduring Farms.*
52. FAO, *Save and Grow.*
53. Five Year Freeze, "Feeding or Fooling the World?"
54. Badgley, "Organic Agriculture"; Huggins and Reganold, "No-Till: The Quiet Revolution."
55. Huggins and Reganold, "No-Till: The Quiet Revolution."
56. FAO, *Save and Grow.*
57. Mark Rosegrant et al., *Food Security in a World of Natural Resource Scarcity: the role of agricultural technologies* (Washington, D.C.: International Food Policy Research Institute, 2014).
58. Pretty, "Agroecology in Developing Countries."
59. FAO, *Save and Grow.*
60. UNEP, *Options for Decoupling Economic Growth from Water Use and Water Pollution.*
61. FAO, *Save and Grow;* De Schutter, "The New Green Revolution."
62. David Pimentel et al., "Economic and Environmental Benefits of Biodiversity," *BioScience* 47/11 (1997): 747–57; Thomas Cox et al., "Prospects for Developing Perennial Grain Crops"; Lee DeHaan and David Van Tassel, "Useful Insights from Evolutionary Biology for Developing Perennial Grain Crops," *American Journal of Botany* 101/10 (2014): 1801–19; Jerry Glover et al., "Future Farming: A Return To Roots?" *Scientific American* 297/2 (2007): 82–89; David Van Tassel and Lee DeHaan, "Wild Plants to the Rescue," *American Scientist* 101/3 (2013).
63. Thomas Cox et al., "Prospects for Developing Perennial Grain Crops"; Lee DeHaan and David Van Tassel, "Useful Insights from Evolutionary Biology"; Glover, "Future Farming: A Return To Roots?," all in Mark Rosegrant, *Food Security in a World of Natural Resource Scarcity: the role of agricultural technologies* (Washington, D.C.: International Food Policy Research Institute, 2014).
64. Cox, "Prospects for Developing Perennial Grain Crops"; DeHaan and Van Tassel, "Useful Insights from Evolutionary Biology"; Glover, "Future Farming: a return to roots?"
65. UNCTAD, *Evolution of the International Trading System.*
66. De Schutter, "The New Green Revolution."
67. Pretty, "Agroecology in Developing Countries."
68. FAO, *Save and Grow.*
69. Olivier de Schutter, "The New Green Revolution"; Jules Pretty, "Agroecology in Developing Countries."
70. FAO, *Save and Grow.*

71. Marian Lawson et al., "The Obama Administration's Feed the Future Initiative," Congressional Research Service, 7-5700, January 29, 2016, www.crs.gov.

72. Ibid.

73. FOEI, "A Wolf in Sheep's Clothing? An Analysis of the 'Sustainable Intensification' of Agriculture," *Friends of the Earth International*, 2012, www.foei.org.

74. Ibid.

75. Ibid.

76. FAO, *Save and Grow.*

77. GACSO, *Climate-Smart Agriculture, Site-Specific Nutrient Management: Implementation Guidance for Policy Makers and Investors,* 2014, www.fao.org/gacso.

78. Perfecto, "Synergies between Agricultural Intensification and Climate Change."

79. Rosegrant, *Food Security in a World of Natural Resource Scarcity.*

80. Ibid.; Gattinger, "No-Till Agriculture."

81. Gattinger, "No-Till Agriculture"; FOEI, *Fueling Destruction in Latin America.*

82. UNEP, *Towards a Green Economy;* World Bank, "Double Jeopardy: Responding to high food and fuel prices" (Washington, D. C.: World Bank, 2008).

83. Stefan Bringezu et al., *Assessing Global Land Use: Balancing Consumption with Sustainable Supply* (Nairobi: The International Panel, UNEP, 2014).

84. IRENA (International Renewable Energy Agency), *Renewable Energy and Jobs: Annual Review 2015,* www.irena.org.

85. Tim Searchinger and R. Heimlich, "Avoiding Bioenergy Competition for Food Crops and Land," Working Paper, Installment 9, of Creating a Sustainable Food Future (Washington, DC: World Resources Institute, 2015).

86. IRENA, *Renewable Energy and Jobs.*

87. Mark S. Jaobson et al., "Examining the Feasibility of Converting New York State's All-Purpose Energy Infrastructure to One Using Wind, Water, and Sunlight," *Energy Policy* 57 (2013): 585–601.

88. Mark Z. Jacobson et al., "A Roadmap for Repowering California for All Purposes with Wind, Water, and Sunlight," *Energy Policy* 73 (2014): 875–89.

89. Tim Dickinson, "The Dirty War on Solar Power," *Rolling Stone,* February 25, 2016.

90. Ibid.

91. Greenpeace USA, *Koch Industries 2011 Update,* www.greenpeace.org.

92. Ibid.; Jane Mayer, *Dark Money: The Hidden History of the Billionaires Behind the Rise of the Radical Right* (New York: Penguin Random House, 2016); Michael Mechanic, "Spying on the Koch Brothers," *Mother Jones* 36/6 (Nov.–Dec. 2011); Tim Dickinson, "Inside the Koch Brothers' Toxic Empire," *Rolling Stone,* October 9, 2014; Philip Elliott, "Power Brokers Recharge," *Time,* August 17, 2015.

93. Mayer, *Dark Money*; Mechanic, "Spying on the Koch Brothers"; Dickinson, "Inside the Koch Brothers' Toxic Empire," *Rolling Stone;* Elliott, "Power Brokers Recharge."

94. Mayer, *Dark Money*; Dickinson, "Inside the Koch Brothers' Toxic Empire," *Rolling Stone.*

95. Mayer, *Dark Money*; Dickinson, "Inside the Koch Brothers' Toxic Empire," *Rolling Stone;* Daniel Schulman, *The Sons of Wichita: How the Koch Brothers Became America's Most Powerful and Private Dynasty* (New York: Grand Central Publishing, 2014).

Index

ADM, *See* Archer Daniels Midland
advanced countries: decrease in arable
    land in, 111; increased food pro-
    duction in, 117; *See also* Global
    North
Africa: agricultural workers in, 249;
    expected water shortages in, 215;
    indigenous fruits consumed in,
    269; land grabs in, 68, 69, 103, 212;
    oil imported by, 288; poverty in,
    110; stem borers (insects) in, 272
Agency for International
    Development, U.S (USAID),
    280–81
agrarian reform, 106
Agricultural Biotechnology Council,
    282
agriculture: in Global South, 252;
    increased food production in,
    30–31; organic and agroecology,
    257–58; small farms in, 29–30; sub-
    sidies for, 277; workers in, 248–49;
    See also agroecology
Agriculture, U.S. Department of:
    Biopreferred Program of, 152–53;
    Conservation Reserve Program

of, 166–68; genetic use restriction
    technology developed by, 222;
    Mississippi River Basin Healthy
    Watershed Initiative of, 180
Agrilife Research, 79, 80
agroecology, 16, 254–55, 257–65;
    corporate opposition to, 279–80,
    284–85; in Cuba, 266–67; FAO
    symposium on, 282–84; in Latin
    America, 267–70; no-till farming
    in, 273, 285–87; perennial grain
    crops in, 274–75; rainwater har-
    vesting in, 278–79; of soil, 270–72;
    water in, 273–74, 277–78
agroforestry, 254, 259, 268, 269
air pollution, 100; from ethanol plants,
    173
algae, 124, 177, 179
Altieri, Miguel, 257
Amazon River basin, 41; Congo basin
    connected with, 49; deforestation
    of, 28, 202
American Jobs Creation Act (US,
    2004), 141
American Petroleum Institute (API),
    148

ammonia, 39; emissions of, 38
Amstutz, Daniel, 118, 119
Amyris (firm), 124
Andreas, Dwayne, 123
annual crops, 275
Archer Daniels Midland (ADM; firm),
    14; in Brazil, 201; corn converted to
    biofuel by, 122–23, 135–36; ethanol
    produced by, 100–101; as omnipo-
    tent global conglomerate, 219;
    subsidies for, 138
Argentina: biofuel production in, 208;
    genetically-modified crops in, 128
atrazine (herbicide), 183
Australia: coal production in, 85;
    increased food production in, 117;
    shale oil and gas in, 84
automobile industry, biofuels and,
    90–92, 137
automobiles, See cars

Badgley, Catherine, 263
Bangladesh, 254, 290
banks, 211
Barclays Bank, 97
Barclays Capital (firm), 211
BASF (firm), 217
Battell (firm), 151
Baucum, Scott, 222
Bharucha, Zareen, 256
biodiesel fuel: carbon released by,
    241–43; global production of, 10;
    Koch brothers' interests in, 295;
    U.S. production of, 140; water
    needed for, 235
biodiversity, 37
bioenergy: carbon neutral, 237; geog-
    raphy of, 68–69; International
    Energy Agency predictions for, 72
bioethanol, 140
biofuel-biotechnology industrial com-
    plex, 15–16, 134
biofuels, 12–13; as alternative to fossil
    fuels, 72; automobile industry

and, 90–92; carbon costs of,
    240–41; competition between
    food production and, 34–35, 208;
    corn converted into, 122; crops
    engineered for, 129–30; eco-
    logical depletion linked to, 26–27;
    environmental impact of, 173;
    federal subsidies for, 123; food
    consequences of production and
    consumption of, 164–73; food
    production and, 31; genetically-
    modified organisms and, 124;
    geoeconomics in America of,
    135–54; greenhouse gas emissions
    from, 239; impact on forest ecol-
    ogy of, 187–89; investments in, 75;
    oil industry control over, 78–79;
    oligopolies and, 92–104; prince
    increases in food tied to, 205–7;
    production competition with food,
    32–33; second-generation, 74; solar
    energy compared with, 289; water
    consequences of production and
    consumption of, 154–64, 235
bioinformatics, 131
biology, 104
Biomass Power Louisiana (firm), 191
bioplastics, 187
Biopreferred Program, 152–53
biorefineries, 153
biotechnology, 95–96, 150–52, 282; for
    engineering crops, 129–30; export-
    ing, 128; genomics applied to, 131;
    promise of, 216; purpose of, 126
Biotechnology Industry Organization
    (BIO), 18, 79, 150
Bolan, Dan, 145
Borlaug, Norman, 107
Bovard, James, 123
BP (firm), 77–80; in Brazil, 200–201;
    forms Butamax with DuPont, 124
Brazil, 28, 34; commercialization of
    agriculture in, 111; competition
    between livestock and growers in,

165; deforestation in, 240; ethanol produced in, 200–202, 208; food imported into, 249; genetically-modified crops in, 128; livestock in, 120; no-till farming in, 286; as soybean producer, 199–200; transnational corporations in, 219

Bremer, Paul, 118–19

Brown University, 59–60

Bunge Limited (firm), 96, 101

Burkina Faso, 278

Bush, George W., 60; in Latin America, 134–35, 200; national energy task force under, 71–72

Bush, Jeb, 135

Bush administration (GHWB), 123

Bush administration (GWB): Iraqi agriculture restructured by, 118–19; on link between ethanol production and food crisis, 94

Butamax (firm), 124

Cabrera, Antonio, 201

California: clean energy legislation in, 294–95; renewable energy in, 291

Camacho, Manuel Avila, 106–7

Campbell, Tom, 80

Canada, 117, 208–9

cancers, tied to herbicides, 186–87

canola, 209

capitalism: accumulation by dispossession in, 66; communism versus, 246–47; expansion of accumulation essential to, 54, 104; Polanyi on, 21; state welfarism and, 245–46; use value becoming exchange value under, 29

carbon: in fossil fuels, 238; no-till farming and, 287; sequestration by agriculture and forests of, 139–40; sequestration by soil of, 44–45; sequestration in rainforests, 49; stored in peatland rainforests, 45–46, 242–43

carbon dioxide: benefits of, 61, 62; released by burning tropical trees, 49–50

carbon dioxide emissions: from bioenergy, 237–38; from biofuels, 241; Clean Power Plan on, 189; International Energy Agency predictions for, 72; linked to livestock production, 38, 39

Cardenas, Lázaro, 106

Cargill (firm), 96, 101, 118, 219; in Brazil, 201; Renessen and, 129

Carlyle Group (firm), 200

cars (automobiles), 56; fuel for, 90–92

Catskill Mountains, 185

cattle, 120, 253; *See also* livestock

cellulosic ethanol, 148–49

Central America, 269

cereals, 105–6, 214; corporate control over seeds for, 223–24; decline in varieties of, 255; green revolution and, 110–11

Cheney, Dick, 71

Chesapeake Energy (firm), 88

Chevron (firm), 76–77; Australian operations of, 84; biofuels research by, 80

children, malnutrition among, 198–99, 210–11, 262

China, 105; African land bought by, 69; coal consumed in, 84–85; economic growth of, 25; genetically-modified crops in, 128; livestock in, 120; shale gas in, 83; solar power in, 289–90; synthetic fertilizer used in, 262; water relocation in, 234

Christie, Chris, 295

Citizens United v. FEC (U.S., 2010), 203

Clapp, Jennifer, 264–65

Clean Power Plan, 189

climate, impact of loss of rainforests on, 49

climate change: biofuels as answer to, 12; corporate lobbying on, 81; crop yields impacted by, 214; denial of, 293–95; hunger increased by, 215; natural gas causing, 87; organizations urging denial of, 61–62
Clinton administration, 123
coal, 84–85; being replaced by wood pellets, 189, 191
coffee, 268
Colorado River, 158–61
Columbia River, 170
Committee on World Food Security, 250
communism, 246–47
Congo River basin, 49
Conservation Reserve Program (CRP), 142, 165–68
Consultative Group for International Agricultural Research (CGIAR), 281–82
coral reefs, 53
corn, 99; converted into biofuel, 122; cotton growing shifting to, 162; dependent upon synthetic agrochemicals, 166; diverted to biofuel production, 197–98; land diverted to soybeans from, 199; price increases for, 102, 103; soil degradation caused by, 173–75; soybean growing shifting to, 165; subsidies for, 137; used for livestock feed, 34; used in ethanol, 135–37, 143; water required for, 155, 156; *See also* maize
Costanza, Robert, 51
cotton, 162
Cowen, Deborah, 64
cropland, 42, 164; climate change's impact on, 214; Conservation Reserve Program on, 166–68; diverted to corn from soybeans, 199; wetlands converted to, 169–70
Crouch, Martha, 224

Cuba, 265–67

D1 Oils (firm), 78
Daly, Herman, 22–23, 27–28, 50, 51
dams, 112
Danisco (firm), 124
Davenport, Doug, 168
decoupling, 56–57
Deere & Co., 219
Defense, U.S. Department of (Pentagon), biofuels used by, 144–45
deforestation, 228–29; in Brazil, 202; greenhouse gas emissions from, 238; linked to livestock production, 37; linked to paper industry, 44; soybean production and, 103
Delta and Pine Land Company, 222, 223
Democratic Republic of Congo (DRC), 69
Deutch, John, 89
developing countries: as food importers, 249; genetically-modified crops introduced in, 128, 132; increase in arable land in, 111; poverty in, 250; rice production in, 108; *See also* Global South
Dow AgroSciences (firm), 217
Drax Power (firm), 190, 191
Dreyfus (firm), 219
drinking water, 175–78, 215; for New York City, 185; pesticide pollution of, 183
drought-tolerant crops, 19
Dudley, Susan, 60
DuPont (firm), 79, 119; forms Butamax with BP, 124; genetic engineering by, 171; proprietary seed market controlled by, 218

E4tech (consulting company), 91
earth, as thermodynamically closed system, 50

Earth Council (organization), 63–64
Easum, Donald, 216
ecological economics, 52–58
economy: contribution of biotechnology to, 152; ecological versus neoclassical, 52–55; as part of ecosystem, 23; states' role in, 57; thermodynamics of, 25
Ecuador, 28
Egypt, 249
ejidos (collective farms in Mexico), 106
electric vehicles, 90
employment: in biofuels, 146; in biotechnology, 151; in chemical and plastics industries, 149
energy, 288; biomass needed to generate, 227; from coal, 84–85; national energy task force on, 71–72; solar, 289–93
Energy Independence and Security Act (U.S., 2007), 141–42, 193
Energy Policy Acts (U.S., 2005; 2007), 141
Energy Security Act (U.S., 1980), 136
Energy Tax Act (U.S., 1978), 136
Engdahl, F. William, 126
Enova Energy Group (firm), 191
entropy, 23–24
environmental organizations, 137
Environmental Protection Agency (EPA), 58; on cellulosic ethanol, 148–49; ethanol production requirements of, 164; on hypoxia, 182–83
Enviva (firm), 190–91, 193
ethanol: from algae, 124; blended with gasoline, 148; BP's production of, 78; in Brazil, 200–202; carbon dioxide emissions from use of, 241; corn used in, 102, 135–37, 197–98; energy input to produce, 143; environmental impact of production of, 173; EPA's production requirements

for, 164; food crisis and, 94; fossil energy needed to produce, 243–44; greenhouse gases released by, 238; increased production of, 140; mandatory consumption of, 138; oligopoly production of, 100; tax credits for, 141; water used in production of, 155–56
Ethiopia, 98, 264–65, 278–79
Europe: agricultural surpluses in, 113; genetically-modified organisms blocked in, 92, 127; wood pellets used in, 190–92
European Commission, 191–92
European Parliament, 92
European Union (EU), 113; increased food production in, 117, 208; resistance to genetically-modified crops in, 128; sustainable intensification of agriculture policy of, 281; wood pellets used as fuel by, 189–90
exchange value, 29
Exxon-Mobil (firm), 61; on biofuels, 77; Synthetic Genomics and, 124

Fargione, Joseph, 241–42
Farm Bill (Public Law 480; U.S.), 114
farms: agroecological, 259, 262–64, 266; decline in, 113; small, 253–54
fascism, 245
feedstocks, 138–39; land required for, 230
Feed the Future Initiative, 280–81
fertilizers, 176; dependency on, 113; food price increases caused by, 261; nitrogen used in, 206; oligopolies controlling, 93
firewood, 288–89
first-generation biofuels, 237
fish and aquatic species, 196–97
Florida, 292–93
food: biofuels and price increases for, 102; competition between biofuel production and, 208; consequences

of biofuels production on, 164–73; exported by U.S., 114–17; green revolution's impact on, 93, 109; increase in production of, 30–32; livestock production for, 33–34; organic, 257–58; price increases for, 94–99, 205–7; production competition with biofuels, 32–33; unequal distribution of, 250; wasted, 119–21; wild plants and animals for, 256

Food and Agriculture Organization (FAO), 94–96, 109; agroecology symposium of, 282–84

Food and Drug Administration, U.S. (FDA), 220

food commodity derivatives market, 99

food crisis (2008), 94–97

food miles, 264–65

food riots, 102

food security, 250–51, 264

food versus fuel debate, 47

forest fires, 194

forests, 29; agroforestry, 268, 269; in Brazil, 202; carbon stored in, 239; deforestation of, 228; impact of biofuel production on, 187–89; lost to livestock production, 37; temperate forests, 229; tree plantations compared with, 233; tropical forests, 229–30; varieties of life in, 256; water captured by, 235–36; wood pellets from, 189–96

fossil energy, 243–44

fossil fuels: biofuels as alternative to, 72; carbon content of, 238; coal as, 84–85; government subsidies for, 81; imported into Global South, 288; price of fertilizers tied to, 206

fracking (hydraulic fracturing), 82, 85–88

gasoline, 100; ethanol blended with, 138, 148; replaced by ethanol, 142

Gates Foundation, 282

gene revolution: agroecology versus, 260; dangerous effects of, 220; green revolution transitions to, 121–22, 125, 216–17; promoted by Rockefeller Foundation, 123

genetically engineered (GE) crops, biofuels derived from, 47

genetically-modified organisms (GMOs), 19; as answer to global hunger, 95; for biofuels production, 124, 129–30; blocked in Europe, 92; deregulation of, 123; food crisis and, 99; genetic use restriction technology for, 222–25; hazards of, 220; health risks associated with, 127–28; in India, 64; Monsanto's domination of, 217; revenues from, 127

genetic trait control, 223

genetic use restriction technology (GURT), 222–25

genomics, 96; applied to biotechnology, 131; Rockefeller Foundation promotion of, 126

George C. Marshall Institute, 61

Georgescu-Roegen Nicholas, 22

Georgia Biomass (firm), 191

Georgia Institute of Technology, 80

Georgia-Pacific (firm), 295–96

Gill, Stephen, 247–48

Gliessman, Steve, 257, 258–59

Global Alliance for Climate-Smart Agriculture, 284

Global Association of Corporate Sustainability Officers (GACSO), 284–85

globalization, environmental costs of, 53

Global North: abundant food in, 109; food waste in, 120; livestock production in, 34

Global South: accumulation by dispossession in, 67; agricultural workers in, 248–49; agriculture in, 252; biofuel production in, 13; biofuels countries in, 68–69; in corporate markets, 64; food exported from U.S. to, 116–17; food gap between Global North and, 211; food production in, 30–31; food waste in, 120; gene revolution causing dependency on U.S. in, 126–27; green revolution in, 113; land grabs in, 67–68; meat consumption in, 33; neoliberalism in, 65–66; poverty and malnutrition in, 109–10, 249–51

glyphosate herbicide, 183

Goldman Sachs (firm), 97, 200

Gore, Al, 12, 137

grain: corporate control over seeds for, 223–24; green revolution and surpluses of, 92–94; oligopolies selling, 99–101, 218, 219; perennial grain crops, 274–75; price increases for, 94; U.S. exports of, 114–18; used as feed for livestock, 33–34, 120; *See also* cereals

Gramsci, Antonio, 59

greenhouse gas emissions (ghgs): from coal, 85; from ethanol, 238; from livestock, 35

green revolution, 43–44; agroecology versus, 260–61; becomes gene revolution, 121–22, 125, 216–17; decline in varieties of crops after, 255; land and water needed for, 110–12; limits reached for, 212–13; neoliberalization of, 113; Rockefeller Foundation in, 104–9; surplus food created by, 93

Green River (U.S.), 82

Greenwood, James C., 150–51

Groat, Charles C., 89

gross domestic product (GDP), 52

Grupo Cabrera (firm), 201

Guatemala, 268

Gulf of Mexico, 178–82

Haiti, 249

Harvey, David, 20, 65–67

Heimlich, Ralph, 227, 290

herbicides, cancers tied to, 186–87

Howarth, Robert, 87–88

Hubbert, King, 10–11

Hubbert peak, 10–12, 71, 72, 76

Humphrey, Hubert, 114

hunger, 121; genetically-modified crops as solution to, 95; in Global South, 14, 250; green revolution's impact on, 109–10

Hurricane Mitch, 269

hydraulic fracturing (fracking), 82, 85–88

hydroelectric projects, 288

hypoxia, 179–83

Iceland, 26

index funds, 98

India: coal consumed in, 84–85; economic growth of, 25; genetically-modified crops in, 128; land needed for food production in, 43; processing mustard seed oil banned in, 64; shale gas in, 83; wheat production in, 108; wild plants eaten in, 256

Indonesia, 28; carbon dioxide emissions from, 243; catastrophic fire in, 239; green revolution rice in, 125; peatland rainforests in, 45–46; shale gas in, 83

Ingraffea, Anthony, 87–88

Inhofe, James, 61–62

insecticides, 186

insect pests, 272

InterAmerican Development Bank (IDB), 135, 200, 202

Inter-American Ethanol Commission, 135

International Center for the

Improvement of Maize and Wheat (CIMMYT), 107–8
International Energy Agency (IEA): on biofuels, 10, 226–27; on demand for coal, 85; on exhaustion of fossil fuels, 72–73; World Energy Outlook by, 11
International Finance Corporation, 200
International Fund for Agricultural Development (IFAD), 282
International Labour Organization (ILO), 251
International Monetary Fund (IMF), 134
International Program on Rice Biotechnology, 125
International Resource Panel, 289
International Rice Research Institute (IRRI), 108–9
Iowa, 168
Iran, 279
Iraq, 118–19
irrigation, 111–12; for corn, 156

Jacobson, Mark, 290, 291
Japan, 117
jatropha, 78, 124
jet fuel, 129
Jevons, William Stanley, 56
Johnson administration (LBJ), 114

Kenya, 277–78
Keynesian economics, 245–47
Kissinger, Henry, 114, 115, 224
Koch, Charles, 58–62, 292–96
Koch, David, 58–62, 292–96
Koch Industries, 58–59, 292, 295–96
Kyoto CDM (Clean Development Mechanism), 287

land: diverted to corn from soybeans, 199; land-grabs, 67–69, 103, 212; needed for green revolution,

110–11; required for food crops and feedstocks, 230–31; speculation in, 168; *See also* cropland
Land Institute, 276
Latin America: agroecology in, 267–70; G.W. Bush in, 134–35, 200; increase in arable land in, 111; U.S. outsourcing feedstock production to, 203
lignin, 130
lignocellulosic ethanol, 79–80, 139
livestock, 33–41; cost of feed for, 209–10; grain used as feed for, 120; in Latin America and Caribbean, 253; soybean feed for, 140
Louis Dreyfus (firm), 101
Lula da Silva, Luiz Inácio, 94
Lutzenberger, Jose, 262–63

maize, 105–8; attacked by stem borers, 272; ethanol made from, 238, 241; genetically modified, 217; varieties of, 267; *See also* corn
malnutrition, 198–99, 210–11, 214, 262
Malthus, Thomas Robert, 28
manure, 184–85
Martin, John P., 89
Marx, Karl, 66, 133
Mauritania, 98
Mayan civilization, 27
meat: consumption of, 33; global production of, 35
Meggs, Anthony, 88
Mercatus Center (George Mason University), 60, 294
methane emissions, 252–53; from natural gas, 87–88; from shale, 88
metropolitan states: domestic functions performed by, 133–34; *See also* states
Mexico, 34, 106–7; maize imported by, 209; no-till farming in, 273; tortilla prices in, 198; water scarcity in, 234; weeds in, 268–69

micro-propagation techniques, 131
milk, 35
Millennium Ecosystem Assessment, 42
millet, 255–56
Minnesota, 136, 183
miscanthus, 79
Mississippi-Atchafalaya River basin, 172–73, 177–82
Mississippi River, 162–63
Mississippi River Basin Healthy Watershed Initiative, 180
Mississippi River Valley Alluvial (MRVA) aquifer, 162–63, 169
MIT Energy Initiative (MITEI), 86–88
Moniz, Ernest, 88
Monsanto (firm), 19, 96, 219; in Brazil, 202; control over seeds by, 221–22; European market abandoned by, 127–28; genetically modified crops by, 217; genetic use restriction technology bought by, 222–23; glyphosate herbicide by, 183; proprietary seed market controlled by, 218; Renessen and, 129; Sapphire Energy and, 124; seeds from, 119
Moreno, Luis Alberto, 135
Morocco, 83
Mozambique, 85

National Sugar and Alcohol (CNAA) company (Brazil), 201–2
natural gas (methane), 87–88
Natural Resources Defense Council (NRDC), 192
Negroponte, John, 95
Nelson, Willie, 137
neoliberalism, 65–66; international intergovernmental network supporting, 134; new constitutionalism and, 247–48
Nessler, Craig, 80
new constitutionalism, 247–48
New York City, 185

New York State, 290–91
Niger, 278
Nigeria, 98, 233
nitrates, 184
nitrogen: linked to livestock production, 38, 39; used in fertilizers, 206, 261–62; water pollution caused by, 178–86
nitrous oxide, 252; emissions of, 38
no-till farming, 273, 285–87

Obama, Barack, 248, 280
Obama administration: on biotechnology, 151–53; Clean Power Plan of, 189; cropland policies of, 167–68
Odari, Joyce, 277–78
Ogallala aquifer, 156–58
oil; *See also* petroleum
oil industry, 58–59; academics tied to, 88–90; agriculture dependent on, 113; biofuels investments and research by, 76–81; in Brazil's ethanol sector, 200–201; climate change denial organizations funded by, 61; control over biofuels by, 78–79; on fracking's environmental and health risks, 86–88; government subsidies for, 81–82
Oliver, Melvin J., 224
Orbiach, Raymond, 89
organic agriculture (OA), 257–58, 264
orphan crops, 105, 255
ozone levels, 58

palm oil, 99; plantations for, 46; used for biodiesel fuel, 242
Palouse region (Washington State), 270–71
paper, consumption of, 29
paper industry, 44
patents, 217; on seeds, 221; on terminator technology, 224
Patzek, Tadeusz W., 243
Paul, Donald, 76–77

peatland rainforests, 45–46; carbon
    stored in, 242–43
Pelletier, Nathan, 35
Penn State University, 87
perennial grain crops, 274–76
Perrings, Charles, 25
Perry, Rick, 164
Peru, 267
pesticides, 176, 254, 272; nitrogen
    and phosphorus pollution of water
    caused by, 183; oligopolies control-
    ling, 93
petroleum (oil): exhaustion of reserves
    of, 12; Hubbert peak in produc-
    tion of, 10–11; national energy task
    force on, 71–72; price increases for,
    98–99
petroleum industry, See oil industry
Phelps, Willard, 224
phosphorus pollution, 178–86
Pimentel, David, 142, 243
Plains Exploration and Production
    (firm), 89
Polanyi, Karl, 21
population, 18; demands on ecology
    made by, 28–29
potatoes, 171; varieties of, 267
poverty, 32; biofuel production and,
    12–13; in Global South, 249–51;
    green revolution's impact on,
    109–10; integrity of the ecological
    system and, 51; in Mexico, 209
Pretty, Jules, 256, 263
primitive accumulation, 66
production, impacts on ecosystem
    of, 27
Public Law 480 (Farm Bill; U.S.), 114
pulp and paper industry, 187–88
punctuated equilibrium, 226

rainfall, 49
rainforests: climate impact of loss of,
    49; peatland, 45–46
rainwater harvesting, 278–79

Raizen (firm), 201
Reagan administration, 123
Reganold, John, 270
Renessen (firm), 129
renewable energy, 290–91
Renewable Energy Directive, 191
Renewable Fuel Standards (RFS), 138,
    164
Rentech Inc., 129
rice: decline in varieties of, 255; fertil-
    izers used on, 262; International
    Rice Research Institute, 108–9;
    Rockefeller Foundation promotion
    of, 125–26; speculation on price of,
    97; varieties of, 267; water needed
    by, 274
Rifkin, Jeremy, 34
road biofuels, 72–73
Rockefeller Foundation: food crops
    central to, 104–9; gene revolution
    promoted by, 123; rice technology
    promoted by, 125–26
Rodrigues, Roberto, 135
Rosset, Peter, 257
Routs, Rob, 77
Rubin, Robert, 211
RWE (firm), 191

Saccharomyces cerevisiae, 130
Sachs, Jeffrey, 25
salinization, 160–61
salmon, 170
Salton Sea (California), 160–62
Sapphire Energy (firm), 124
Saudi Arabia, 83
Scalia, Anthony, 60
Searchinger, Timothy, 227, 239, 240, 290
second-generation biofuels, 47, 74,
    143; deforestation caused by, 44;
    genetically-modified organisms
    and, 124, 130
seeds: corporate control of, 218,
    221–23; genetic engineered,
    172; introduced into Iraq, 119;

oligopolies controlling, 93; for perennial and annual crops, 275; sold by Monsanto, 127–28
Senegal, 210–11
Shale and Society Institute, 89
shale oil and gas, 82–84; academic research on, 88–90; environmental and health risks of, 85–86; increased production of, 11
Shell (firm), 77; Australian operations of, 84; in Brazil, 201
shipping industry, 53
Sierra Club (organization), 88
Smith, Neil, 64, 122
Soddy, Frederick, 22
soil, 38; agroecology of, 270–72; degradation of, 173–74; sequestration of carbon by, 44–45
solar energy, 289–93
sorghum, 34, 137–38, 255–56
South Africa: coal production in, 85; genetically-modified crops in, 128, 132; tree plantations in, 233–34
South Asia, agricultural workers in, 249
Southern Alliance for Clean Energy, 293
South Korea, 69
Soviet Union, 105
soybean oil, 64
soybeans, 103, 140, 165, 209; diverted to biofuel production, 197; land used for corn diverted to, 199; nitrogen fixation by, 174; produced in Brazil, 199–200
Standard Oil Company, 106, 107
states: intervention in markets by, 63; responsibility for ecological system of, 51; role in economy of, 57; in service to corporate markets, 64; *See also* metropolitan states
State University of New York at Buffalo, 87, 89–90
state welfarism, 245–46

stem borers (insects), 272
sugarcane, 200, 240; in Cuba, 265; used in ethanol, 201, 202, 235
Sumerian civilization, 27
Summers, Lawrence, 211
supermarkets, 219–20
Supreme Court (U.S.), 203
sustainability, thermodynamics of, 25
switchgrass, 144
Syngenta (firm), 218
Synthetic Genomics (firm), 124
synthetic nitrogen fertilizers, 113, 261, 272
Syria, 279

Tanzania, 256, 273
tar sands oil, 82
temperate forests, 229
terminator technology (genetic use restriction technology; GURT), 222–25
Texas AgriLife Research, 80
Texas A&M University, 79–80
Thailand, 256
thermodynamics, laws of, 23–25, 239; applied to livestock production, 36
Thomas, Clarence, 60
Tillerson, Rex, 77
Togo, 99
tortilla prices, 198, 209
tourism, 56
trade, environmental costs of, 53
transnational corporations (TNCs), 46; on biofuels, 12; on solutions to climate change, 9–10
transport ethanol, 10
tree plantations, 232–34; carbon stored by, 241; water requirements of, 235, 236
tropical forests, 229–30, 241
Tudge, Colin, 39
Tyedmers, Peter, 35

United Kingdom (UK), 281

United Nations (UN): "Electricity for All" declaration by, 288; on food security, 250, 251
United Nations Environment Program (UNEP), 55–56
United States (US): agriculture dependent on fertilizers in, 113; biofuels subsidized by, 123; Feed the Future Initiative of, 280–81; food exports from, 114–18; food insecurity in, 262; gene revolution making Global South countries dependent on, 126–27; genetically-modified crops in, 92; geoeconomics of biofuels in, 135–54; increased cropland in, 164; increased oil and gas production in, 83; outsourcing feedstock production to Latin America by, 203; petroleum consumption in, 11; post-World War II hegemony of, 105; subsidies for oil companies in, 81–82
University of Texas at Austin, 87, 89
urban farms, 266
use value, 29
utility companies, 293

Vilsack, Tom, 168
Volkswagen (firm), 90–91
Volkswagen commission, 90

wastes, 48, 226; food as, 93, 119–21; linked to livestock production, 37; thermodynamics of, 50; used for biofuel production, 141

water: in agroecology, 273–74, 277–78; captured by forests, 235–36; consequences of biofuels production on, 154–64; contamination of, 175–78; expected shortages of, 215; irrigation projects for, 111–12; needed for green revolution, 110–11; nitrogen and phosphorus pollution of, 178–86; rainwater harvesting of, 278–79; scarcity of, 234–35; shortages of, 31; used in livestock production, 39–40
weeds, 268–69
wetlands, 168–69; in Corn Belt, 183–84; wood pellets from, 193–96
wheat, 107–8; fertilizers used on, 262
wild food sources, 258; wild plants, 256
wood pellets, 189–96
Woodworth, Elizabeth, 190
World Bank, 94, 111, 134
World Development Movement (Global Justice Now; organization), 97
World Food Program, 210
World Trade Organization (WTO), 134

Yapa, Lakshman, 27
Yazoo River (Mississippi), 162–63

Zoellick, Robert, 94